Anxiety in Childbearing Women

Anxiety in Childbearing Women

Diagnosis and Treatment

Amy Wenzel

With contributions by Scott Stuart

American Psychological Association • Washington, DC

Published by
American Psychological Association
750 First Street, NE
Washington, DC 20002
www.apa.org

To order
APA Order Department
P.O. Box 92984
Washington, DC 20090-2984
Tel: (800) 374-2721; Direct: (202) 336-5510
Fax: (202) 336-5502; TDD/TTY: (202) 336-6123
Online: www.apa.org/pubs/books
E-mail: order@apa.org

In the U.K., Europe, Africa, and the Middle East, copies may be ordered from
American Psychological Association
3 Henrietta Street
Covent Garden, London
WC2E 8LU England

Typeset in Goudy by Circle Graphics, Columbia, MD

Printer: Edwards Brothers, Inc., Ann Arbor, MI
Cover Designer: Mercury Publishing Services, Rockville, MD

The opinions and statements published are the responsibility of the authors, and such opinions and statements do not necessarily represent the policies of the American Psychological Association.

Library of Congress Cataloging-in-Publication Data

Wenzel, Amy.
  Anxiety in childbearing women : diagnosis and treatment / Amy Wenzel. — 1st ed.
     p. ; cm.
  Includes bibliographical references and index.
  ISBN-13: 978-1-4338-0900-2
  ISBN-10: 1-4338-0900-1
  ISBN-13: 978-1-4338-0901-9 (e-book)
  ISBN-10: 1-4338-0901-X (e-book)
  1. Anxiety in women. 2. Mental illness in pregnancy. 3. Postpartum psychiatric disorders. 4. Pregnant women—Mental health. 5. Childbirth—Psychological aspects. I. American Psychological Association. II. Title.
  [DNLM: 1. Anxiety Disorders—diagnosis. 2. Anxiety Disorders—therapy. 3. Postpartum Period—psychology. 4. Pregnancy—psychology. 5. Pregnancy Complications. WM 172 W482a 2011]
  RG588.W46 2011
  618.7'6—dc22
                                        2010019775

British Library Cataloguing-in-Publication Data

A CIP record is available from the British Library.

Printed in the United States of America
First Edition

CONTENTS

ACKNOWLEDGMENTS

What a delight this book was to write! When I proposed this volume, I thought I knew most of what there was to know about prenatal and postpartum anxiety disorders. Over the past year, I was pleased (and, at times, horrified, for I am diligent about keeping deadlines!) to see just how much has been written on this topic over the past 30 years, perhaps even longer. This project led me on a journey to explore literatures from my own discipline, psychology, as well as from the disciplines of psychiatry, nursing, obstetrics and gynecology, and neuroscience. Although these bodies of literature do not exist in isolation, they have not yet been integrated fully into a complete conceptualization of the phenomenon of anxiety that occurs during the transition to parenthood. It is a privilege to bring together this literature, and I thank the authors of the high-quality research and critical analyses that have been published. I became a better scholar and thinker because of their work, and I eagerly await advances in this field over the next decade.

I thank many individuals with whom I have worked over the years to develop an expertise in perinatal anxiety and depression. I am grateful to my mentors at the University of Iowa—Michael O'Hara and Scott Stuart—for having faith in my ability as a research assistant and inviting me to serve on their project on interpersonal psychotherapy for postpartum depression, funded by the National Institute of Mental Health. It was on this project that I discovered the impetus to initiate a program of research on perinatal anxiety disorders, as many of the hundreds of women whom I interviewed in order to ascertain a diagnosis of depression spontaneously described their struggles with anxiety.

I also thank the many graduate and undergraduate research assistants at the University of North Dakota who helped me to make this program of research a reality. In addition, this program of research would not have been possible without several internal grants awarded through various funding mechanisms from the University of North Dakota. Finally, I am grateful for Karen Kleiman's continuing collaboration and support. As the founder and director of the Postpartum Stress Center in the Greater Philadelphia area and the author of several books, she has been a leader in this field for many years.

I also have appreciated the support and encouragement from Susan Reynolds, acquisitions editor at APA Books. She makes the process of developing and writing scholarly books smooth, enjoyable, and gratifying. It has been a pleasure to work with her, and I look forward to continued collaboration on future projects. In addition, I express my sincere gratitude to my development editor, Beth Hatch; to Kathleen Kendall-Tackett; and to an anonymous reviewer for their comments and encouragement on the first draft of this volume.

Finally, I thank my husband for his unwavering support and for being with me every step of the way as I prepare to take on a new role that will undoubtedly inform my scholarly work on the transition to parenthood—that of being a mom. I learned I was pregnant with my first child about 4 months into the contract for this book. Although we lost our son at 21 weeks' gestation, during his short life he made quite a contribution to the professional world by influencing my writing as this volume unfolded. Conversely, my research on this topic had a positive effect on the manner in which I handled the loss. I dedicate this book to his memory and eagerly await another attempt at parenthood.

Anxiety in Childbearing Women

INTRODUCTION: ISN'T IT NORMAL FOR NEW MOTHERS TO BE ANXIOUS?

Perhaps no life event brings as many intense (and extreme and conflicting) emotional experiences as pregnancy and childbirth. Although most expectant parents are filled with joy and eager anticipation for the new addition to their family, they also experience episodes of sadness (e.g., grief over the loss of previous roles) and anxiety (e.g., concern about the baby's health). There is a vast literature on the nature, causes, and consequences of depression associated with pregnancy and childbirth (e.g., O'Hara, 1995; O'Hara & Swain, 1996). In contrast, much less attention has been devoted to anxiety associated with pregnancy and childbirth. Since the 1970s, many research studies have examined the association between maternal anxiety during pregnancy and birth outcomes, infant behavior, and child development. However, the past decade has witnessed a substantial increase in research on the diagnosed anxiety disorders that women experience in pregnancy and the postpartum period.

The term *postpartum depression* can encompass a variety of postpartum mood and anxiety disorders (C. T. Beck & Driscoll, 2006), and some researchers have advocated for broadening the term to *postnatal mood disorder* to include both depression and anxiety (Matthey, Barnett, Howie, & Kavanagh, 2003). However, evidence is accumulating that many aspects of the phenomenology of anxiety experienced during this time period are distinct from depression.

Thus, the time is ripe to bring together a volume that describes, evaluates, and extends the literature on prenatal and postpartum anxiety, which I refer to as *perinatal anxiety* (cf. Bennett & Indman, 2006) and define as anxiety symptoms and disorders that occur during pregnancy and the postpartum period. The postpartum period has been defined in the literature as anywhere between 4 weeks (*Diagnostic and Statistical Manual of Mental Disorders*; 4th ed., text revision [*DSM–IV–TR*]; American Psychiatric Association, 2000) and 1 year (C. T. Beck & Driscoll, 2006; Bennett & Indman, 2006; Kleiman, 2009; Kleiman & Raskin, 1994). To be as inclusive as possible and to account for the biological, emotional, and relational changes that occur for several months after having a baby, I join my fellow scholars and regard the postpartum period as the 1st year following childbirth.

The material presented in this Introduction was written to accomplish four main aims. First, I describe the boundary between normal and clinically significant instances of anxiety in pregnant and postpartum women. Second, I discuss the significance of scholarly investigation and clinical consideration of anxiety that occurs during this time period. Third, I compare and contrast clinical aspects of anxiety and depression and consider the implications of focusing only on depression. Finally, I orient the reader to the organization of the book.

NORMAL VERSUS CLINICALLY SIGNIFICANT ANXIETY

When I discuss my scholarly work on this topic with others, their first response is, "Isn't it normal for new mothers to be anxious?" The quick response to this question is yes, it is absolutely normal for new mothers to be anxious. As I describe in Chapter 2, I surveyed approximately 150 new mothers about the degree to which they worried about different topics such as relationships, their jobs, finances, the appearance of themselves and their babies, and household duties. On average, these women reported that they worried a moderate amount, or approximately 20% to 50% of the time. In other words, their worry did not necessarily take over their lives, but it certainly was in their minds a good amount of time. I regard this level of anxiety as normal and to be expected during pregnancy and the postpartum period.

In contrast, there is a small percentage of women who have difficulties with anxiety symptoms or disorders and who become pregnant, and their condition must be monitored to determine whether intervention is necessary during this time of transition. Although these women have struggled with anxiety well before their pregnancy, they are usually counted in statistics examining the prevalence of perinatal anxiety disorders because they are exhibiting symptoms during this time period. Some researchers regard these women as having a *recurrence* of a previous episode (e.g., Cooper & Murray, 1995; Matthey et al., 2003). There is another small percentage of women, different from the first subset of women, who were well-adjusted before pregnancy but who develop anxiety symptoms or an anxiety disorder during pregnancy or following childbirth. These women are regarded as having a *de novo* episode of anxiety (Matthey et al., 2003). The literature on perinatal anxiety gives fairly equal coverage to both of these categories of women. The key issue for all of these women is that they are regarded as having clinically significant levels of anxiety, or anxiety that is persistent and/or severe enough that it causes life interference and/or substantial distress. The majority of this volume is focused on clinically significant manifestations of anxiety symptoms and disorders. However, normative instances of perinatal anxiety are pointed out when relevant.

One straightforward way to identify a clinically significant manifestation of anxiety is to determine whether the person has received a psychiatric diagnosis. Diagnoses of anxiety disorders are made when a trained professional verifies that a person meets criteria for one of these diagnoses according to the *DSM–IV–TR*. At times, anxiety experienced during pregnancy and/or the postpartum period is overlooked because some symptoms of anxiety disorders are also experienced by nonanxious women during this time period (e.g., sleep disturbance, fatigue; Nonacs, Cohen, Viguera, & Mogielnicki, 2005). Thus, it is important that health care professionals assess the degree to which these symptoms present in excess of that which would be experienced by most pregnant women or new mothers. To qualify for a diagnosis, not only must a person endorse and/or exhibit certain symptoms described in the *DSM–IV–TR*, she also must provide evidence that these symptoms cause life interference and/or substantial distress. Notice that this is the second time I have referred to life interference and distress. Whenever I am asked to distinguish between normal and problematic instances of anxiety during pregnancy and the postpartum period, I look for life interference and personal distress. If one or both of these are present, the likelihood increases that the person is suffering from a perinatal anxiety disorder; if one or both of these are absent, the likelihood increases that the person is suffering from unpleasant but relatively normal anxiety associated with being a new parent. Consider the follow case descriptions, which illustrate the difference between normal and problematic levels of anxiety.

Esther is a 38-year-old Asian American woman who is 5.5 months pregnant with her first child. During the 1st trimester, she experienced a moderate amount of bleeding and went to the emergency room twice because she suspected that she was having a miscarriage. Although in both instances it was determined that the baby was fine, Esther continued to worry and became tearful at times, believing that she was doomed to miscarry because statistics show that miscarriage is more frequent in women over age 35. The bleeding stopped when she was approximately 11 weeks pregnant, and her nurse–midwife determined that the cause was a polyp on her cervix, which did not pose a threat to the pregnancy. Esther felt a tremendous sense of relief and no longer worried that she was at great risk of miscarrying. She experienced an increase in anxiety again when she was 4 months pregnant, as she was waiting for the results of her amniocentesis. Although she knew, rationally, that the risk of a genetic abnormality was less than 1%, she frequently wondered if she would be the "one" who would have problems. Once she received news that the results of the amniocentesis were negative, her anxiety dissipated, and for the remainder of her pregnancy she eagerly anticipated the birth of a healthy baby boy.

Robin is a 30-year-old Caucasian woman who gave birth to her second daughter approximately 3 months ago. Robin's daughter sleeps in a crib in the same room as her and her husband. Robin checks on her daughter every 20 to 30 minutes to ensure that her she is still breathing. As a result, Robin is chronically sleep deprived and describes herself as being a "zombie" throughout the day. She often catches herself yelling at her 4-year-old daughter for things that would not have agitated her before having her second child. Moreover, she is so preoccupied with whether her baby is still breathing that, at times, she does not provide adequate supervision for her older daughter, who was found playing with dangerous objects, such as knives and cleaning supplies, in a few instances of this lapse in supervision. Her husband offers to help care for both children, but Robin quickly becomes frustrated with him, saying that he does not do things as carefully as she does. Recently, her husband has been spending more and more time away from the home, indicating that he cannot take the tension that has developed between the two of them and that he is tired of being told that he cannot do anything right.

The description of Esther illustrates an instance of normal prenatal anxiety, and the description of Robin illustrates an instance of problematic postpartum anxiety. Both women could point to times in which their anxiety was all consuming. However, Esther's intense anxiety was short term and time limited, always associated with an external stimulus such as vaginal bleeding or the impending results of the amniocentesis. Her anxiety dissipated as soon as she had evidence that the fetus was in good health. Even though she was anxious, she was able to redirect her attention to tasks that required her focus, such as responsibilities at work and around the house. In contrast, Robin's anxiety seemed never ending. Each time she checked her baby, there was evidence that the baby was breathing and was not in distress. Yet, Robin did not accept this evidence at face value and felt compelled to check again soon thereafter, to the detriment of her physical and emotional health (e.g., her sleep) and at the expense of supervising her older daughter and attending to the relationship with her husband.

Nearly all providers of obstetric and mental health care would say that some degree of anxiety during pregnancy and the postpartum period is normal. Indeed, when Esther expressed how anxious she was at her second prenatal visit, her nurse–midwife validated that any woman who experienced the degree of bleeding that she did would be fearful of a pregnancy loss. Perinatal anxiety such as this is not particularly problematic when the woman can still function in her major responsibilities and relationships; is able to gain some perspective on her anxiety (even if she is still unsettled); and can still take care of herself by eating, sleeping, and relaxing when appropriate. In fact, it could be argued that anxiety in reasonable doses might be adaptive (cf. Affonso, Liu-Chiang, & Mayberry, 1999) in that it could mobilize the woman to gather information about the source of her anxiety, ways to take care of herself and her unborn child, and ways to prepare for the future. Perinatal anxiety becomes problematic when it consumes a significant proportion of a woman's time, takes away from her ability to fulfill major role responsibilities, and interferes with her ability to take care of herself. This volume describes many manifestations of problematic levels of perinatal anxiety and its effects on the woman's and child's well-being during pregnancy, labor and delivery, and the postpartum period.

SIGNIFICANCE OF PERINATAL ANXIETY

Why is it important to write a book that focuses exclusively on perinatal anxiety? I maintain that there are three reasons why this topic warrants attention: (a) the high prevalence of anxiety symptoms and disorders that have been documented to date in pregnant and postpartum women, (b) the nature of the changes that women experience during this time period that increase the likelihood of experiencing anxiety, and (c) the effects of perinatal anxiety that have already been described in the literature.

Epidemiology of Perinatal Anxiety

It is logical to expect that anxiety would be prevalent in childbearing women. It is known that approximately 10% to 13% of women experience perinatal depression (Bennett, Einarson, Taddio, Koren, & Einarson, 2004; O'Hara & Swain, 1996) and that even more childbearing women report depressive symptoms but do not necessarily qualify for a diagnosis of depression (e.g., Matthey, Barnett, Ungerer, & Waters, 2000). Because there is a significant overlap (or a *comorbidity*) between depression and anxiety, one would expect that a substantial percentage of women who experience depression associated with childbirth would also experience symptoms of anxiety. However, anxiety symptoms and disorders are also prevalent in their own right and occur in the absence of depression, particularly in women (Brown, Campbell, Lehman, Grisham, & Mancill, 2001). Moreover, the mean time of onset of most of the anxiety disorders considered in this volume in women is their early to mid-20s, a time during which many women contemplate childbirth (Kessler, Ruscio, & Shear, 2009). Thus, from an epidemiologic standpoint, one would expect perinatal anxiety to be a common occurrence.

Childbirth-Related Changes

Boyce and Condon (2000) outlined five reasons why childbirth is a stressful and potentially anxiety-provoking event: (a) the large array of psychosocial stressors experienced by new mothers, (b) the dramatic physiological and hormonal changes that accompany pregnancy and childbirth, (c) the physical demands and pain associated with pregnancy and childbirth, (d) the possibility of having to undergo physically and psychological stressful obstetric interventions, and (e) the fact that preexisting psychiatric disturbance will likely be exacerbated during this time of transition. In other words, the confluence of the biological, physical, emotional, and psychological changes that a woman experiences during pregnancy and the postpartum period makes her vulnerable to develop problems with anxiety, especially if she is predisposed to develop an anxiety disorder because of a personal or family history of emotional disturbance. In the following sections, I comment briefly on each of these factors.

Stress

It is well established that people with anxiety disorders report significantly more life stress than people without anxiety disorders (Sandin, Chorot, Santed, & Valiente, 2004), which suggests that the time surrounding childbirth would create a context that is ripe for the emergence of anxiety symptoms. For example, the physical changes that accompany this time period often make it difficult for women to maintain their prepregnancy level of energy and effectively meet numerous professional and personal demands. A new addition to the family requires financial resources for supplies and day care, which creates extra pressure for families that are already stretching their paychecks. After the baby is born, there is often a dramatic decrease in the amount of time women are able to spend with their spouses or partners. Moreover, many women find the transition back to work difficult when their maternity leave has ended (Holtzman & Glass, 1999). Mothers of multiples may be at particular risk of life stress because their babies often have problems, such as slow and frequent feeding and/or irritability (Choi, Bishai, & Minkovitz, 2009; Leonard, 1998). Any one of these stressors could be enough to prompt or exacerbate emotional disturbance in women, particularly in women who are vulnerable to developing an anxiety disorder. When they are experienced simultaneously at a time in which women's emotional resources are low because of sleep deprivation and fatigue, the results can be especially devastating.

Biological Changes

The physiological and hormonal changes that women experience during pregnancy and the postpartum period are profound. Table 1 displays hormones that are elevated during this time period, along with their typical function and an indication of the manner in which they might affect mood in child-bearing women. During pregnancy, progesterone levels increase 10- to 30-fold, and various hormones in the estrogen family increase 100- to 1,000-fold (Cowley & Roy-Byrne, 1989). Corticotropin-releasing hormone is produced in the placenta and released into the bloodstream, which causes cortisol levels to rise about halfway through pregnancy and by the end of pregnancy reach levels comparable with those in people with severe depression (Glover & Kammerer, 2004). There is evidence from animal studies that adverse maternal and child outcomes in the postpartum period resulting from prenatal stress emerge through the action of cortisol (Weinstock, 2001). In addition, there are increases in the levels of many other hormones, such as prolactin, oxytocin, adrenocortical hormones, human chorionic gonadotropin, human placental lactogen, human chorionic corticotrophin, and human chorionic thyrotropin (Cowley & Roy-Byrne, 1989). Changes in levels of these hormones can affect the hypothalamic–pituitary–adrenal (HPA) axis, which is the stress system in the brain that is often implicated in explaining symptoms of anxiety and depression (Altemus, 2001; Jolley & Spach, 2008).

Levels of these hormones plummet in the first 2 days following childbirth (Nonacs, 2005) and reach prepregnancy levels around the 5th day postpartum (Jolley & Spach, 2008). It is not surprising that the sudden drop in hormone concentrations has the potential to facilitate dysregulation of the HPA axis—the expression of which might resemble symptoms of anxiety and depression. The body of research on hormonal changes associated with postpartum mood disturbance has failed to identify consistent results; both increasing and decreasing levels of hormones have been associated with emotional disturbance (Brace & McCauley, 1997). Instead, researchers have speculated that there is a subset of women who are particularly sensitive to rapid changes in hormonal levels and who are likely to experience emotional difficulties as a result (Altemus, 2001; Glover & Kammerer, 2004; Nonacs, 2005).

TABLE 1
Hormonal Changes Associated With Childbirth and Mood

Substance	Function in childbirth	Function in mood
Estrogens (including estriol, estrodiol, estrone)	• Regulate production of progesterone and other hormones • Stimulate development of many fetal organs • Maintain endometrium during pregnancy • Regulate blood flow in the uterus • Protect female fetus from effects of androgens (i.e., substances that promote masculine features) in the mother's system	• Stimulate the HPA axis • Stimulate the serotonergic system • Increase dopamine and serotonin receptors • Act on regions of the brain known to have a large concentration of neurotransmitters involved in the control of mood, such as the locus coeruleus and the dorsal raphe • Reduce MAO levels, which increases the availability of monoamines
Progesterone	• Stimulates development of endometrium • Maintains the functions of and protects the placenta • Prevents the uterus from making spontaneous movements • Strengthens the mucus plug covering the cervix • Prepares the body for labor by strengthening the pelvic walls • Prevents the uterus from contracting before it is time for birth • Helps the baby to use foods	• Exerts anxiolytic effects by increasing the activity of adenosine • Decreases plasma carbon dioxide levels • Works on GABA-binding receptor sites • Increases MAO levels, which reduces the availability of monoamines • Increases amygdala reactivity
Cortisol	• Determines the length of gestation and the timing of labor	• Dysregulates the HPA axis • Prepares the body for danger (e.g., increases blood pressure)
Corticotropin-releasing hormone	• Plays a role in uterine contractions	• Releases cortisol
Prolactin	• Regulates the mother's metabolism during pregnancy • Prepares the breasts for breastfeeding • Promotes growth of the fetus	• Decreases responsivity of the HPA axis • Associated with irritability and anger
Oxytocin	• Promotes contractions • Stimulates mammary glands to produce milk	• Stimulates the HPA axis

Note. HPA = hypothalamic–pituitary–adrenal; MAO = monoamine oxidase; GABA = gamma-aminobutyric acid. Data are from Brace and McCauley (1997); Glover and Kammerer (2004); Jolley and Spach (2008); Steiner, Dunn, and Born (2003); Torner, Toschi, Pohlinger, Landgraf, and Neumann (2001); Sichel and Driscoll (1999); and van Wingen et al. (2008).

Lactating women do not experience as dramatic a drop in many of these hormones, as some hormones remain elevated to stimulate milk production and mother–infant bonding through breastfeeding. Thus, Altemus and Brogan (2004) speculated that lactation and gradual weaning protects some women against postpartum emotional disturbance. For example, research has shown that lactating women have lower levels of hormones associated with anxiety as well as a lower heart rate and a blunted galvanic skin response, which are indicators of low anxiety (Altemus, Deuster, Galliven, Carter, & Gold, 1995; Weisenfeld, Malatesta, Whitman, Grannose, & Vile, 1985). Moreover, lactation is associated with suppressed HPA axis response to mental stress (Heinrichs et al., 2001). The implications of this research are that it is important to assess for breastfeeding status in women at risk of perinatal emotional disturbance and carefully monitor their symptoms when they discontinue breastfeeding.

In addition, an intriguing line of research has suggested that postpartum anxiety and depression are triggered by an inflammatory response (Maes et al., 2000), which could in turn disrupt HPA axis functioning and increase cortisol levels (Kendall-Tackett, 2008). Specifically, the inflammatory response system is activated in late pregnancy and continues through the early postpartum period, which correlates with both state anxiety and depressive symptoms in the first few days following delivery (Maes et al., 2000). Empirical research has suggested that this response is amplified in women with a history of major depression (Maes, Ombelet, De Jongh, Kenis, & Bosmans, 2001), although research has not yet been conducted to determine whether this is also the case with women who have a history of anxiety. The inflammatory response system facilitates the degradation of tryptophan, which is a precursor to serotonin, a neurotransmitter that is closely related to anxiety and depression (Maes et al., 2002). Thus, postpartum mood disturbance might not only be affected by the dramatic changes in hormone levels but also influenced by an activated inflammatory response system. With all of these biological shifts, it is no wonder that new mothers are vulnerable to anxiety and depression associated with childbirth.

Childbearing women also undergo many biological and physical changes that do not involve hormones and inflammatory responses but that have just as much potential to provoke symptoms of anxiety. For example, pregnant women often experience increases in their heart rate as their bodies work harder to circulate blood and oxygen to the fetus. As the uterus expands, it often presses up against the diaphragm, which can cause women to take shorter, shallower breaths (March & Yonkers, 2001). Increased heart rate and shallow breathing are symptoms of anxiety, as well as uncomfortable physical sensations that can signal danger or distress to women who are vulnerable to experience emotional distress.

Physical Demands

Childbearing women usually find that pregnancy, labor, and delivery are physically demanding events that involve some degree of pain. The physical demands associated with childbirth can consume women's energy and psychological resources that they would normally direct toward managing symptoms of emotional distress. Moreover, some women develop a pronounced aversion to the experience of pain, at times to the extent that they develop a phobia of childbirth because they fear the pain associated with labor. There is no doubt that most women who have vaginal deliveries report a great deal of pain. In research I conducted with my colleagues at the University of Iowa, nearly all 37 women in our sample described their pain during labor as "excruciating" (Larsen, O'Hara, Brewer, & Wenzel, 2001). However, this research also demonstrated that women's expectations about their ability to implement pain management strategies (e.g., relaxation, breathing, distraction) explained about 20% of the variance in pain ratings during the early and active phases of labor. It has been known for some time that a significant cognitive aspect of anxiety is the person's perception that she will not be able to cope with danger or adversity (A. T. Beck & Emery, 1985); thus, it is possible that fears of the physical pain associated with labor and delivery can be explained, in part, by a woman's prediction that she will not be able to handle it.

Possibility of Complications

Pregnancy and childbirth go hand in hand with ambiguity. Approximately 15% to 20% of conceptions result in miscarriage (Puscheck & Pradhan, 2006). Although the vast majority of babies are born healthy, pregnant women face the small possibility that their children will be born with birth defects or that they will need to undergo stressful obstetric interventions in the event that there are complications during labor and delivery. These possibilities would make any childbearing woman anxious or nervous (see the case of Esther); however, in the case of a woman who is vulnerable to emotional distress, the ambiguity could create the context for clinically significant symptoms of anxiety to emerge. Indeed, a growing body of research has suggested that people who are characterized by an intolerance of uncertainty have an increased likelihood of regarding ambiguous situations as distressing (e.g., Koerner & Dugas, 2008). It is possible that the intolerance of uncertainty is one vulnerability factor for the development of an anxiety disorder during a stressful period of time, such as pregnancy and the postpartum period.

Preexisting Psychiatric Disturbance

There is a great deal of evidence that women with a preexisting psychiatric history are especially likely to develop emotional disturbances during the transition to parenthood. In my writing to this point in the Introduction, I have noted on several occasions that stressors, pain, and the possibility of undergoing difficult obstetric interventions are particularly likely to evoke anxiety reactions in *vulnerable* women. I regard a woman as being vulnerable for the development of perinatal anxiety symptoms and disorders if she has had previous episodes of anxiety or depression. I also regard a woman as being vulnerable if she has a family history of an anxiety or mood disorder. Although there is little research on the degree to which a family history of anxiety or depression is a risk factor specifically for perinatal anxiety, there is evidence that a family history of these types of psychiatric disturbance makes women vulnerable to postpartum depression (C. T. Beck, 2001; Nonacs & Cohen, 1998). Moreover, research has shown that a family history of anxiety and depression is a risk factor for the development of anxiety disorders in women who are not necessarily pregnant or in the 1st year postpartum (Barlow, 2002).

Thus, I adopt a diathesis-stress model to explain the onset of perinatal anxiety, such that perinatal anxiety disorders are most likely to manifest in women who have some sort of vulnerability or predisposition (cf. Gunthert et al., 2007), usually in the form of a personal or family history or anxiety or depression. In these women, it might take only a small amount of stress to prompt the expression of the anxiety disorder. Perinatal anxiety disorders may also be evident in women who have little, if any vulnerability, but this is most likely to be the case when they experience a great deal of stress during pregnancy or the postpartum period.

Effects of Perinatal Anxiety

As is evident in many of this volume's chapters, the effects of perinatal anxiety have the potential to be substantial. As is discussed in Chapter 1, some research has suggested that excessive anxiety during pregnancy is associated with changes in fetal behavior, pregnancy complications, and difficulties in maternal and child postpartum adjustment (e.g., Field et al., 2003). Other studies have indicated that anxiety that persists following childbirth has the potential to disrupt the mother–infant relationship; in fact, case studies of women with severe postpartum posttraumatic stress disorder (PTSD) have indicated that some women avoid caring for their baby altogether (e.g., Ballard, Stanley, & Brockington, 1995). In addition, there is evidence that the effects of postpartum anxiety on the child can persist years later, as shown by lower scores on measures of motor, intellectual, social, and emotional development and elevated rates of childhood psychiatric diagnoses (e.g., Van den Bergh & Marocen, 2004). Thus, having an understanding of the nature of perinatal anxiety disorders is a first step in identifying women at risk of these emotional disturbances and offering anxiety-management strategies in order to avoid these deleterious consequences.

An unfortunate reality of perinatal anxiety is that when expectant and new mothers are provided with information about the possibility of short- or long-term harm coming to their babies, they often become more anxious as a result. The addition of this burden to an already anxious woman would be contraindicated. Thus, professionals who work with childbearing women must have a sense of the degree to which research supports and does not support the notion that anxiety is associated with adverse outcomes, as not every investigation has found that perinatal anxiety is associated with negative outcomes (cf. Istvan, 1986). In fact, even in studies that found a significant association between prenatal anxiety and adverse effects in the child, most of the children in the sample were not affected. Approximately 15% of the variance in child outcomes, such as behavioral problems, can be attributed to maternal anxiety during pregnancy (Glover, Bergman, & O'Connor, 2008), which suggests that many other variables can exacerbate or prevent problems in child development.

Short bouts of anxiety that do not affect a woman's ability to take care of herself are not likely to be associated with problems in labor, delivery, and child development. However, chronic, untreated anxiety has the potential to activate biological mechanisms that could dysregulate the fetal environment and create a context that is ripe for pregnancy complications. If this level of anxiety continues into the postpartum period, it has the potential to disrupt mother–infant attachment, which in turn would increase the likelihood that cognitive, emotional, and social problems in children would be observed. Although these consequences are of concern, it is important for women and the clinicians who treat them to understand that they can be prevented with efficacious treatments for anxiety disorders. Part II of this volume describes some of these treatments.

PERINATAL ANXIETY VERSUS PERINATAL DEPRESSION

How does one differentiate between perinatal anxiety and perinatal depression, and why is it important to do so? This issue is considered in a number of the chapters in Part I of this volume. The reader will quickly see that, in many instances, there is substantial overlap. According to the *DSM–IV–TR* (American Psychiatric Association, 2000), a person must endorse five of nine symptoms to qualify for a diagnosis of major depressive episode. These symptoms are (a) depressed mood, (b) anhedonia (i.e., the inability to experience pleasure from activities that are normally enjoyable), (c) sleep disturbance, (d) appetite disturbance, (e) psychomotor agitation or retardation, (f) fatigue, (g) worthlessness and/or inappropriate guilt, (h) concentration difficulties and/or indecisiveness, and (i) suicidal thoughts and/or behavior.

Some of these symptoms are also included in the diagnostic criteria for various anxiety disorders. For example, people who are diagnosed with generalized anxiety disorder (GAD) and PTSD often report sleep disturbance and concentration difficulties. Thus, there is a relatively high likelihood that women with some anxiety disorders will also meet diagnostic criteria for depression simply because of the overlap in symptoms. This also means that much of what is known about perinatal depression is also relevant to the understanding of perinatal anxiety. This being said, it will also become evident that some women with perinatal anxiety disorders do not meet the criteria for depression. Focusing solely on the identification of women with perinatal depression, then, would have the effect of missing women with perinatal anxiety who experience few, if any, depressive symptoms.

Another important reason for correctly diagnosing perinatal anxiety versus depression is so that the woman can get the appropriate treatment. As is described in greater detail in Chapter 10, cognitive behavioral therapy (CBT) is an efficacious form of psychotherapy for the treatment of both depression and anxiety. Clinicians who use CBT often engage in a procedure called *cognitive restructuring*, in which they work with patients to develop the skills to identify and evaluate thoughts and images that might be exacerbating their symptoms. This procedure is usually incorporated in CBT for anxiety disorders as well as CBT for depression. However, clinicians who use CBT with depressed patients might also incorporate *behavioral activation*, which is a strategy for actively engaging patients in their environment by ensuring that they are participating in pleasurable and meaningful activities (M. E. Addis & Martell, 2004). In contrast, clinicians who use CBT with anxious patients will likely incorporate *exposure*, which is a systematic set of procedures that help anxious patients face their fears either in their daily lives (i.e., in vivo exposure) or imaginally (Moscovitch, Antony, & Swinson, 2009). Researchers have determined that the exposure component of CBT is critical in ensuring this treatment's efficacy (cf. Riggs & Foa, 2009); thus, if a clinician proceeds to treat an anxious woman under the umbrella label of perinatal depression, he or she might omit a crucial component of treatment.

ORGANIZATION OF THIS VOLUME

Whereas perinatal depression is a relatively straightforward condition to identify and define, perinatal anxiety is observed in many forms. Part I of this volume is geared toward the description of various manifestations of perinatal anxiety disorders and an evaluation of empirical research conducted to date. Part I opens with a chapter on research examining the association between anxiety symptoms, rather than diagnoses, and maternal and infant well-being during pregnancy, labor, delivery, and the postpartum period. This chapter was included because the majority of research on perinatal anxiety has defined this construct on the basis of high scores on questionnaires measuring anxiety symptoms. Moreover, much of this research predates research on the diagnoses of perinatal anxiety disorders that are described in the remaining chapters of this section. Many of the questions answered by the research described in this chapter have not been investigated adequately using samples of childbearing women who have been diagnosed with anxiety disorders. Thus, one can view the literature evaluated in this chapter as an agenda for future researchers to conduct with each of the anxiety disorders described in subsequent chapters.

There are several types of anxiety disorders described in the *DSM–IV–TR*, many of which are beginning to receive attention in childbearing women. Chapter 2 describes perinatal symptoms of worry and diagnoses of GAD, which is characterized by excessive worry that occurs more of the time than not and that is accompanied by symptoms such as restlessness, muscle tension, and difficulty sleeping. Chapter 3 describes symptoms of perinatal obsessions and compulsions and diagnoses of obsessive–compulsive disorder (OCD). *Obsessions* are unwanted thoughts, images, and/or impulses that people rec-ognize as being distressing and have trouble getting out of their mind, and *compulsions* are repetitive behaviors that people must do over and over, often to neutralize the obsessions. Chapter 4 examines panic attacks that occur during pregnancy and the postpartum period and associated diagnoses of panic disorder. A *panic attack* is the sudden experience of anxiety symptoms that come out of the blue (e.g., racing heart, sweating, feeling as if one were going to die) and that peak within 10 to 15 minutes. Chapter 5 examines symptoms of perinatal social anxiety and diagnoses of social anxiety disorder, which center on fears of being rejected, judged, disliked, or embarrassed. Finally, Chapter 6 presents information on perinatal fears and posttraumatic stress as well as diagnoses of childbirth-related specific phobia and PTSD. A *specific phobia* is a persistent, irrational fear of a particular object or situation (in this case, childbirth) that results in avoidance or extreme distress when one is exposed to the feared stimulus. Women who are diagnosed with PTSD experience symptoms in three domains: (a) intrusive memories of the event (e.g., night-mares, flashbacks), (b) emotional numbing and avoidance of reminders of the event, and (c) increased arousal. Most of the research described in this chapter pertains to women who develop posttraumatic stress symptoms following a difficult or traumatic delivery experience.

Chapter 7 does not focus on one particular anxiety disorder but integrates information across the various manifestations of anxiety to provide the begin-nings of a biopsychosocial model to capture the etiology, maintenance, and exacerbation of perinatal anxiety. The model is informed by integrating the implications of empirical research for many of types of anxiety associated with childbirth as well as research that has not yet been carried out on childbearing women but that pertains to people in general who suffer from anxiety disorders. It accounts for the hormonal and biochemical changes associated with pregnancy, childbirth, and lactation and the interplay of these factors with genetic and psychological vulnerability factors to facilitate the onset of perinatal anxiety disorders.

Part II of this volume focuses on the clinical implications of the many types of perinatal anxiety symptoms and disorders described in Part I. Chapter 8 summarizes approaches to the assessment of perinatal anxiety, describing inventories specific to manifestations of anxiety that are observed during pregnancy and/or the postpartum period and ways to adapt existing measures to be relevant to this population. Chapter 9 evaluates the empirical research on pharmacotherapy for childbearing women who suffer from anxiety disorders. I am pleased to include my friend and former mentor, Scott Stuart, MD, as a coauthor in this chapter. We describe various classes of medications that are efficacious for anxiety disorders and consider the degree to which these medications affect fetal and infant development and well-being. Chapter 10 describes psychotherapeutic approaches in the treatment of perinatal anxiety and evaluates the small amount of research that has been conducted with pregnant and postpartum samples. Finally, Chapter 11 presents self-help approaches for managing perinatal anxiety symptoms, which I view as an important but often overlooked topic, given that many postpartum women have difficulty attending regular doctor's appointments in addition to the host of new responsibilities that they are trying to manage. The Conclusion to the volume highlights important themes that emerge across chapters and proposes an agenda for future research.

CONCLUDING THOUGHTS

Researchers have made tremendous progress in identifying and describing the nature and phenomenology of perinatal anxiety. Symptoms of anxiety have been studied in relation to birth outcomes for more than 30 years, and diagnoses of perinatal anxiety disorders have been the subject of much empirical research particularly over the past decade. Various manifestations of perinatal anxiety are being linked with increasing frequency to the biological and psychological changes that accompany pregnancy and the postpartum period. Moreover, there is an increasingly large body of literature that identifies factors that have the potential to make women vulnerable to developing perinatal anxiety. Research pertaining to these and other related issues is brought together here in one volume for the first time. I invite readers to join me on an exploration and critical evaluation of this important and, until recently, neglected topic.

I

ANXIETY IN
CHILDBEARING WOMEN:
NATURE AND PREVALENCE

1

ANXIETY SYMPTOMS DURING PREGNANCY AND THE POSTPARTUM PERIOD

A comprehensive book on perinatal anxiety would not be complete unless it summarized and interpreted the vast literature that has examined anxiety symptoms measured by nonspecific self-report inventories and their relation to childbearing. Studies that define anxiety as high scores on these inventories tell us little about the phenomenology of anxiety disorders that might have their onset or be exacerbated during pregnancy and the postpartum period. Nevertheless, they give us a starting point to begin to understand the anxiety symptoms that pregnant and postpartum women experience that do not fit so neatly into our diagnostic system. Thus, this chapter describes what is known about the association between self-reported anxiety symptoms and aspects of pregnancy, childbirth, and functioning in the postpartum period, and the chapters that follow consider specific domains of anxiety that correspond with our current diagnostic system.

Before proceeding, it is worth noting that there is an even more expansive literature on the relation between prenatal stress and labor, delivery, and post-partum outcomes. In fact, most animal research that has relevance to this volume examines postpartum variables associated with maternal stress because it is difficult to assess the subjective experience of anxiety in animal subjects. There are many similarities between stress and anxiety in that both involve the activation of the sympathetic nervous system and activity of similar neuro-transmitters. Some people regard anxiety and stress as being one and the same; others regard stress as a more general construct that encompasses a range of negative emotions, including anxiety, anger, and frustration. According to the website of the American Institute of Stress (http://www.stress.org/topic-definition-stress.htm), there is no one definition of stress that is accepted by scientists, and stress has different meanings for different people because everyone has his or her own unique way of responding to things that cause stress (i.e., stressors). Moreover, at times stress can occur in response to a situation that would generally be regarded as positive, such as winning an election. Thus, I regard stress as the body's physiological, emotional, and/or cognitive response to an internal or external situation that causes a shift in the body's homeostasis, or the body's consistent, stable condition. Although research on the effects of stress on labor, delivery, and postpartum outcomes has relevance to the understanding of perinatal anxiety, I limit the focus in this chapter to research that has specifically measured one or more forms of anxiety. I do this for two reasons: (a) to make this scholarly analysis as targeted as possible and (b) to acknowledge research on this topic that measures both anxiety and stress, as some findings suggest that they are differentially associated with certain outcomes.

The majority of the studies that I review in this chapter used the State–Trait Anxiety Inventory (STAI; Spielberger, Gorsuch, & Lushene, 1970) to measure symptoms of anxiety. Thus, it is worthwhile to take a moment to appreciate the nature of the items that make up this instrument. The STAI consists of two 20-item scales. One scale measures *trait anxiety*, which reflects the degree to which a person generally experiences broad symptoms of anxiety. Items on the trait anxiety scale (i.e., STAI-T) include items similar to "Little things often bother me" and "I can handle difficulties that come my way." The other scale measures *state anxiety*, which reflects the degree to which a person experiences discomfort at the moment he or she is completing the questionnaire. Items on the state anxiety scale (i.e., STAI-S) include items similar to "I feel distressed" and "I am satisfied." Items on both scales are rated on a scale of 1 to 4 (1 = *not at all*; 4 = *very much so*). Positively worded items, such as some of those provided in the examples, are reverse scored so that higher ratings are reflective of higher ratings of anxiety. Scores on all 20 items are summed to obtain an overall score of trait or state anxiety. Whenever I refer to trait anxiety or state anxiety in this chapter, the reader can assume that these constructs were assessed using the STAI.

PREVALENCE

It is difficult to estimate the prevalence of state and trait anxiety in pregnant and postpartum women. Most studies that have used the STAI have either (a) examined associations between scores on these scales with other indices of symptoms or birth outcomes without identifying women high or low in anxiety, or (b) defined high and low anxiety in a predefined manner on the basis of the unique sample under consideration, such as by assigning women who scored one standard deviation above the mean on one or both scales to a "high anxiety" group. The former approach is referred to as *correlational*, which means that it takes the full continuum of scores on an anxiety measures and associates them with the full continuum of values pertaining to the outcome under consideration. Correlational research is not designed to yield prevalence rates. When researchers define high and low anxiety according to the latter approach, they predetermine the percentage of women in their sample who would be regarded as anxious. In these cases, prevalence rates are arbitrary and are dependent on the definition specified by the researcher.

The authors of the most commonly cited study on the prevalence of perinatal anxiety symptoms (Stuart, Couser, Schilder, O'Hara, & Gorman, 1998) administered the STAI to the study's sample of postpartum mothers but instead calculated the prevalence of anxiety using the Beck Anxiety Inventory (BAI; A. T. Beck & Steer, 1990). The BAI is a 21-item self-report inventory that measures the severity of various physical symptoms of anxiety (e.g., racing heart, sweating, difficulty breathing) and subjective experiences of fear and terror. Stuart et al. (1998) regarded women as having clinically significant symptoms of anxiety if they scored 10 or higher on this measure. Using this definition, they determined that 8.7% of their sample experienced clinically significant symptoms of anxiety at 14 weeks postpartum and that 16.8% of their sample experienced clinically significant symptoms of anxiety at 30 weeks postpartum. Not only do their findings suggest that anxiety symptoms are quite common in the postpartum period, but they also indicate that many new cases of anxiety can develop as the postpartum period progresses. However, it is important to recognize that this conclusion pertains only to anxiety defined as physical symptoms and subjective experiences of fear. These manifestations of anxiety are most relevant to the understanding of panic symptoms and panic disorder (see Chapter 4, this volume). Unfortunately, results from this study do not speak to the prevalence of other manifestations of anxiety, such as worry, anxious apprehension, and women's perceptions of their ability to cope with adversity.

EFFECTS

Much research has examined the degree to which trait anxiety and state anxiety are associated with specific maternal and child outcomes. There are several possible explanations for the proposed relation between anxiety and adverse outcomes associated with birth and postpartum adjustment. From a biological perspective, anxiety stimulates the release of neurotransmitters called catecholamines (e.g., norepinephrine). In pregnant women, catecholamines constrict blood vessels, which reduces the rate of blood flow to the fetus and restricts the amount of oxygen and nutrients the fetus absorbs. This process has the potential to disrupt the development of the fetus's central nervous system (Hirshfeld-Becker et al., 2004; Lobel, Dunkel-Schetter, & Scrimshaw, 1992; Monk et al., 2000), which, in turn, has the potential to adversely affect fetal and child development. Anxiety also stimulates a biochemical pathway that leads to the release of cortisol, 10% to 20% of which is passed onto the fetus and could affect the development of the fetal brain (Kinsella & Monk, 2009). In addition, mood disturbance during pregnancy is associated with engagement in poor maternal health behavior (e.g., poor nutrition, smoking; Hirshfeld-Becker et al., 2004; Lobel et al., 1992), which could also adversely affect fetal and child development. Another explanation for poor outcomes associated with maternal anxiety invokes a psychological mechanism, in that mothers who are anxious during pregnancy are likely to be anxious in the postpartum period, and postpartum anxiety could prevent a new mother from providing the stimulation and interaction that infants need to thrive. Finally, it could be that an interaction among these factors best explains the association between maternal anxiety and poor birth outcomes, such that the biological effects of intrauterine exposure to increased levels of neurotransmitters and hormones could be exacerbated after the child is born by exposure to a suboptimal environment (cf. Brouwers, van Baar, & Pop, 2001b).

In the following section, several categories of mother and child outcomes are considered, including (a) those relevant to the intrauterine environment and fetal behavior before birth; (b) those relevant to the health and well-being of the infant soon after delivery; (c) those relevant to complications during pregnancy, labor, and delivery; (d) those relevant to maternal birth experiences; and (e) those relevant to maternal and child functioning in the postpartum period and beyond.

Intrauterine Environment and Fetal Behavior

Studies examining the relation between anxiety and fetal behavior have the potential to identify biological mechanisms for this association, as the mother has not yet had the opportunity to interact directly with the infant. Both state and trait anxiety have been linked to abnormal uterine and fetal blood flow, which could in turn cause low birth weight (Teixeira, Fisk, & Glover, 1999) or be a sign of fetal hypoxia (i.e., insufficient oxygen in the blood and/or tissue; Sjöström, Valentin, Thelin, & Maršál, 1997). Results from these studies are consistent with the biological mechanism described previously, such that increased activity of catecholamines stimulated by anxiety restricts the rate of blood flow to the fetus. In addition, both trait and state anxiety have been associated with decreased fetal growth rate (i.e., lower fetal weight, lower abdominal circumference; Field et al., 2003), which can be accounted for by elevations in maternal cortisol levels (Field, Diego, & Hernandez-Reif, 2006). Groome, Swiber, Bentz, Holland, and Atterbury (1995) found that, relative to fetuses of low-trait anxious mothers, fetuses of high-trait anxious mothers spent more time in active sleep and moved around less frequently during active sleep after statistically controlling for other variables known to affect fetal behavior in analyses (e.g., food and caffeine intake). In all, this body of literature points to several differences in the development and behavior in the fetuses of anxious and nonanxious women.

Infant Outcomes Soon After Delivery

The empirical research on the association between maternal anxiety and birth outcome is decidedly mixed. For example, several studies failed to find evidence that a high level of state or trait anxiety is associated with lowered 1-min or 5-min Apgar scores (Barnett & Parker, 1986; Brouwers et al., 2001b; Cox & Reading, 1989), whereas one older study using a different measure of anxiety (i.e., the IPAT Anxiety Self-Analysis Form; Cattell & Scheier, 1963) revealed a large difference between the 5-min Apgar scores of anxious and nonanxious women (i.e., 5.83 vs. 9.00; Crandon, 1979b). In addition, many studies found no differences in the size of the newborn (e.g., head circumference, length, weight) between trait or state anxious and nonanxious mothers (Barnett & Parker, 1986; Groome et al., 1995; Sjöström et al., 1997). However, work by Tiffany Field and her colleagues has indicated that the decreased fetal growth rate detected in fetuses of anxious mothers in utero extends to low birth weight and shorter gestational age (Field, Hernandez-Reif, et al., 2006). Moreover, results from Field et al.'s 2003 study suggested that newborns of trait anxious mothers were characterized by a number of other differences from newborns of nonanxious mothers, such as lowered dopamine and serotonin levels, greater right frontal electroencephalogram activation, lower vagal tone, less time alert and active, lower motor organization, lower autonomic stability, and more pronounced withdrawal symptoms.

Perhaps the most comprehensive analysis of the relation between anxiety and abnormal birth outcomes was conducted by Istvan (1986). Although this analysis was published over 20 years ago, it is still cited frequently today. Istvan included studies that measured anxiety not only using the STAI but also using other measures of anxiety (and a few measures of stress) that were commonly administered in the 30-year time period between the mid-1950s and the mid-1980s. When obstetric outcomes were conceptualized using global variables such as "normal" or "abnormal" and combined a large array of problematic birth outcomes, approximately one third of the studies confirmed an association between high levels of anxiety and poor obstetric outcomes. When he examined studies that targeted specific obstetric outcomes as dependent variables (e.g., low birth weight), Istvan found that a significant association between anxiety and a particular poor birth outcome found in one study often was not replicated in other studies. He attributed the lack of a clear pattern to researchers' failure to take into account the complexity of the social, psychological, structural, endocrinological, and metabolic changes that women experience during pregnancy. That is, this conclusion indicates that there is likely not a direct correspondence between anxiety experienced during pregnancy and problematic birth outcomes, but instead that poor birth outcomes likely arise from the confluence of many factors.

Pregnancy, Labor, and Delivery Complications

Maternal anxiety also has the potential to affect infant health indirectly by increasing the likelihood of complications during pregnancy, labor, and delivery. For example, maternal anxiety has been associated with an increased likelihood of preeclampsia (i.e., a hypertensive disorder during pregnancy; Crandon, 1979a; Kurki, Hiilesmaa, Raitasalo, Mattilla, & Ylikorkala, 2000), spontaneous preterm labor (Dayan et al., 2002; Glynn, Dunkel-Schetter, Hobel, & Sandman, 2008; Kramer et al., 2009), and difficulties during labor (e.g., prolonged labor, shortened labor, forceps delivery, postpartum hemorrhage; Crandon, 1979a). In a comprehensive analysis of STAI scores taken at each trimester, Kalil, Gruber, Conley, and LaGrandeur (1995) found that trait anxiety assessed in the 1st trimester predicted maternal pregnancy complications (e.g., hypertension; cervical or vaginal problems) and that trait anxiety assessed in all 3 trimesters predicted labor and delivery complications (e.g., operative delivery; birth canal trauma). Furthermore, they found that both state and trait anxiety assessed in the 3rd trimester were associated with maternal postpartum complications (e.g., urinary tract problems, breast problems); although these complications are not relevant to the physical health of the infant, they have the potential to affect infant well-being if they prevent the mother from providing adequate care. It should be noted, however, that although anxiety was associated with a host of negative outcomes in this study, the number and intensity of life stressors were even stronger predictors, suggesting that pregnant women would be wise to focus more energy on reducing stress rather than on modifying their anxious temperament.

Not all studies have confirmed this pattern of results, as some research has shown that state and trait anxiety during pregnancy are not associated with premature birth (Barnett & Parker, 1985) or the length of labor (Cox &

Reading, 1989). In an investigation of maternal anxiety throughout pregnancy, Perkin, Bland, Peacock, and Anderson (1993) measured anxiety using the General Health Questionnaire (Goldberg & Hillier, 1979) in 1,515 pregnant women at 17, 28, and 36 weeks' gestation. Anxiety items on the General Health Questionnaire are similar to "Been feeling constantly anxious or tense" and "Been feeling wound up or on edge." They found that anxiety was not associated with preterm delivery, nonspontaneous onset of labor, major analgesia in the first stage of labor, or nonspontaneous vaginal delivery. Although anxiety correlated with the use of major analgesia in the second stage of labor in this study, it accounted for only 0.1% of the variance in this outcome variable, which suggests that this finding has little practical significance.

One group of researchers suggested that it is variability in state anxiety, or changes in STAI-S scores, rather than absolute levels of anxiety as measured on any one occasion, that predicts a range of maternal pregnancy and delivery complications, such as preeclampsia, premature birth, and prolonged labor (Rizzardo, Mangi, Cremonese, Rossi, & Cosentino, 1988). It is possible that variability in anxiety prevents the mother and fetus from achieving a sort of biological homeostasis, such that the mother and the fetus would have to tolerate a widely variable neurochemical environment. This research underscores the need to measure anxiety on multiple occasions throughout pregnancy, as a single assessment might not capture the clinical profile of women who are experiencing emotional distress. At present, however, we can generally conclude that maternal anxiety during pregnancy is moderately associated with a host of problems during pregnancy, labor, and delivery, as some but not all studies confirm these relations.

Maternal Birth Experiences

Evidence suggests that anxious women may also have more negative birth experiences than nonanxious women. For example, trait anxious women are more likely than nonanxious women to report negative experiences with hospital staff (Barnett & Parker, 1986). Using scales from the Prenatal Self-Evaluation Questionnaire II (Lederman, Lederman, Work, & McCann, 1979) to measure anxiety (i.e., preparation for labor; fear of pain, helplessness, and loss of control in labor; concern for well-being of self and baby), Beebe, Lee, Carrieri-Kohlman, and Humpherys (2007) found that anxious mothers were less likely than nonanxious mothers to have confidence that they would be able to perform relaxation techniques during labor, a finding that supports the notion proposed in the Introduction to this volume that the pain associated with labor and delivery is particularly daunting for anxious women. When trait anxious mothers return home, they are less likely to perceive that they are coping well and report more doubts about parenting (Barnett & Parker, 1986).

All of the birth experiences described in this section are perceptions reported by new mothers rather than objective measures of the birth and post-partum experience. According to cognitive behavioral theory, our perceptions often have a great influence on our emotions and mood, as well as our subsequent behavioral responses (cf. A. T. Beck, 1970). As is described in Chapter 10, cognitive behavioral therapy (CBT) was developed, in part, to help people identify and evaluate perceptions associated with emotional disturbances. Thus, women who report distress associated with their birth experience and adjustment to parenthood in the immediate postpartum period would be well suited for CBT.

Postpartum Functioning

Researchers also have assessed the degree to which anxiety is associated with various indices of maternal and child postpartum functioning in the months and years following childbirth. This body of literature suggests that maternal anxiety during pregnancy is more strongly associated with longer term sequelae in the child than it is with the shorter term outcomes described in the previous sections.

Maternal Functioning

Women who experience significant anxiety during pregnancy are at risk of poor postpartum adjustment. For example, Barnett, Schaafmsa, Guzman, and Parker (1991) found that trait anxious women were less confident in their parenting abilities, had fewer hobbies, and were less satisfied with their social support network than nonanxious women approximately 5 years following childbirth. In addition, anxiety experienced during pregnancy also increases the risk of postpartum depression (Austin, Tully, & Parker, 2007; Barnett et al., 1991; C. T. Beck, 2001; Heron et al., 2004; O'Hara & Swain, 1996; Sutter-Dallay, Giaconne-Marcesche, Glatigny-Dallay, & Verdoux, 2004). Thus, anxious women are not only at risk of poor adjustment during labor, delivery, and the immediate postpartum experience, as described in the previous section, they also are at risk of longer term emotional distress.

Child Functioning

There has been much interest in examining the relation between maternal anxiety and child development. Some research has indicated that trait anxious mothers report more concerns about their children than do nonanxious mothers (e.g., Gunter, 1986). For example, Barnett et al. (1991) found that trait anxious mothers rated their children as lower in social competence than did their nonanxious counterparts. Interestingly, teacher ratings did not confirm these reports. Results from these studies raise the possibility that their anxious symptoms bias mothers' judgments of their children. Despite the fact that anxious mothers may have the tendency to cast their children's behavior in an excessively negative light, it could very well be that their children do indeed exhibit some physical, cognitive, emotional, and/or social sequelae of their emotional disturbance. The soundest research that examines the relation between maternal anxiety and child development uses objective instruments and/or raters to measure child outcome.

Some studies using objective measurements of outcome have demonstrated that maternal anxiety during pregnancy is associated with lower scores on measures of cognitive and motor development. Brouwers et al. (2001b) reported that women who were designated as either state anxious or trait anxious had infants with lower "orientation" scores on the Neonate Behavioral Assessment Scale conducted at 3 weeks, lower scores on the Bayley mental and motor scales at 1 year, and lower scores on "task orientation" and "motor coordination" scales of the Infant Behavioral Record of the Bayley at 1 year. Regression analyses revealed that maternal anxiety during pregnancy, low maternal education, and male sex of the child predicted low scores on an overall Mental Development Index, which includes indices of sensory-perceptual skills, memory, learning, problem solving, understanding of object consistency, vocalizations, and language development, assessed when children were 2 years old. Results from this study raise the possibility that infants of mothers who experienced anxiety during pregnancy have reduced attentional capacity, relative to infants born to nonanxious mothers, at least through their 1st year, and have blunted cognitive development after 2 years.

The most comprehensive investigation of maternal anxiety on child outcome was conducted within the context of the Avon Longitudinal Study of Parents and Children (ALSPAC), which is a longitudinal study of child-bearing women, their partners, and the child to whom they gave birth during the course of the study (Golding et al., 2001). Approximately 85% to 90% of pregnant women who lived in Avon, England, were enrolled in the study across a period of 21 months, and analyses that were specifically relevant to maternal anxiety were conducted with data supplied by over 7,000 women. Maternal anxiety was measured using the anxiety items from the Crown-Crisp Experiential Index (Birtchnell, Evans, & Kennard, 1988), which included items about feeling restless, uneasy, and worrying, as well as items assessing instances of somatic anxiety, similar to those included on the BAI. Scores on this measure correlate strongly with scores on the STAI (O'Connor, Heron, Glover, & the ALSPAC Study Team, 2002), which suggests that results from this series of studies can be compared with those from other studies that use the STAI to measure anxiety. Women who scored in the top 15% on this index were regarded as being anxious. Anxiety and depression were assessed at 18 and 32 weeks' gestation, as well as at 8 weeks, 8 months, 21 months, and 33 months postpartum. Child outcomes were assessed on multiple occasions as the children matured, and data collection is still ongoing for children as they go through puberty (Golding et al., 2001).

One series of studies using the ALSPAC database examined the relation between maternal anxiety during pregnancy and children's behavioral and emotional problems (i.e., conduct problems, hyperactivity, internalizing symptoms) at 47 months and again at 81 months. The authors controlled for a host of other variables, such as obstetric risks (e.g., low birth weight, smoking during pregnancy, drinking alcohol during pregnancy); psychosocial variables (e.g., mother's educational attainment, crowding in the household); and most important, anxiety reported in the postpartum period. Results indicated that women who scored in the top 15% on the Crown-Crisp index during pregnancy had an approximately two-fold increased risk of having children with significant behavioral and emotional problems at 47 months (i.e., approximately 4 years old; O'Connor, Heron, Golding, Beveridge, & Glover, 2002; O'Connor et al., 2003). There was a slight decrease in the risk of behavioral and emotional problems in boys at 81 months (i.e., almost 7 years old), but there was no decrease in the risk of behavioral and emotional problems in girls at this age (O'Connor et al., 2003).

O'Connor et al. (2003) were particularly interested in examining the influence of anxiety during pregnancy, rather than the postpartum period, to investigate a *programming hypothesis,* which they defined as occurring when "biological systems adapt to input from the environment during particularly sensitive periods of development" (p. 1033). They hypothesized that maternal anxiety "programs" the activity of the hypothalamic–pituitary–adrenal (HPA) axis in the fetus in a way that makes this system particularly reactive in later years, persisting into adulthood. Behavioral and emotional problems in childhood and beyond would be evidence of an overactive HPA axis. Problems are especially likely to arise when the environment changes later in life and the programmed set points do not easily adapt.

Although there are much data suggesting that maternal stress and anxiety are associated with lasting HPA axis dysfunction in nonhuman research subjects (for reviews, see Maccari et al., 2003; Schneider & Moore, 2000), O'Connor and his colleagues were the first to examine this systematically using a measure of anxiety, rather than an general index of stress, in a large sample of human research participants. They predicted that anxiety assessed at 32 weeks' gestation would be the best predictor of children's emotional and behavioral problems during childhood because the fetal HPA axis does not become active until midgestation (Gitau, Fisk, Cameron, Teixeira, & Glover, 2001). With the exception of one finding—that maternal anxiety assessed at 18 weeks' gestation predicted behavioral and emotional problems in girls at

81 months (O'Connor et al., 2003)—that is exactly what they found. In a subsequent report, O'Connor et al. (2005) examined the degree to which maternal anxiety at 32 weeks' gestation predicted cortisol levels in a subsample of 74 ten-year-old children who completed more rigorous assessments. Cortisol levels are commonly regarded as an index of HPA axis functioning. In support of their biological model, they found that maternal anxiety in late pregnancy predicted children's awakening and afternoon cortisol levels 10 years later, even after controlling for obstetric risk, psychosocial risk, and maternal post-partum mood variables.

Although much of their research was conducted to support a biological mechanism to explain the association between anxiety during pregnancy and child outcomes, O'Connor and his colleagues were mindful of the great body of literature indicating that postpartum depression adversely affects children's cognitive, social, and emotional development through impairment in the mother–child relationship (e.g., Murray, Fiori-Cowley, Hooper, Stein, & Cooper, 1996). Indeed, supplementary analyses indicated that anxiety during pregnancy and postpartum depression independently accounted for variance in children's behavioral and emotional problems (O'Connor, Heron, Glover, & the ALSPAC Study Team, 2002; O'Connor et al., 2003). O'Connor et al. (2003) acknowledged that both biological and psychosocial mechanisms may operate in explaining these adverse child outcomes. As stated previously, pre-natal anxiety is strongly associated with postpartum depression; thus, it could be that prenatal anxiety affects child outcome directly through biological mechanisms and indirectly through psychosocial mechanisms, such as through the onset of postpartum depression.

Other investigations have provided additional evidence that maternal anxiety during pregnancy is associated with children's behavioral and emotional problems later in childhood. Van den Bergh and Marcoen (2004) reported that state anxiety predicted children's symptoms of attention-deficit/hyperactivity disorder, externalizing problems, and self-reported anxiety in a sample of 71 mothers and their 72 firstborn children. Although in many ways their results replicated those reported by O'Connor and his colleagues, one sub-stantial difference is that it was maternal anxiety assessed early in pregnancy (i.e., 12–22 weeks' gestation) that was the significant predictor, not anxiety that was assessed later in pregnancy (i.e., 32–40 weeks' gestation). Anxiety expe-rienced by mothers early in pregnancy predicted salivary cortisol when the children reached ages 14 to 15 years, which was in turn associated with depression in girls (Van den Bergh, Van Calster, Smits, Van Huffel, & Lagae, 2008). The authors attributed this finding to the fact that early pregnancy is a time when there is rapid development of neurons in the fetal brain, and alterations in this process early in development have the potential for wide-spread effects on HPA axis functioning. Because this explanation is different from that proposed by O'Connor and his colleagues, it will be important to test these competing hypotheses in the same design by examining markers of neuronal development and maternal and fetal HPA axis activity at various points during pregnancy.

In addition, Davis et al. (2004) reported that maternal state anxiety and depression during pregnancy were associated with behavioral reactivity in infants who were 4 months old. *Behavioral reactivity* was defined as infants' motor reactions and crying in response to a range of potentially startling situations, such as tasting a drop of lemon juice or hearing a balloon popped behind their heads. Infants who demonstrate reactivity in these tests are vulnerable to becoming behaviorally inhibited as young children (Kagan, Snidman, & Arcus, 1998), which can in turn increase the likelihood of an anxiety disorder during adolescence (Schwartz, Snidman, & Kagan, 1999). Moreover, O'Connor et al. (2007) used the ALSPAC sample to determine that maternal anxiety at 18 weeks' gestation and maternal depression at 32 weeks' gestation predict sleep problems in infants at 18 and 30 weeks. Thus, regardless of whether children are assessed in infancy, toddlerhood, early childhood, or midchildhood, there is robust evidence that maternal anxiety during pregnancy is associated with children's emotional reactivity.

CORRELATES

The clinical implications of the research described here are clear: It is important to identify women who are at risk of experiencing anxiety, particularly when they are still pregnant, so that they can develop strategies for managing their distress. A reduction in perinatal anxiety has the potential to reduce the offspring's vulnerability to behavioral and emotional problems during childhood, as well as to increase the likelihood that the mother will have a positive birth experience and favorable adaptation to parenthood. How, then, can psychologists identify women who would be most appropriate for such intervention? In this section, research that has identified correlates of anxiety symptoms associated with childbirth is reviewed so that we might construct a profile of the woman who might be vulnerable to developing or experiencing perinatal anxiety.

It is important to acknowledge that the word *correlate* means that there is an association between a particular variable and symptoms of perinatal anxiety. In other words, there is no evidence that the variable causes perinatal anxiety. Ideally, we would identify women at risk of developing perinatal anxiety symptoms by determining variables that are present before the onset of anxiety and establishing that they statistically predict symptoms of perinatal anxiety (cf. Kraemer et al., 1997). The body of research on perinatal anxiety has not yet progressed to this point. Thus, we can regard the correlates described in this section as hypotheses of the variables that put women at risk of perinatal anxiety, to be tested in future, prospective research.

Sociodemographic Correlates

When I describe my interest in this topic to people, the first correlate they identify is parity, with the logical reasoning that women who have never given birth (i.e., nulliparous women) would be more anxious than women who have had previous children (i.e., parous women). It is interesting that my own research, as well as research conducted by many others, suggests that there is no relation between parity and self-reported anxiety. However, Maes, Bosmans, and Ombelet (2004) found that state anxiety increased 3 days after delivery in nulliparous women, but not in parous women, and that this increase in anxiety was associated with greater activation of the inflammatory response system. Moreover, Canals, Esparó, and Fernández-Ballart (2002) reported that older mothers endorsed lower levels of anxiety than younger mothers, regardless of whether they were having their first child. Many explanations can be speculated for this intriguing finding; perhaps older mothers are more settled in their careers, finances, partner relationships, or even just their senses of self, and they are more prepared than younger mothers for the responsibility that awaits them. Other sociodemographic variables associated with perinatal anxiety include being unmarried, low income, and low educational attainment (Glazer, 1980; Kalil, Gruber, Conley, & Sytniac, 1993). These correlates are understandable, as they pose barriers to providing ideal child care and obtaining support during this transition. Because they cause stress, I regard them as making women vulnerable to perinatal anxiety.

Psychological Correlates

Identification of sociodemographic variables associated with psychiatric symptoms is useful for screening purposes, but they do not provide enough direction to support speculation about specific individuals who are vulnerable. It is often useful to identify psychological variables that characterize individuals who are vulnerable for psychiatric distress—not only do they allow for a rich characterization of vulnerable individuals, but they also might provide clues about the most effective method of intervention. Two main domains of psychological variables that serve as correlates and predictors of perinatal anxiety have been considered: those pertaining to a woman's psychiatric profile and those related to relationship functioning.

As might be expected, women who report current depression and/or a history of depression or anxiety are more likely to experience anxiety symptoms associated with childbirth than women without this profile of psychiatric symptoms (Breitkopf et al., 2006), particularly if they have discontinued psychotropic medication (Nonacs, Cohen, Viguera, & Mogielnicki, 2005). Such a history suggests that these women are vulnerable to clinically significant expressions of emotional distress and less likely than women without such a history to respond adaptively to a major life transition. Although one's psychiatric history cannot be altered with treatment, current psychiatric symptoms associated with anxiety can be.

Research has also found that perinatal anxiety is associated with the quality of relationships with close others, particularly with the spouse or partner. High levels of intimacy with one's partner and perceptions of having an emotionally supportive partner are associated with lower levels of state and trait anxiety (Hobfoll & Leiberman, 1989; Kalil et al., 1993). Interestingly, Hobfoll and Leiberman (1989) found that greater intimacy with one's family immediately after delivery was associated with higher levels of state anxiety 3 months later, particularly in women with low perceptions of mastery. It is possible that women who lack confidence in their ability to effect change in their environment perceive family members as being particularly intrusive. In her master's thesis, my former student found that negative social interactions with others, but not positive social support, predicted a composite of anxiety symptoms (i.e., worry, physical symptoms of anxiety, social anxiety, obsessions, compulsions; Haugen, 2003). This group of findings has significant implications for partners and family members of childbearing women, as it suggests that a negative communication style with close others could adversely affect the woman's well-being.

Environmental Correlates

Finally, there is some evidence that stressful environmental variables outside of a woman's control can exacerbate her level of anxiety. For example, Mantz and Britton (2007) conducted a study in which a subset of their sample gave birth when the hospital was under construction, forcing women to endure noise and unpleasant odors during delivery and share rooms when they would not otherwise do so. They found that the women who gave birth during the time of hospital construction reported more state anxiety than the women who gave birth when the hospital was not under construction. Other research has shown that, understandably, women whose babies spent prolonged periods of time in a neonatal intensive care unit reported particularly high levels of state anxiety (Zanardo, Freato, & Zacchello, 2003). Thus, unexpected and negative environmental conditions exacerbate state anxiety. It is important for future research to identify the degree to which state anxiety that arises from these stressors persists over time, elevates women's baseline levels of trait anxiety, and affects longer term maternal and child postpartum adaptation.

PRACTICAL IMPLICATIONS

Health care professionals who work with childbearing women must be educated about the nature and prevalence of perinatal anxiety so that vulnerable and symptomatic women can be identified and referred for appropriate prevention or intervention efforts. Unfortunately, research shows that only 44% of obstetricians routinely screen for depression, most of whom do not follow a standardized procedure (LaRocco-Cockburn, Melville, Bell, & Katon, 2003), and even fewer routinely screen for anxiety (Coleman, Carter, Morgan, & Schulkin, 2008). Thus, the task of implementing systematic screening and achieving early detection for perinatal emotional distress in general remains formidable, let alone differentiating between the specific emotional experiences of depression and anxiety.

Nevertheless, I advocate for items primarily assessing anxiety symptoms to be integrated into general screens for perinatal emotional distress. Examples of such questions might include the following: (a) Have you been especially nervous, on edge, anxious, or fearful since the time you became pregnant (or since you gave birth to your child)? (b) Do you have concerns about the amount of anxiety that you've been experiencing? or (c) Have you had any anxiety or worry that has interfered with one or more aspects of your life? Practitioners could administer the three anxiety items of the Edinburgh Postnatal Depression Scale (Cox, Holden, & Sagovsky, 1987; Kabir, Sheeder, & Kelly, 2008), which identifies with high accuracy instances of postpartum depression that has a significant anxiety component. Expectant mothers who are young, have a low income, have current depression or a history of depression or anxiety, and have frequent negative interactions with close others might be especially vulnerable to the development of perinatal anxiety and would therefore be good candidates for screening of this nature. I say more about screening for perinatal anxiety disorders in Chapter 8.

2

WORRY AND GENERALIZED ANXIETY

Carla is a 28-year-old Caucasian woman who has three children and is due to give birth in 2 months. Her husband is a heating and air conditioning repairman, and she is a stay-at-home mother. Carla indicates that she has always been a worrier but that she has been more consumed by her worry over the past several months, as she and her husband are experiencing financial problems, and she wonders whether they will be able to keep their home. Carla estimates that she worries over 90% of the day and that her worrying has impaired her relationships with her family. She states that she is easily distractible when she is watching the children because she is worrying about money, where the family will live if they lose their house, and how she will manage caring for a newborn in addition to her other young children. Alongside these major issues, Carla worries about small things; for example, she planned a birthday party for her son and worried so much about minor details that she was miserable throughout the entire event. Carla reports that it takes her several hours to fall asleep each night, which she attributes more to worries running through her mind than to discomfort because of her size.

This case example illustrates prenatal generalized anxiety, the hallmark feature of which is excessive and uncontrollable worry. Although Carla had a predisposition to excessive and uncontrollable worry, as evidenced by her statement that she has always been a worrier, her symptoms became clinically significant during pregnancy. It is important to note that most of her worries are in the realm of normality—she and her husband are indeed experiencing financial problems, there is a real threat that they will face foreclosure, and it will be a challenge to take care of an infant along with three young children. However, she meets criteria for generalized anxiety disorder (GAD) because of the impact that her worry is having on her functioning, especially her relationships with her husband and her children.

DEFINITION AND NATURE OF WORRY

According to Borkovec, Robinson, Pruzinsky, and DePree (1983), *worry* is a "chain of thoughts and images, negatively affect-laden, and relatively uncontrollable. The worry process represents an attempt to engage in mental problem solving on an issue whose outcome is uncertain but contains the possibility of one or more negative outcomes" (p. 10). Worry is associated with (a) concerns about the future rather than on a focus on the present, (b) cognitive contents that are vague and abstract, (c) feelings of apprehension and tension, and (d) low confidence and perceptions of control in situations that require problem solving (Hazlett-Stevens, Pruitt, & Collins, 2009).

As stated in the Introduction to this volume, frequent worry is a common emotional experience in pregnant and postpartum women. During pregnancy, one of the most common worries reported by women pertains to uncertainty about the baby's well-being—approximately two thirds of pregnant women worry about having an "abnormal" baby, and approximately half of pregnant women worry about having a pregnancy with complications (Searle, 1996). Following childbirth, women worry about how they will be able to care for the baby, including breastfeeding and soothing their infant when he or she is crying. Other common worries include weight gain, employment and maternity leave, and changes in the partner relationship (Affonso, Liu-Chiang, & Mayberry, 1999; Arizmendi & Affonso, 1987). My students and I examined the typical domains of worry reported by women at 8 weeks, 6 months, and 12 months postpartum (cf. Wenzel, Haugen, Jackson, & Robinson, 2003). At all three assessments, the most common worries were finances, their appearance, household duties, and the cleanliness of their surroundings. However, the extent to which these women worried about these issues declined steadily across the 1st year postpartum. Specifically, ratings of worry in these four domains dropped from an average rating of "moderate," defined as worrying 20% to 50% of the time, to an average rating in between "a little" (i.e., 10%–20% of the time) and moderate.

This decline demonstrates that most women adapt to the demands of the 1st year postpartum.

> Carla reports some degree of worry about nearly all of these domains. Although she indicates that her most substantial worry is about finances, she also worries about the health and well-being of all of her children. Carla worries about her ability to manage the rearing of four young children and predicts that she will not be able to take care of the household. She often focuses on "what if" questions—What if the baby has Down's syndrome? What if the baby consumes so much of her attention that her older children will be permanently "scarred?" What if she needs to get a job—how will they pay for day care for multiple children? When Carla is consumed by these worries, she often "shuts down" and sits in front of the television. This style of coping only exacerbates her symptoms, as she then becomes overwhelmed and chastises herself for not getting anything done.

If a woman continues to worry more than 50% of the time about many issues as pregnancy and the postpartum period progress, then it is possible that that she is struggling with perinatal GAD and should see a professional who can confirm this diagnosis. A diagnosis of GAD should be considered in instances in which it is clear that the woman is worrying more than do most pregnant women and new mothers, when she cannot be reassured, when she cannot control the worry, when the worry generalizes to many domains of her life, and when the worry occurs without an identifiable trigger (Ross & McLean, 2006; Weisberg & Paquette, 2002). The core diagnostic feature of GAD is the report of excessive and uncontrollable worry that is present more often than not. In addition, the individual must endorse three of the following six associated symptoms: (a) restlessness, (b) easily fatigued, (c) concentration difficulties, (d) irritability, (e) muscle tension, and/or (f) sleep disturbance (*Diagnostic and Statistical Manual of Mental Disorders* [4th ed., text revision; *DSM–IV–TR*]; American Psychiatric Association, 2000).

> In addition to experiencing uncontrollable worry approximately 90% of the time, Carla reports symptoms of fatigue, concentration difficulties, irritability, and sleep disturbance. Her fatigue and concentration difficulties interfere with household duties, such as paying the bills and managing her children's schedules. Her irritability manifests itself when she snaps at her husband and her children. In particular, she finds herself resenting her children's laughter, wondering how they can experience positive emotions when life is so difficult for the family. Carla is usually exhausted when she goes to bed after she puts her oldest child down, but she experiences a barrage of thoughts about finances and paying the bills when she tries to fall asleep. She has received a diagnosis of migraine headaches in the past, and she finds that she experiences migraines more frequently as her worry has increased.

Another aspect of the *DSM–IV–TR* diagnosis of GAD is that the individual must report uncontrollable worry for a period of at least 6 months. However, my clinical experience is that pregnancy and childbirth are life-changing events that can prompt a rather sudden onset of GAD. Many childbearing women report having clinically significant levels of worry, the associated symptoms such as muscle tension, and corresponding life interference, but they do not fulfill the 6-month criterion. I have chosen to assign a diagnosis of GAD in my research because these women otherwise exhibit the central features of this anxiety disorder. Research has shown that broadening the definition of GAD to include people who report uncontrollable worry and associated symptoms for only 1 month, rather than for 6 months, actually increases the specificity of the diagnosis because it reduces the degree to which it is comorbid with other disorders (Ruscio et al., 2007). Furthermore, people who are diagnosed with GAD but only report uncontrollable worry for 1 month share many of the same clinical features as people who are diagnosed with GAD after worrying for a full 6 months, such as the degree of disability associated with their anxiety disorder and the rate at which they seek treatment (Kessler, Brandenburg, et al., 2005). In fact, Rickels and Rynn (2001) argued that GAD is a chronic condition that presents in brief, repeated episodes. A sudden onset of worry associated with the transition to parenthood could easily fall into this conceptualization of GAD.

However, it is important to note that other scholars who have conducted research on perinatal anxiety have handled this issue differently. For example, some other experts in the field (e.g., C. T. Beck & Driscoll, 2006; Matthey, Barnett, Howie, & Kavanagh, 2003; Ross & McLean, 2006; Rowe, Fisher, & Loh, 2008) have recommended assigning diagnoses of adjustment disorder with anxious mood for women who do not meet the 6-month criterion. As various samples of new mothers are described in this chapter, I point out explicitly whether they met diagnostic criteria for GAD (and the length of time they were required to experience clinically significant worry symptoms), were diagnosed with adjustment disorder with anxious mood, or reported high levels of worry on a self-report inventory.

PREVALENCE

The following section summarizes the epidemiological literature on the rates of GAD during pregnancy and the postpartum period. Throughout this section, the reader can compare the rates of GAD in various samples of pregnant and postpartum women with the prevalence of current diagnoses of GAD in women who are not necessarily pregnant or postpartum. These rates range from a 4-week prevalence of 1.5% (Jacobi et al., 2004) to a 1-year prevalence of 2.1% to 2.7% (Jacobi et al., 2004; Vesga-López et al., 2008).

Pregnancy

Only a few studies have examined the prevalence of GAD in pregnant samples. In an investigation designed to identify variables during pregnancy that predict postpartum depression, Sutter-Dallay, Giaconne-Marcesche, Glatigny-Dallay, and Verdoux (2004) recruited 497 women in their 3rd trimester from a university antenatal clinic and found that 8.5% of women met criteria for GAD according to *DSM–IV–TR* criteria, which presumably means that women were diagnosed with GAD only in instances in which they reported uncontrollable worry for at least 6 months. Unfortunately, the investigators did not include a control group of women who were not pregnant, so the degree to which this prevalence was elevated as compared with women representative of the general population in this community is unclear. However, this rate is clearly in excess of the prevalence rates of GAD in women who participate in epidemiological research (i.e., Jacobi et al., 2004; Vesga-López et al., 2008).

Two studies indeed included nonpregnant control groups in their research designs. Adewuya, Ola, Aloba, and Mapayi (2006) compared the prevalence of GAD in 175 women in late pregnancy (i.e., 32 weeks or longer) and 172 nonpregnant women who were matched for age, marital status, parity, and social class. GAD was operationalized according to *DSM–IV–TR* (American Psychiatric Association, 2000) criteria, which again suggests that the researchers were incorporating the 6-month criterion into their diagnostic decisions. Pregnant women were recruited from antenatal clinics in a semi-urban African town. Approximately 10.5% of the pregnant women met criteria for GAD, compared with 5.2% of the nonpregnant women. Although this difference reached only a trend level of statistical significance ($p = .071$), I mention it here because the rate of GAD was essentially doubled in the pregnant sample.

Mota, Cox, Enns, Calhoun, and Sareen (2008) examined the prevalence of GAD in pregnancy in the National Epidemiologic Survey on Alcohol and Related Conditions, a survey of 43,093 adults living in the United States. They compared the rates of GAD in women between the ages of 18 and 44 who were pregnant at the time of the survey, pregnant at some point in the past year, and not pregnant. Like Adewuya et al. (2006), they operationalized GAD according to strict *DSM–IV–TR* criteria. Rates of GAD in currently pregnant ($n = 451$), pregnant in the past year ($n = 1,061$), and nonpregnant women ($n = 10,544$) were 1.9%, 2.3%, and 3.4%, respectively. There were no significant differences among groups. These rates are much different from those reported by Sutter-Dallay et al. (2004) and Adewuya et al. (2006).

Thus, the small literature on the prevalence of GAD during pregnancy yields conflicting results. Results from two studies that recruited pregnant women from obstetric clinics yielded rates of 8.5% to 10.5%, whereas the rate of GAD in a large sample of community women who happened to be pregnant at the time of the interview was a little less than 2%. It is important to note that both of the former studies recruited women when they were in their final trimester of pregnancy, whereas pregnant women in the Mota et al. (2008) investigation were interviewed at any point in their pregnancy. One could speculate that rates of GAD increase substantially during the 3rd trimester of pregnancy, as women anticipate the imminent births of their babies and as they have had 6 or more months of pregnancy to exhibit clinically significant symptoms of worry. This pattern of results highlights the need to conduct a prospective study of worry throughout the course of pregnancy, with a focus on the degree to which worry symptoms increase near the end of pregnancy and are associated with life interference and distress in each trimester.

Postpartum Period

In the first comprehensive epidemiological study of postpartum anxiety, I examined the prevalence of a number of anxiety disorders, including GAD, at various points in the postpartum period (Wenzel, Haugen, Jackson, et al., 2005). I describe the results of this research in each of the subsequent chapters on specific types of anxiety disorders. In this chapter, I also summarize the methodology that I used to achieve these rates so that the reader will have an understanding of the nature of the sample and the measures used to determine diagnoses.

My research team and I identified women who had recently given birth through the birth announcements in the local newspaper. When women were approximately 6 weeks postpartum, those for whom we could find contact information were sent letters inviting them to participate in the study. We followed up with a telephone call soon thereafter, and women who agreed to participate scheduled a telephone interview when they were approximately 8 weeks postpartum so that trained clinical psychology graduate students could establish *DSM–IV–TR* diagnoses of anxiety disorders and depression. The clinical interviewers also identified *subsyndromal* cases of anxiety disorders and depression, defined as instances in which (a) women endorsed the majority, but not all, of the criteria for a disorder, and the symptoms caused life interference and/or distress, or (b) they fulfilled all of the *DSM–IV–TR* criteria for a disorder, but the symptoms did not cause life interference or distress. In addition, women were mailed a battery of questionnaires that assessed different manifestations of anxiety symptoms. They completed the interview and self-report inventory assessments at 8 weeks, 6 months, and 12 months postpartum.

My results indicated that GAD was the most prevalent anxiety disorder, with 8.2% of the sample meeting diagnostic criteria at 8 weeks postpartum, 7.7% at 6 months postpartum, and 7.0% at 12 months postpartum. In addition, 19.7% of the sample were subsyndromal for GAD at 8 weeks postpartum, 15.5% at 6 months postpartum, and 18.3% at 12 months postpartum (Wenzel, 2005; Wenzel, Haugen, Jackson, et al., 2005). It is important to keep in mind that we modified the duration criteria for a diagnosis of GAD to be 2 months, rather than 6 months, because the first assessment occurred approximately 2 months after women had their babies. Ruscio et al. (2007) determined that the prevalence of GAD increases by 50% to 60% when a 1-month duration is used. If one applies that rule of thumb to the values identified in epidemiological research by Jacobi et al. (2004) and Vesga-López et al. (2008), then it can be estimated that the maximum prevalence of GAD in women who participate in epidemiological research using a shorter duration criterion would be 2.4% to 4.3%. These values are still much lower than the rates of GAD observed in my sample of women across the 1st year postpartum. Interestingly, GAD diagnoses were approximately twice as prevalent as depression diagnoses, and subsyndromal cases of GAD were approximately 3 times as prevalent as subsyndromal cases of depression.

The most comprehensive epidemiological investigation of postpartum anxiety disorders was conducted by Navarro and her colleagues in Spain (Navarro et al., 2008). In a large sample of women who attended follow-up visits at 6 weeks postpartum ($n = 428$), they found that the prevalence of women meeting criteria for GAD, using the 6-month duration criterion, was 0.6%. The prevalence of women meeting criteria for anxiety disorder unspecified, which included women who otherwise met the criteria for GAD minus the 6-month duration criterion as well as women who had subsyndromal expressions of fear (e.g., fears of the health or breathing of the newborn), was 1.3%. Unlike those in my longitudinal study, rates of depression were substantially higher than rates of GAD or anxiety disorder unspecified (major depression = 9.8%; minor depression = 3.3%). It is difficult to explain the difference in rates of GAD and depression between my study and that by Navarro et al. (2008), as both used the Structured Clinical Interview for DSM–IV Disorders (Non-Patient Edition; First, Spitzer, Gibbon, & Williams, 1997) to assign diagnoses.

In contrast, Matthey et al. (2003) identified the prevalence of adjustment disorder with anxious mood in two samples of first-time mothers who were recruited from antenatal classes to participate in a program designed to prevent postpartum depression. Women completed diagnostic interviews when they were approximately 6 to 8 weeks postpartum. In their first sample of 216 women, 1.9% met criteria for adjustment disorder, and in their second sample of 192 women, 3.1% met criteria for adjustment disorder. These rates are much lower than the rate I observed at 8 weeks postpartum in my sample. The authors speculated that rates were low because women had been participating in a prevention program; it is possible that the women were using the strategies that they learned in this program to manage symptoms of emotional distress, thereby reducing their psychiatric symptoms.

Finally, two studies examined rates of GAD in samples who were at higher risk of distress than women in the community studies described previously. In a study of high-risk women admitted to a residential parenting program for "mothers of infants with caretaking difficulties," Rowe et al. (2008) found that 10.9% of their sample met *DSM–IV–TR* criteria for GAD at an average of 10.3 weeks postpartum. Ballard, Davis, Handy, and Mohan (1993) examined the prevalence of GAD in women who were 6 months postpartum, many of whom scored high on a self-report inventory of depression. Diagnoses were made according to Research Diagnostic Criteria (RDC). RDC is a precursor to our current diagnostic system, and the definition of GAD is much less specific and does not include reference to the key feature of excessive and uncontrollable worry. Instead, it indicates that a diagnosis of GAD is made when a person presents with "anxious mood" for at least 2 weeks and has at least two of the following associated features: (a) difficulty falling asleep; (b) sweating, dizziness, palpitations, or shortness of breath; (c) muscle tension or tremors; (d) persistent worry; or (e) fidgeting or an inability to sit still (Wolk, Horwath, Goldstein, Wickramaratne, & Weissman, 1996). Out of 148 mothers interviewed, Ballard and his colleagues identified nine cases of GAD (6.1%)—six of whom had scored high on the self-report inventory of depression and who met RDC criteria for depression, two of whom had scored in the midrange on the self-report inventory of depression, and one of whom scored in the low range on the self-report inventory of depression.

In summary, the body of literature on the prevalence of GAD in the postpartum period suggests that rates of GAD range from 0.6% to 10.9% at 6 to 10 weeks postpartum. Rates of adjustment disorder and anxiety disorder unspecified range from 1.3% to 3.1% at 6 to 8 weeks postpartum. These estimates represent a wide range, so it will be important for future research to address this in a prospective design that clearly defines the parameters of GAD as well as adjustment reactions with anxiety. In contrast, the two studies that have examined the rates of GAD at 6 months postpartum yielded remarkably consistent estimates: 7.7% and 6.1%. The one estimate of the prevalence of GAD at approximately 12 months postpartum is 7.0%.

EFFECTS

The most targeted investigation to date examining a specific area of dysfunction associated with perinatal GAD came from my own research laboratory. My students and I examined sexual adjustment in 10 women with postpartum

GAD and 70 women without postpartum GAD (Wenzel, Haugen, & Goyette, 2005). Women completed the Brief Index of Sexual Functioning for Women (BISF; Taylor, Rosen, & Leiblum, 1994), the Body Image Self-Consciousness Scale (BISC; Wiederman, 2000), and the Sexual Fear and Avoidance Questionnaire (SFAQ; Mills, Antony, Purdon, & Swinson, 2001). Contrary to expectation, responses on the BISF indicated that women with and without postpartum GAD endorsed similar levels of desire, arousal, activity, and orgasm in the context of sexual intercourse. However, relative to women without postpartum GAD, women with postpartum GAD reported higher levels of body image self-consciousness on the BISC and higher levels of sexual fear and avoidance on the SFAQ. These results refuted our a priori prediction that postpartum GAD would be associated with sexual dysfunction, but they suggest that generally anxious women experience elevated levels of distress regarding sexual activity. On reflection, I realized that these findings supported something I often observe in my clinical practice: that women with perinatal GAD are usually engaging in the types of activities that are normative for women at their stage of pregnancy or postpartum, but often at the expense of their emotional well-being. I encourage future researchers to test this observation in domains other than sexual functioning, including parenting; relationships with other family members; completion of household responsibilities; and for those women who have completed their maternity leave, occupational functioning.

There is a dearth of empirical research on the effects of GAD and worry associated with childbirth. However, GAD is often regarded as a nonspecific anxiety disorder (Barlow, 2000), so it is likely that much of the research described in Chapter 1, which used general questionnaires to assess anxiety symptoms, would be relevant in generating hypotheses about the effects of perinatal GAD. In addition, we can make reasonable speculations about the manner in which perinatal GAD would affect the lives of new mothers on the basis of research conducted on people with GAD who are not necessarily going through the transition to parenthood. For example, GAD is associated with overall impairment in social and emotional functioning (Grant et al., 2005), marital distress (Whisman, 2007), lowered general health status (Revicki, Brandenburg, Matza, Hornbrook, & Feeny, 2008), increased health care utilization (Revicki et al., 2008; Wittchen, 2002), impairment in major life roles (e.g., work; Revicki et al., 2008; Wittchen, 2002), and lower quality of life (Revicki et al., 2008). On the basis of this research, it would be reasonable to formulate the following hypotheses about women with perinatal GAD:

- GAD is likely to be associated with impairments in close relationships during pregnancy and the postpartum period, particularly the marital or partner relationship.

- GAD is likely to be associated with pronounced emotional reactivity during pregnancy and the postpartum period.
- GAD is likely to be associated with health concerns during pregnancy and the postpartum period (e.g., hypertension, gestational diabetes). A corollary of this hypothesis is that childbearing women with GAD would utilize more health-care services than childbearing women without GAD.
- GAD is likely to be associated with difficulty adjusting to pregnancy and new motherhood.

Carla experiences many adverse effects as a result of her worry. As stated previously, her relationship with her husband is strained. She views herself as taking out her anxiety and irritability on her children, and she wonders whether these unpleasant interactions will have lasting effects on their emotional well-being. She frequently scans the Internet for ways to consolidate their bills, often at the expense of providing supervision to her children. She snaps at store clerks and customer service agents when she perceives that they are not giving her what she needs or are trying to hassle her. At times, she is so paralyzed by her worry that she is unable to perform basic household functions, such as preparing dinner for the family. This, in turn, causes further strife with her husband, who perceives that he is being forced to take on more and more responsibilities that Carla had previously handled.

COMORBIDITY WITH DEPRESSION

Much evidence points to a substantial overlap between generalized anxiety and depressive symptoms in childbearing women. For example, in my epidemiological research, at 8 weeks postpartum approximately 75% of the women were diagnosed with GAD and 50% of the women who were subsyndromal for GAD were either diagnosed with a depressive disorder (i.e., major depressive disorder or dysthymic disorder) or were regarded as being subsyndromal for a depressive disorder (Wenzel, Haugen, Jackson, et al., 2005). From a different perspective, Austin, Tully, and Parker (2007) found that women who scored high on a worry inventory were 2.6 times more likely to have postpartum depression than women who scored low on this inventory.

This pattern of results mirrors the overlap between generalized anxiety and depression that is seen in samples of women who are not necessarily pregnant or postpartum. Epidemiological research has indicated that 40% of people are diagnosed with concurrent GAD and major depressive disorder at the time they are assessed; this value increases to 59% when one considers the percentage of people with GAD who met criteria for major depressive disorder at some point during the past year (Wittchen, Carter, Pfister, Montgomery, & Kessler, 2000). Pregnancy and childbirth would be logical events that could prompt the expression of both of these disorders simultaneously, as many women experience them as stressful, and elevated hormone levels in turn affect many neuro-chemicals that have the potential to exacerbate symptoms of both of these emotional disorders. These findings suggest that professionals who diagnose GAD or depression in their patients should be cognizant for symptoms of the other disorder, as research has shown that comorbid anxiety and depression is associated with less improvement and a lower remission rate, relative to a single anxiety or mood disorder (van Balkom et al., 2008).

> Carla reports depressive symptoms in addition to her chronic worry. She experiences at least one episode of tearfulness per day when she becomes overwhelmed with her household responsibilities. She no longer engages in activities that she once found enjoyable, such as talking to her two closest girlfriends on the telephone, meeting up with her mother's group, and maintaining her Facebook page. She has little appetite, and her obstetrician is concerned that she is not gaining enough weight in her pregnancy. When she is asked how she is feeling about herself, she describes herself as a "worthless piece of shit" and states that it is "pathetic that I am a stay-at-home mom and can't even keep the house clean." Carla denies any suicidal ideation, although she admits that there are times in which she would like to "disappear" and that, lately, she has been wondering if her family would be better off without her.

POSSIBLE ETIOLOGY

There is a paucity of empirical research designed to identify variables that contribute to the etiology of perinatal GAD. In the following sections, I describe some variables that were associated with worry in my sample of women who were 8 weeks postpartum (Wenzel, Haugen, Jackson, et al., 2005). In addition, I discuss research with nonperinatal samples that has identified possible etiological factors and consider the manner in which it applies specifically to childbearing women.

Sociodemographic Factors

In my longitudinal study, I examined the degree to which four sociodemographic variables (i.e., mother's age, baby's age, number of children in the household, socioeconomic status) predicted scores on the Penn State Worry Questionnaire (PSWQ; Meyer, Miller, Metzger, & Borkovec, 1990), which is a self-report inventory that assesses the severity of chronic worry.

Contrary to expectation, none of these variables predicted PSWQ scores at 8 weeks postpartum. I also determined that diagnoses of GAD and symptoms of worry as assessed by the PSWQ were not associated with the mother's age, the skill level of the mother's job, the mother's level of education, the baby's father's age, the skill level of the baby's father's job, the level of education that the baby's father had attained, the mother's ethnicity, the baby's father's ethnicity, socioeconomic status, or income.

However, in subsequent exploratory analyses, I found that PSWQ scores correlated negatively with the length of time the woman was in a relationship with the baby's father. This means that women who were in their relationships for a shorter amount of time reported a higher level of worry. I also found that women who were not married to the father of their child reported more worry than women who were married to the father of their child. How can we explain these associations? It is possible that that women who have been in a relationship with the father of their child for a relatively short amount of time are less secure in their relationship than women who have been in a relationship with the father of their child for a longer period of time. This insecurity could be associated with an array of worries, such as whether the relationship would last, whether the father would provide the necessary support, and so on. Furthermore, it is logical to speculate that women who were not married to the father of their children (many of whom were no longer in a relationship with that individual) would worry about meeting the multiple demands that are required of new mothers.

In addition, a diagnosis of GAD was more frequent in women who endorsed a past history of emotional disturbances (i.e., anxiety or depression). However, women with a family psychiatric history were no more likely than women with no family psychiatric history to receive a diagnosis of GAD. There are several reasons why psychiatric history variables can explain anxiety symptoms experienced during the transition to parenthood. A personal history of anxiety or depression could signal a biological vulnerability that is activated during times of stress, such as the time surrounding childbirth. Further, a family history of depression or anxiety could point to a genetic predisposition for emotional disturbance. Yet, psychological mechanisms could also account for the manner in which a personal or family history of anxiety or depression could make a woman vulnerable to experience a perinatal anxiety disorder. A previous episode of anxiety or depression could form certain ways of processing information and viewing the world that are invoked in situations that are stressful or difficult. Women could learn maladaptive or unhelpful ways of managing emotions and life stress from family members who struggled with anxiety or depression. Because the mechanism associated with a personal and family history of anxiety and depression is unclear, in this and in subsequent chapters, I make note of these psychiatric history variables in this section on sociodemographic factors, rather than in the sections on possible biological or psychological etiological factors.

> Carla has been in the relationship with her husband since they were 17 years old, and they were married at age 20. Thus, Carla has been in the relationship with her husband for quite some time. Nonetheless, she expresses insecurities about whether their relationship will last. She views herself as driving her husband away because she is irritable and complains all the time. She wonders whether he will leave her with all four children and no money. Thus, Carla is not characterized by the sociodemographic variables associated with GAD in my research, but she has similar insecurities as women who have been in their relationship for only a short period of time.

Biological Factors

In general, there is a surprising dearth of empirical investigation into the neurobiology of GAD, let alone GAD that has its onset or is exacerbated during pregnancy and the postpartum period. In their discussion of the neurobiology of GAD, Connor and Davidson (1998) described evidence suggesting that people with GAD are characterized by decreased sensitivity in some receptors to which norepinephrine binds and reduced cerebrospinal levels of serotonin. It is possible, then, that women who are vulnerable to experience GAD are especially sensitive to hormonal changes that affect these neurochemicals. It will be important for future research to determine the degree to which changes in hormone levels associated with pregnancy exacerbate decreased norepinephrine receptor sensitivity and serotonin activity.

Breastfeeding status is an important variable to consider in understanding anxiety disorders in the postpartum period because various hormones remain elevated until a woman weans her child. However, results from my longitudinal study revealed that breastfeeding status was not related to scores in the PSWQ or the diagnosis of GAD at 8 weeks, 6 months, or 12 months postpartum (Wenzel, Haugen, Jackson, et al., 2005). However, more research is needed to replicate this finding before we can draw the definitive conclusion that breastfeeding and postpartum GAD are unrelated. Moreover, finer grained analyses of breastfeeding status should be considered (e.g., the degree to which worry is elevated in women who breastfeed exclusively vs. those who breastfeed only a couple of times a day).

Psychological Factors

No known studies have examined psychological factors that make women vulnerable to develop GAD during pregnancy or the postpartum period.

However, the larger literature on GAD can provide some clues. Dugas, Gagnon, Ladouceur, and Freeston (1998) identified four cognitive factors that make people vulnerable to the development of GAD: (a) intolerance of uncertainty, (b) inaccurate beliefs about the benefits of worry, (c) poor problem orientation, and (d) cognitive avoidance. Each of these constructs is discussed in turn, with an emphasis on the manner in which they might play a role in the development, maintenance, and exacerbation of perinatal GAD.

Intolerance of uncertainty reflects cognitive, emotional, and behavioral overreactions to situations that are uncertain or ambiguous (Ladouceur, Talbot, & Dugas, 1997). People characterized by intolerance of uncertainty believe that uncertainty is extremely negative and cannot be managed (P. L. Fisher & Wells, 2009). People who have difficulty tolerating uncertainty ask many "what if?" questions that cannot be answered (Dugas et al., 1998), and they focus their attention on the possibility of negative outcomes, no matter how remote they are. Because some degree of ambiguity and uncertainty is unavoidable, people with an intolerance of uncertainty spend a good bit of time worrying and are not adept at handling everyday situations that are unexpected (P. L. Fisher & Wells, 2009). As stated in the Introduction, women experience a great deal of uncertainty during pregnancy and the postpartum period, so it is logical to predict that women who are characterized by an intolerance of uncertainty would struggle during pregnancy and the postpartum period, which could influence the onset of clinically significant symptoms of GAD.

Many people with GAD also exhibit inaccurate beliefs about the benefits of worry (Freeston, Rhéaume, Letarte, Dugas, & Ladouceur, 1994). Examples of these beliefs include "worrying helps to find better ways of doing things" and "worrying can prepare me for bad things that might happen." In pregnant and postpartum women, these beliefs might take the form of "worrying will protect me from disappointment in the event that something goes wrong" and "worrying will help me to detect something wrong at the earliest possible time." These beliefs are maintained by both positive and negative reinforcement. Positive reinforcement occurs whenever there is a desired outcome to a situation about which one was worrying (which erroneously allows the individual to conclude that worrying was beneficial), and negative reinforcement occurs in the absence of the feared catastrophic outcome (P. L. Fisher & Wells, 2009).

Problem orientation includes the abilities to perceive when problems exist, make attributions for the causes of problems, appraise the parameters of the problem, have confidence in one's ability to solve problems, and make appropriate emotional responses (Dugas et al., 1998). Dugas et al. (1998) weighed most heavily one's confidence to solve problems in problem orientation, viewing poor problem orientation as being closely associated with low confidence in one's ability to solve problems. Their research demonstrated that, relative to people without GAD, people with GAD have lower confidence in their problem-solving ability despite the fact that they demonstrate similar knowledge of problem-solving skills (Dugas, Freeston, & Ladouceur, 1997). Given their lack of confidence in their ability to solve problems, one might expect that people with GAD would report a strong sense of helplessness and engage in behaviors such as excessive reassurance seeking. In pregnant and postpartum women, this might manifest in a high number of calls and visits to the doctor.

Cognitive avoidance refers to the process of focusing on the verbal aspects of worry at the expense of acknowledging threatening mental images that are associated with physiological arousal. The unfortunate consequence of this process is that mental images recur quickly and with increased strength (Freeston, Dugas, & Ladouceur, 1996), which perpetuates the cycle of worry (Borkovec & Lyonfields, 1993). As is described in the next chapter, some postpartum women have scary images of harm coming to their baby (e.g., dropping their babies down the stairs). It is conceivable that women engage in worry to prevent these images from occurring as well as to provide a false sense of confidence that they are preventing a tragic event like this from occurring.

> Carla has had long-standing difficulties in tolerating uncertainty in ambiguous situations. For example, when her second child was 6 months old, he developed a persistent cough. Carla was convinced that something terrible was wrong with her baby and that he would die despite the fact that otherwise, he appeared to be a happy and healthy baby. She made three trips to her pediatrician and called numerous times between visits. It was clear that her doctor and his medical staff were becoming annoyed by her. Her worry also caused difficulties in her relationship with her husband, as she became extremely frustrated with his response that they should trust the doctor's opinion that it was just a cough and that they should wait and see before jumping to dire conclusions. However, Carla was persistent in attending to her worries, stating that if she did not take the time to notice subtle changes in her baby's condition, then she might miss something important that would make a difference in whether he lived or died. Four days later, her baby's cough had subsided, and there were no adverse long-term effects.

There is a large body of research demonstrating that these four psychological variables are characteristic of individuals with GAD, and some research has shown that people with these characteristics are vulnerable to developing clinically significant generalized anxiety symptoms. There is no reason to believe that these constructs do not operate in women with perinatal GAD, although it will be important for scholars to test this in future empirical research. Thus, these constructs are integrated into the biopsychosocial model of perinatal anxiety that I describe in Chapter 7.

PRACTICAL IMPLICATIONS

Results from my longitudinal study indicate that GAD is the most common type of emotional disturbance that women experience in their 1st year postpartum; thus, it is imperative that health professionals assess for worry in addition to depression when they are screening for postpartum mood disorders. It also is important to assess for concurrent symptoms of GAD and depression, as research has shown that the syndromes are highly comorbid, and when comorbidity occurs, it is associated with higher levels of dysfunction than are associated with either disorder alone. Clinicians should treat comorbid presentations of GAD and depression particularly aggressively in order to prevent declines in functioning in major life roles and in quality of life.

Because I found that worry was associated with length of time in the partner relationship and women's subjective assessments of the quality of that relationship, it makes sense that in some cases an intervention involving both parents would be warranted. Such a conjoint intervention might focus on problem solving to ensure that the needs of the baby and the household are being met, as well as strategies for enhancing the partner relationship during this period of time when the relationship typically gets little attention. For women who are no longer in a relationship with the father of their newborn, it is imperative that interventions focus on ways to obtain quality social support.

> Carla began psychotherapy for her emotional distress, claiming that she did not want to take medications because she did not want to hurt the baby. It became clear that most of her worries centered on issues over which she and her husband disagreed. Thus, Carla's husband was invited to a few sessions, which were focused on problem solving to address the current life stressors that they were facing and communication skills. Psychotherapy was discontinued temporarily when Carla gave birth to a healthy baby girl. She resumed treatment at approximately 8 weeks postpartum. She admitted that the postpartum period was "rough" and that many of her worries were realized (e.g., she could not provide as much supervision as she would have liked for her three older children, she and her husband needed to refine their budget because of new expenses for the newborn). On the other hand, she indicated that she and her husband had been communicating about their challenges more frequently and more effectively than they had in the past. Carla continued with psychotherapy throughout the 1st year postpartum.

The psychological factors associated with GAD that I described in this chapter—intolerance of uncertainty, inaccurate beliefs about the benefits of worry, poor problem orientation, and cognitive avoidance—are all issues that can be addressed in psychotherapy. I recommend that mental health professionals who treat pregnant and postpartum women with GAD or clinically significant symptoms of worry assess their patients' standing on these four constructs and the degree to which they manifest in relation to childbirth or parenting. These cognitive characteristics orient the new mother to the future, rather than allowing her to be present in the moment, and are associated with absolute, negative judgments (e.g., "I won't be able to handle this," "Uncertainty is too risky, and I must get answers"). Cognitive behavioral therapy (CBT) would be a logical choice to treat pregnant and postpartum women who exhibit these characteristics, as a large focus of CBT for GAD is on the identification and evaluation of cognitions that are associated with distress. This approach to treating GAD is described at greater length in Chapter 10.

Although CBT is efficacious in reducing symptoms of GAD, it is less efficacious than it is in the treatment of other anxiety disorders, and many patients treated with GAD achieve only partial remission (Ninan, 2001). In the past 5 to 10 years, researchers have been developing mindfulness and acceptance-based approaches to treating GAD, with the rationale that mindfulness training helps patients with GAD to focus intentionally on the moment, rather than the future (Roemer & Orsillo, 2002), and to accept uncertainty without judging it as aversive. Preliminary research has found that mindfulness and acceptance-based treatments reduce anxiety and depressive symptoms from pre- to posttreatment (Evans et al., 2008) and that these gains persist 3 and 9 months following treatment (Roemer, Orsillo, & Salters-Pedneault, 2008). It is important to acknowledge that neither CBT nor mindfulness training has been tested in women who suffer from GAD during pregnancy and/or the postpartum period. However, there is nothing about the clinical presentation of perinatal GAD that would suggest that these treatments are contraindicated.

3

OBSESSIONS AND COMPULSIONS

Diane is a 36-year-old Caucasian woman who gave birth to her first child 4 months ago. Before giving birth, she worked in investment banking and was regarded as efficient and level-headed in handling the stress that she encountered on a daily basis. After giving birth, she has wondered if she is going crazy. Diane frequently has violent images of throwing her baby down the stairs or smothering him when she and her husband let him sleep with them at night. Diane reports that her images are becoming increasingly graphic, and as a result she has been finding more and more reasons to let others take over child-care duties. Although she had planned to breastfeed for the first 6 months of her child's life, she recently discontinued because she was afraid that she would be overcome by an urge to strangle her baby during feeding. When she is alone with the baby and is forced to provide child care, she counts to five before touching him, believing that this ritual will protect her baby and keep her from harming him.

This case illustrates obsessive–compulsive disorder (OCD) that had its onset following the birth of a child. Diane's obsessions consisted of fears and violent images of hurting her baby. As a result, she engaged in extensive avoidance behavior and compulsive counting when she could not avoid caring for him. Her obsessive–compulsive symptoms resulted in substantial life interference, as she discontinued breastfeeding, and she was beginning to feel increasingly detached from her child (which could adversely affect mother–infant attachment). Moreover, the symptoms began to cause some burden to her extended family members, as they rearranged their schedules to take shifts in helping Diane to care for her child.

DEFINITION AND NATURE OF OBSESSIONS AND COMPULSIONS

To qualify for a *Diagnostic and Statistical Manual of Mental Disorders* (4th ed., text revision; American Psychiatric Association, 2000) diagnosis of OCD, a person must endorse the presence of either obsessions or compulsions. Characteristics of *obsessions* include (a) recurrent thoughts, images, or impulses that are intrusive and cause marked distress; (b) the thoughts, images, or impulses are not simply excessive worries; (c) the person makes repeated attempts to ignore, suppress, or neutralize the thoughts, images, or impulses; and (d) the person is aware that the thoughts, images, or impulses are coming from her own mind, rather than being inserted by external forces. Characteristics of *compulsions* include (a) repetitive behaviors or mental acts that the person feels driven to perform in response to an obsession, rigid rules, or standards; and (b) the fact that the repetitive behaviors or mental acts are performed with the intent of reducing distress or preventing an awful event from occurring and that they either are not related to the obsessions in a meaningful way or are excessive. People who are diagnosed with OCD recognize that their obsessions and compulsions are unreasonable, and their symptoms cause a great deal of distress, consume at least an hour of the person's day, or interfere with the person's functioning (APA, 2000).

Published case studies have documented a diverse array of obsessive–compulsive symptoms that occur during pregnancy (e.g., religious obsessions, contamination obsessions accompanied by cleaning compulsions; Chemlow & Halfin, 1997; Kalra, Tandon, Trivedi, & Janca, 2005). In many cases, the contents of the obsessive–compulsive symptoms during pregnancy echo the contents of obsessive–compulsive symptoms experienced at other times in a woman's life (Brandt & MacKenzie, 1987). In contrast, empirical research and clinical observation have suggested that something is different about the nature of obsessive–compulsive symptoms that emerge in the postpartum period. For example, some postpartum women have reported significant impairment because of obsessions but few, if any, compulsions. Many women experience a rapid onset of postpartum obsessive–compulsive symptoms, whereas the typical onset at other times in people's lives tends to be more gradual (Abramowitz, Schwartz, Moore, & Luenzmann 2003; Sichel, Cohen, Rosenbaum, & Driscoll, 1993). The content of obsessions is usually targeted toward possible harm coming to the infant or aggression toward the infant (Sichel, Cohen, Dimmock, & Rosenbaum, 1993; Wisner, Peindl, Gigliotti, & Hanusa, 1999), and in turn women often avoid the situations that evoke those obsessions (Abramowitz, Moore, Carmin, Wiegartz, & Purdon, 2001).

Obsessions Versus Psychosis

Before proceeding, it is important to differentiate postpartum OCD from postpartum psychosis, a rare condition experienced by one or two women per 1,000 births (Kendell, Chalmers, & Platz, 1987). In both conditions, new mothers can experience intrusive thoughts about harming their infant. However, there are many differences that can be used as heuristics to distinguish between the two conditions. Table 3.1 summarizes the key differences between postpartum OCD and postpartum psychosis. Perhaps the most substantial difference is that intrusive thoughts of harming the newborn in women with postpartum OCD are *ego-dystonic*. This means that the thoughts are inconsistent with the new mother's reality, and she is mortified that she is having them. As a result, she experiences a great deal of distress, is uncomfortable talking with others about her thoughts, and usually avoids at

TABLE 3.1
Key Differences Between Postpartum OCD and Postpartum Psychosis

Postpartum OCD	Postpartum psychosis
Ego-dystonic (i.e., inconsistent with the mother's reality)	Ego-syntonic (i.e., consistent with the mother's reality)
Associated with distress	Not associated with distress
Avoids newborn	Does not avoid newborn, and instead experiences impulses to act on the thoughts
Decreased likelihood that woman will act on the intrusive thoughts	Increased likelihood that woman will act on the intrusive thoughts
In touch with reality	Not in touch with reality
Absence of associated symptoms that often co-occur with psychosis	Presence of associated symptoms that often co-occur with psychosis (e.g., loose associations, labile mood, agitation)
More common (e.g., up to 91% of new mothers experience intrusive thoughts)	Less common (e.g., 1–2 women out of 1,000 experience psychotic symptoms)
Usually occurs throughout the first several months following childbirth	Usually occurs within the first few days following childbirth

Note. Data from Abramowitz, Schwartz, Moore, and Luenzmann (2003); Altemus (2001); Brandes, Soares, and Cohen (2004); Fairbrother and Abramowitz (2007); Kleiman (2009); Ross and McLean (2006). OCD = obsessive–compulsive disorder.

all costs circumstances that she believes will allow her to act on her thoughts. In contrast, the intrusive thoughts of harming the newborn in women with postpartum psychosis are *ego-syntonic*. This means that these thoughts are viewed as consistent with the new mother's reality, such that she does not experience distress when she has the thoughts, she is able to talk about them with others, and there is a high likelihood that she will act on her thoughts, perhaps because she carries through with hallucinations and delusions that instruct her to harm her child (Spinelli, 2004). Women with ego-syntonic thoughts of harming the baby often believe that doing so is a way to save the baby from danger (Altemus, 2001).

Andrea Yates, the Texas mother who drowned her five children in 2001, stated on more than one occasion that she heard voices telling her to harm others, including her children, and that harming her children would punish her for being a bad mother. Andrea Yates was experiencing a postpartum psychotic episode. Because cases like that of Andrea Yates are sensationalized by the media, women who experience ego-dystonic intrusive thoughts of harming their infants are gravely concerned that they, too, are on the verge of a post-partum psychotic episode. However, the mere facts that these women are concerned about their thoughts and go to great lengths to avoid them suggest that they are experiencing obsessions, rather than psychotic symptoms. Intrusive thoughts of harm coming to the infant are quite common in the postpartum period, and there is no evidence to suggest that women with these ego-dystonic thoughts will actually do anything to harm their babies (Barr & Beck, 2008).

Obsessions Versus Worries

Another construct that often overlaps with OCD (particularly obsessions) is that of worry, and many clinicians have difficulty differentiating between the two. Table 3.2 displays the differences between obsessive thoughts and worries that have been documented in empirical research. Obsessions are viewed by people as out of character and often reflect themes of contamination, sex, and aggression (Turner, Beidel, & Stanley, 1992). In contrast, worries tend to focus on everyday issues such as the health of family members and safety of children (Hazlett-Stevens, Pruitt, & Collins, 2009). Obsessive thinking is characterized by cognitions that are less realistic than worries but that represent more deleterious consequences. Whereas worries mainly occur in a verbal format, obsessions are frequently experienced in the form of images or impulses (Langlois, Freeston, & Ladouceur, 2000a). Many people who endorse obsessions attribute great meaning or significance to them (e.g., "I am going to act on this thought because I am thinking about it"), whereas most people who endorse worry are focused on the possibility of a negative outcome (Hazlett-Stevens et al., 2009). Surprisingly, excessive worry is associated with a greater frequency

TABLE 3.2
Key Differences Between Obsessive Thoughts and Worries

Obsessive thoughts	Worries
Unexpected situations or events (e.g., contamination, sex, aggression)	Everyday life situations or events
Less realistic	More realistic
Viewed as less likely to occur	Viewed as more likely to occur
Consequences more serious if they occur	Consequences less serious if they occur
Contents of cognitions are unacceptable	Contents of cognitions are acceptable
Often include images and impulses	Usually are restricted to verbal content
Close association with perceived meaning	Close association with perceived negative outcomes

Note. Data from Clark and Claybourn (1997); Hazlett-Stevens, Pruitt, and Collins (2009); Langlois, Freeston, and Ladouceur (2000a, 2000b); Turner, Beidel, and Stanley (1992).

of checking behavior than is obsessive thinking (Clark & Claybourn, 1997). Thus, it would be a mistake for clinicians to conclude that a childbearing woman has OCD solely on the basis of her checking behavior.

The case of Robin described in the Introduction in this volume most clearly illustrates worry about harm coming to the infant, whereas the case of Diane described in this chapter most clearly illustrates obsessions about harm coming to the infant. The perceived consequences are serious in both instances. However, Robin's thoughts are mainly verbal, catastrophic worries about harm coming to her baby when she is not monitoring, whereas Diane experiences vivid images of causing harm to her baby when she is in the baby's proximity. As a result, the two have very different behavioral presentations. Robin closely monitors her baby, especially at night when her baby is sleeping, and she perceives that the baby might die of sudden infant death syndrome. In contrast, Diane avoids her baby or engages in an irrational counting ritual to protect him. Thus, some rules of thumb in differentiating between diagnosis of postpartum OCD and generalized anxiety disorder (GAD) are (a) whether the cognitions come in the form of images/impulses versus verbal activity, (b) the degree to which the contents of the cognitions involve harm coming to the baby specifically by the hands of the mother or an outside source, and (c) the resulting behavioral response (i.e., avoidance vs. excessive checking).

It is important to realize that most clinical presentations will not lend themselves to such clear distinctions. In fact, some research has shown that intrusive thoughts lie on a continuum, with pure obsessions that are not based in reality on one end and pure worries that are indeed based in reality on the other end (Langlois, Freeston, & Ladouceur, 2000b). Most intrusive thoughts reported by patients fall in a gray area in the middle. Thus, it is important to use other clinical information in determining the precise diagnosis (e.g., personal and family history of emotional disturbance, presence of disorder-specific psychological variables [i.e., poor problem orientation for GAD, excessive responsibility for OCD]).

PREVALENCE

Scholars in this field have taken two distinct approaches in examining the prevalence of perinatal OCD. In one approach, clinical samples of women who have been diagnosed with OCD are asked to identify, retrospectively, the circumstances surrounding the onset of their OCD. Researchers then calculate the percentage of women who attribute the onset or exacerbation of their OCD to pregnancy or childbirth. I regard these studies as ones that use clinical samples, as women in these samples are selected because they are seeking psychiatric treatment for their symptoms. In the other approach, samples of women who, presumably, are representative of the population of childbearing women seeking obstetric care at various facilities or recruited from public records are assessed, and the percentage of women with OCD is calculated. I regard these studies as ones that use community samples, as women in these samples are receiving standard obstetric care and are not presenting for concerns specifically related to psychiatric distress. Results from both types of research are described in the following sections.

Clinical Samples

Many retrospective studies have examined the degree to which pregnancy and childbirth are associated with the onset or exacerbation of OCD. In their review of empirical literature on this topic, Albert, Maina, and Bogetto (2000) concluded that childbirth is only one of two life events that differentiate people with and without OCD, such that delivery occurs more frequently in people who have OCD. Retrospective research finds that between 17% (Williams & Koran, 1997) and 39% (Neziroglu, Anemone, & Yaryura-Tobias, 1992) of women with OCD estimate that the onset of their symptoms occurred during pregnancy. Interestingly, both of these studies found no instances of postpartum onset of OCD, although there was postpartum exacerbation of the OCD that had developed during pregnancy. Other retrospective survey research indicates that between 50% and 70% of women with OCD attribute the onset or worsening of their OCD to pregnancy or childbirth (Buttolph & Holland, 1990; Maina, Albert, Bogetto, Vaschetto, & Ravizza, 1999) and that approximately 50% of women with preexisting OCD report a postpartum exacerbation of symptoms (Labad et al., 2005). Of course, a limitation of this research is that these estimates were made retrospectively, such that participants were asked to think back over the course of their illness and identify possible triggering events. Such estimates are vulnerable to biases in memory and to different thresholds of reporting.

This body of literature indicates that pregnancy can serve as a trigger for the onset of OCD, perhaps more frequently than any other single life event. A substantial percentage of women with preexisting OCD become worse during pregnancy, which could occur because they choose to decrease or discontinue their psychotropic medication. Although it appears that the onset of OCD occurs during the postpartum period less frequently than during pregnancy, the postpartum period certainly seems to be a time in which women with preexisting OCD are vulnerable to an exacerbation in their symptoms.

Community Samples

Several groups of researchers have calculated the prevalence of OCD in samples of women who were receiving routine obstetric care or who were recruited from public records during pregnancy or the postpartum period; thus, this section is divided into studies that focus on either one of these time periods. Throughout this section, the reader can compare these rates of OCD with the prevalence of OCD in women who participate in epidemiological research but who are not necessarily pregnant or postpartum. These rates range from 0.6% (4-week rate; Jacobi et al., 2004) to 1.3% (current rate; Torres et al., 2006).

Pregnancy

Two of the studies described in Chapter 2, which investigated the prevalence of GAD in pregnant samples, also examined the prevalence of OCD. In their study of 175 pregnant and 172 nonpregnant women in Africa, Adewuya, Ola, Aloba, and Mapayi (2006) found that 5.2% of their pregnant sample met diagnostic criteria for OCD, relative to 1.7% of their nonpregnant sample. The difference between groups reached statistical significance at only a trend level ($p = .078$) but is highlighted in this chapter because the rate of OCD in pregnant women was approximately 3 times the rate in nonpregnant women. In contrast, Sutter-Dallay, Giaconne-Marcesche, Glatigny-Dallay, and Verdoux (2004) identified a lower rate of OCD (1.2%) in their sample of 497 women in their 3rd trimester of pregnancy.

One study was designed specifically to investigate the prevalence of OCD in pregnant women. In this study, Uguz, Gezginc, et al. (2007) reported that 15 of 434 (3.5%) women in their 3rd trimester of pregnancy met criteria for OCD. Only two of these women indicated that the onset of their OCD occurred during pregnancy; the remaining women stated that OCD was present before they became pregnant. Of the 13 women who had OCD before they became pregnant, six (46.1%) indicated that their symptoms worsened during pregnancy, three (23.1%) indicated that their symptoms improved during pregnancy, and four (30.8%) experienced no change in the severity of their symptoms. The most common obsessions were contamination (80%) and symmetry (60%), and the most common compulsions were cleaning/washing (86.7%) and checking (60%).

On the basis of these three studies, we can estimate that the prevalence of OCD in pregnant women is approximately 1.2% to 5.2%. Two studies reported values that are substantially higher than the rate of 1.3% in women representative of the general population (Torres et al. 2006). It is important to acknowledge that the women in Torres et al.'s (2006) community sample ranged from ages 16 to 74, and that the prevalence of OCD was highest in the 16- to 24-year-old age range and second highest in the 25- to 44-year-old age range. Thus, one factor that could elevate the rate of OCD during pregnancy is the fact that pregnant women fall squarely in the age ranges that are associated with the highest rates of OCD.

Postpartum Period

Abramowitz, Schwartz, and Moore (2003) found that approximately two thirds of new mothers reported that they experience intrusive thoughts that fall into one of seven categories: (a) thoughts of suffocation or sudden infant death syndrome, (b) thoughts of accidents, (c) ideas or urges of intentional harm, (d) thoughts of losing the baby, (e) illness, (f) unacceptable sexual thoughts, and (g) contamination. On average, women reported mild distress associated with these intrusions. In their later research, Abramowitz and his colleagues found that this rate may be as high as 91% (Abramowitz, Khandker, Nelson, Deacon, & Rygwall, 2006). Results from these studies suggest that intrusive thoughts that fall into one or more of these domains and that are associated with only mild distress can be regarded as fairly normative experiences for new mothers. When intrusive thoughts in these domains are associated with moderate to severe distress and are accompanied by avoidance behavior, further assessment by a trained professional is necessary to determine whether the woman meets diagnostic criteria for OCD.

Five studies have examined rates of postpartum OCD in community samples. In my longitudinal study on anxiety disorders in a community sample of postpartum women, 2.7% of the sample met diagnostic criteria for OCD at 8 weeks postpartum (Wenzel, Haugen, Jackson, & Brendle, 2005), 4.2% at 6 months postpartum, and 0.9% at 12 months postpartum (Wenzel, 2005). In addition, 5.4% of the sample was subsyndromal for OCD at 8 weeks postpartum, 4.2% at 6 months postpartum, and 2.6% at 12 months postpartum. My colleagues and I found a similar rate of 3.9% in an earlier study of 788 women recruited when they were between 4 and 7 months postpartum (Wenzel, Gorman, O'Hara, & Stuart, 2001). In their study designed specifically to examine the nature and prevalence of postpartum OCD, Uguz, Akman, Kaya, and Cilli (2007) obtained a rate of 4% in their sample of 302 women who were 6 weeks postpartum. This group of results contrasts with those reported by Navarro et al. (2008), who found that only 0.7% of their community sample of 428 women met criteria for OCD at 6 weeks postpartum. The pattern of findings obtained in these studies is similar to the one discussed in Chapter 2 on GAD, such that higher rates of clinically significant pathology were detected in my study than in Navarro et al.'s study.

Altemus (2001) conducted a unique longitudinal study of the course of OCD that spanned the 3rd trimester of pregnancy through the 1st year postpartum. Specifically, she recruited 100 healthy women with no symptoms of psychiatric disturbance in their 3rd trimester and assessed them at 6 weeks, 16 weeks, and 1 year postpartum. Six women had developed OCD during pregnancy; this was the initial onset of OCD in four of the women, and the remaining two women had experienced transient obsessive–compulsive symptoms during another pregnancy. The OCD symptoms of all of these women pertained to contamination obsessions/cleaning rituals or violent obsessions of harming their infants. By the 1-year assessment, three of the women with OCD had achieved a complete remission. No new cases of OCD in the remaining 94 women developed during the postpartum period, but it is interesting that 25 of these women had subsyndromal obsessive–compulsive symptoms during pregnancy that continued into the postpartum period.

Collectively, results from these studies show that more often than not, women will experience some degree of intrusive thoughts about harm coming to their infants in the postpartum period. Although these thoughts are distressing, it is unlikely that women will act on them, and it is also unlikely that these thoughts will develop into a clinically significant expression of OCD. The research reviewed here suggests that the prevalence of OCD in community samples ranges from 0.7% to 4.0% at 6 to 8 weeks postpartum, is approximately 4.0% around 6 months postpartum, and drops below 1.0% at 12 months postpartum. Thus, it appears that the prevalence of women who meet criteria for OCD during pregnancy for the first 6 months postpartum period is somewhat higher than the percentage of women representative of the general population who meet criteria for OCD.

EFFECTS

The emotional burden of carrying intrusive thoughts of harm coming to the baby can be enormous. Many women are afraid to disclose their obsessions because they are ashamed or because they predict that their child will be taken away from them, which prevents them from getting the help they need (Barr & Beck, 2008; C. T. Beck & Driscoll, 2006). These emotional experiences can cause significant distress in childbearing women, which can in turn interfere with their ability to focus on their parenting (e.g. Chelmow & Halfin, 1997), household responsibilities, and relationships with their partner and other family members (e.g., Brandt & MacKenzie, 1987). Some women develop such extreme concerns about doing harm to their babies that they avoid their infants altogether.

Similar to what was seen in Chapter 2 on GAD, little research has investigated the effects of OCD that occurs during pregnancy and/or the postpartum period. However, the larger literature on functional impairment associated with OCD provides the basis for hypotheses that can be tested in pregnant and postpartum samples. For example, a diagnosis of OCD has been associated with impairment in social functioning (Huppert, Simpson, Nissenson, Liebowitz, & Foa, 2009; Khanna, Rajendra, & Channabasavanna, 1988), marital distress (Emmelkamp & Gerlsma, 1994), impairment in family relationships (Huppert et al., 2009; Khanna et al., 1988), increased health care utilization (Bobes et al., 2001), impairment in occupational duties (Huppert et al., 2009; Khanna et al., 1988), financial difficulties (Bobes et al., 2001), and lowered quality of life (Bobes et al., 2001; Huppert et al., 2009; Norberg, Calamari, Cohen, & Riemann, 2008). Impairment in these domains is particularly pronounced when OCD is comorbid with another disorder (Huppert et al., 2009). On the basis of this research, it would be reasonable to formulate the following hypotheses about women with perinatal OCD:

- OCD is likely to be associated with impairments in close relationships during pregnancy and the postpartum period, particularly in the marital or partner relationship and relationships with family members.
- OCD is likely to be associated with health concerns during pregnancy and the postpartum period (e.g., hypertension, gestational diabetes). A corollary of this hypothesis is that childbearing women with OCD would utilize more health care services than childbearing women without OCD.
- OCD is likely to be associated with difficulty in adjusting to pregnancy; new motherhood; and, in women who work, a return to work after maternity leave.

Diane's obsessive–compulsive symptoms are affecting her in many ways. Most notably, her relationships with close others have deteriorated significantly. Although her husband expressed care and support soon after the onset of her symptoms, his patience has begun to wear thin, and he is fearful that his wife will not return to her usual level of functioning. He is resentful that he has to take over as a full-time care provider for their infant after he has worked long hours at a demanding job. Not surprisingly, Diane and her husband have numerous arguments, and he has fleeting thoughts that he might pursue a divorce if their circumstances do not change. Diane, in turn, experiences substantial distress after these arguments, pleading with her husband to understand what she is going through. In addition, Diane's relationship with her mother is becoming increasingly strained, as her mother cannot understand why Diane does not want to be around her precious child. Diane perceives that her mother is overly critical and that just makes her anxiety worse. She also has isolated herself from friends and acquaintances who are trying to get in contact with her, as she is embarrassed by her perception that she simply cannot handle motherhood. Diane's symptoms have occupational and financial consequences as well. She had been slated to return to work after 3 months of maternity leave. However, she has been so shaken by the severity of her anxiety that she predicts that she would "fall apart" if she experiences any additional stressors. Currently, Diane is on an indefinite hiatus from work without compensation.

COMORBIDITY WITH DEPRESSION

Abramowitz, Schwartz, and Moore (2003) found that postpartum women who reported obsessive thoughts scored in the subclinical range on the Center for Epidemiological Studies Depression Scale (Radoff, 1977). This means that women were not endorsing depressive symptoms at a level of severity that would necessarily require attention from a mental health professional, but that they were noticeable. In my longitudinal study on postpartum anxiety disorders, half of the women who met diagnostic criteria for OCD were diagnosed with major depressive disorder or subsyndromal major depressive disorder at 8 weeks postpartum (Wenzel, Hauger, Jackson, & Brendle, 2005). Many women who develop OCD in pregnancy have a history of severe premenstrual syndrome (Altemus, 2001) or major depression (Diaz, Grush, Sichel, & Cohen, 1997); conversely, a large portion of women who have OCD with a postpartum onset go on to develop secondary depression (Sichel, Cohen, Dimmock, et al., 1993). There is also evidence that depressed women are more likely to experience intrusive thoughts of harming their infant than nondepressed women; for example, Jennings, Ross, Popper, and Elmore (1999) found that 40% of the sample of depressed mothers endorsed these intrusive thoughts compared with 7% of nondepressed mothers in their sample.

As was seen in Chapter 2 on GAD, this pattern of results mirrors the rate of comorbidity observed in samples representative of the general population. Major depression is 10 times more prevalent in people with OCD than in people without OCD (Denys, Tenney, van Megen, de Geus, & Westenberg,

2004). Rates of concurrent diagnoses of major depression and OCD range from approximately 13% (Rush et al., 2005) to 40% (Tükel, Polat, Özdemir, Aksüt, & Türksoy, 2002). People with comorbid OCD and depression have more severe obsessive, compulsive, and depressive symptoms than people with either disorder alone, and they are more likely to have other comorbid disorders and lower quality of life (Besiroglu, Uguz, Saglam, Agargun, & Cilli, 2007). Thus, as was seen in Chapter 2 on GAD, it is important for clinicians to differentiate between symptoms of OCD and major depression in order to arrive at a correct diagnosis, but it would also behoove them to be aware of substantial rates of comorbidity between the two because comorbidity is associated with an especially poor clinical course and outcome.

> Diane experiences depressive symptoms at a level for which she qualifies for a diagnosis of comorbid major depressive disorder. Perhaps the most substantial depressive symptom that she reports is a sense of worthlessness. Diane views herself as a horrible mother and is tormented by her belief that she is failing at parenting her child, when it seems so natural for other women. As a result, she endures constant depressed mood and tearfulness several times a day. She also reports symptoms of anhedonia, sleep disturbance (i.e., fitful sleep, waking up several times in the middle of the night but also spending 10 to 12 hr a day in bed), fatigue, and concentration difficulties. For the first time in her life, she is experiencing suicidal ideation, such that she wonders if life is worth living and is convinced that she would be better off dead. Although she does not have a specific plan for hurting herself, she has fantasies of driving into oncoming traffic or into a tree in order to end it all.

POSSIBLE ETIOLOGY

Although there is a lack of prospective research designed to identify risk factors for perinatal OCD, many scholars have made reasonable speculations about the biological basis of obsessive–compulsive symptoms that emerge specifically in this time period, and other scholars have tested cognitive behavioral aspects of OCD in samples of postpartum women. The current state of the literature on correlates of perinatal OCD is described in the following sections.

Sociodemographic Factors

There is little evidence that most sociodemographic variables differentiate pregnant and postpartum women with and without OCD. For example, Uguz, Gezginc, et al. (2007) compared women in their 3rd trimester with and without OCD and found that groups did not differ in age, educational level, employment status, parity, number of gestational weeks, length of marriage, history of abortion, and pregnancy complications. However, approximately 33% of the pregnant women with OCD endorsed a family history of OCD compared with approximately 2% of the pregnant women without OCD. These researchers also compared their sample of pregnant women with OCD with a sample of nonpregnant women with OCD and found that the two groups were similar in demographic characteristics, frequency of a family history of OCD, and severity and types of obsessive–compulsive symptoms. Results from my longitudinal study with postpartum women (Wenzel, Haugen, Jackson, et al., 2005) support this pattern of results. In fact, the only sociodemographic variable that I found to be significantly related to a diagnosis of OCD was age, such that women who received a diagnosis of OCD or who were subsyndromal for a diagnosis of OCD were younger than those who did not receive a diagnosis of OCD. There was a trend for a diagnosis of OCD to be associated with increased rates of a personal and family psychiatric history.

In contrast, two groups of researchers (Maina et al., 1999; Uguz, Akman, et al., 2007) observed that postpartum OCD was more frequent in nulliparous than parous women in their sample. Thus, two out of four studies that examined the association between parity and perinatal OCD found that primiparous women are more likely to struggle with OCD associated with childbirth. It is important for future research to replicate this and determine the mechanism by which this association is expressed. For example, it is possible that first-time mothers are characterized by a heightened sense of responsibility associated with parenting, as they do not know what to expect and are especially fearful of making a mistake. As is seen in the section on psychological factors, a heightened sense of responsibility is a cognitive characteristic that increases the risk of obsessive thinking.

Biological Factors

C. T. Beck and Driscoll (2006) speculated that the rapid onset of postpartum OCD may be due to the substantial decline in estrogen and progesterone levels following childbirth, which has the potential to disrupt serotonergic functioning. Some evidence suggests that estrogen has anxiolytic effects (e.g., Ditkoff, Crary, Cristo, & Lobo, 1991), so it is possible that a rapid reduction in estrogen would dysregulate the serotonergic system and create a biological pathway for obsessive–compulsive symptoms to emerge. In addition, the high level of oxytocin present near the end of pregnancy and during the postpartum period when women are lactating may trigger or exacerbate OCD (Diaz et al., 1997; McDougle, Barr, Goodman, & Price, 1999). Oxytocin is a hormone that promotes protection, safety, and maternal behavior, and it is possible that an excess in this hormone triggers obsessions about harm coming to the baby (C. T. Beck & Driscoll, 2006). Furthermore, McDougle et al. (1999)

noted that elevated oxytocin is associated with intrusive sexual thoughts and images in nonchildbearing OCD patients, which could explain increases in intrusive thoughts of this nature in postpartum women. Altemus (2001) speculated that women with perinatal OCD are especially sensitive to the high levels of these hormones and the effects of rapid changes in levels of these hormones.

Breastfeeding appears to be associated with improvements in obsessive–compulsive symptoms in women who had subsyndromal manifestations of OCD, but it has no effect on the severity of symptoms in women who had been diagnosed with OCD (Altemus, 2001). It is possible that the neuro-chemical changes associated with lactation, such as increased levels of gamma-aminobutyric acid (GABA), are more relevant to protecting women from other anxiety symptoms (e.g., panic) than obsessive–compulsive symptoms while they are breastfeeding. Indeed, in my longitudinal study of anxiety disorders in postpartum women, breastfeeding status was not associated with a diagnosis of OCD at 8 weeks, 6 months, or 12 months following childbirth (Wenzel, Haugen, Jackson, et al., 2005).

Psychological Factors

Jonathan Abramowitz and his colleagues have proposed a cognitive behavioral model of postpartum OCD and have collected empirical data to validate aspects of the model. The core tenets of their model (see Abramowitz et al., 2001; Abramowitz, Schwartz, Moore, & Luenzmann, 2003; Fairbrother & Abramowitz, 2007) are as follows:

1. Most adults experience intrusive thoughts from time to time.
2. The frequency of the thoughts and associated negative affect increase when people interpret intrusive thoughts as threatening, such as the prediction that they will act on those thoughts.
3. People who misinterpret these thoughts often go to great lengths to avoid situations that trigger the thoughts or situations in which the catastrophes they predict will be realized.
4. Although avoidance reduces distress in the short term, it strengthens obsessional anxiety over the long term through negative reinforcement.
5. It is difficult to control such thoughts, so when they recur, people again misinterpret them as being significant. This, in turn, leads to preoccupation with the thought and the repetitiveness that is often observed in people who struggle with obsessive–compulsive symptoms.

6. Hiding intrusive thoughts has the potential to strengthen them, as it prevents the person from exposure to evidence supporting the notion that having these thoughts is not harmful.

Abramowitz and his colleagues speculated that the postpartum period provides a ripe context for the development of obsessive thoughts because parents have great responsibility for ensuring the safety and well-being of their newborn, who is vulnerable and highly cherished (Abramowitz et al., 2001; Fairbrother & Abramowitz, 2007). In addition, Abramowitz, Schwartz, Moore, and Luenzmann (2003) identified two cognitive biases at work in people who are particularly vulnerable to develop intrusive thoughts. A *probability bias* is demonstrated when people believe that just thinking about something increases the likelihood that it will actually occur. A *morality bias* occurs when people equate thinking about bad things with actually committing a bad behavior. The confluence of these two biases is known as *thought-action fusion* (Shafran, Thordarson, & Rachman, 1996), which captures this tendency to exaggerate the significance and consequences of intrusive thoughts.

Subsequent work by Abramowitz and his colleagues has identified other specific cognitive factors in the development of postpartum OCD. For example, people who hold high moral standards are particularly likely to develop intrusive thoughts, and it is possible that standards for caretaking behaviors are especially high in the time following childbirth (Abramowitz, Schwartz, & Moore, 2003). In addition, three specific dysfunctional beliefs— overestimation of threat/inflated sense of responsibility, beliefs about the importance of and need to control intrusive thoughts, and perfectionism and intolerance of uncertainty—predict symptoms in the domains of compulsive checking, compulsive washing, and obsessions above and beyond symptoms of depression and nonobsessive–compulsive anxiety (Abramowitz et al. 2006). This association is mediated by the tendency to make negative appraisals about the presence and meaning of intrusive thoughts (Abramowitz, Nelson, Rygwall, & Khandker, 2007).

Because intrusive thoughts are so threatening and uncomfortable, many new mothers go to great efforts to neutralize them, such as by avoiding situations that provoke the thoughts, suppressing the thoughts, or engaging in safety behaviors (e.g., checking). These behaviors reinforce obsessional anxiety because they provide temporary relief. Moreover, when the feared outcome does not occur (e.g., nothing bad happens to the baby), mothers often attribute the desired outcome to the fact that they engaged in the safety behavior. Thus, they do not learn that there is no association between their obsessive thoughts, safety behaviors, and the probability of an adverse outcome, and their efforts to avoid or conceal these thoughts prevent them from learning that obsessive thoughts about harm coming to the baby are normal experiences (Fairbrother & Abramowitz, 2007).

The work by Abramowitz and his colleagues has advanced the most comprehensive model of perinatal anxiety to date. Their research has identified a number of vulnerability factors for the development of obsessive–compulsive symptoms associated with childbirth, including (a) the belief that just thinking about something causes it to occur (i.e., probability bias), (b) the belief that thinking about something bad is the equivalent of doing something bad (i.e., morality bias), (c) an overestimation of one's responsibility, (d) the belief that it is imperative to control intrusive thoughts, and (e) the belief that uncertainty is intolerable. It is important that Abramowitz and colleagues have measured each of these constructs in samples of postpartum women and have demonstrated that they account for a significant amount of variance in obsessive–compulsive symptomatology. Thus, clinicians working with women who are near delivery or who have recently delivered should be attune to these vulnerability factors, and if present, assess for OCD.

The astute reader will notice that intolerance of uncertainty is characteristic of both OCD and GAD (Starcevic & Berle, 2006). This could be one reason why clinicians sometimes experience confusion in differential diagnosis between the two disorders. It could be that intolerance of uncertainty is a vulnerability factor for both disorders, or it could be that different aspects of intolerance of uncertainty are unique to each disorder, as the measurement of intolerance of uncertainty in studies examining this construct in GAD is different from that in studies examining this construct in OCD. It will be important for future research to thoroughly measure intolerance of uncertainty in pregnant women, along with other vulnerability factors for both disorders, and examine the pathway by which both GAD and OCD are expressed in the postpartum period.

> Diane is characterized by a number of the psychological vulnerability factors described in this section. Part of her success as an investment banker came from her strong work ethic, perfectionism, and meticulous attention to detail. She has a history of overreacting to perceived threat, regarding it as more dangerous than it really is. For example, when the economy experienced a downslide the previous year, Diane was convinced that she would lose her job and that the lost income would force her and her husband to sell their upscale home at a loss. She maintained this belief despite the fact that the CEO of her company told her that she is one of the most valued employees. As a result, she worked at least 12 hr a day while she was in the early stages of pregnancy, which resulted in substantial fatigue and inattention to self-care. Diane also has a strong sense of responsibility, which is evidenced by her insistence on single-handedly handling the arrangements for her elderly grandmother's nursing care and in taking on the role of mentor for all of her company's summer interns and new trainees.

PRACTICAL IMPLICATIONS

New mothers undoubtedly will be relieved to hear that obsessive thoughts about harm coming to the baby are very common, as these thoughts are often accompanied by a tremendous amount of guilt, shame, and secrecy. It is reassuring that there is no evidence that women who experience obsessive thoughts about harming their infants actually act on their thoughts (Barr & C. T. Beck, 2008). Nevertheless, clinicians would be wise to be alert for variables that signal significant risk for the development of perinatal OCD, as it can cause substantial impairment and distress. Factors that might alert clinicians to the presence of perinatal OCD include the cognitive variables described in the previous section as well as a personal or family history of OCD. Of course, clinicians should be sure to determine whether intrusive thoughts of harming an infant would be better characterized as postpartum psychosis, as a diagnosis of postpartum psychosis is associated with increased risk that a woman will indeed harm her child.

A substantial percentage of women with preexisting OCD experience an exacerbation of the disorder during pregnancy and/or the postpartum period. Clinicians who work with OCD patients who become pregnant should carefully monitor these women's symptoms and weigh the costs and benefits of various treatment options. If some of the cognitive variables described in this chapter emerge as reasons why the transition to parenthood is difficult, then psychotherapy would be a logical option for intervention to modify them. As is described at greater length in Chapter 10, regardless of whether a new mother has preexisting OCD or had an onset of OCD following childbirth, a cognitive behavioral approach to treatment is regarded as the standard in the field for treating obsessions and compulsions.

> Diane's symptoms became severe enough that, in collaboration with her obstetrician, her family encouraged her to seek inpatient care. Diane was in the hospital for a week and was started on a trial of fluvoxamine (Luvox) as well as exposure with response prevention (ERP). Each day, someone from Diane's family brought the baby to the ward, and she engaged in typical activities with him (e.g., changing, playing, holding) instead of avoiding or engaging in her counting ritual. By the end of her hospital stay, her acute symptoms had subsided, although she continued to endorse some depressive symptoms and express concerns about doing something wrong as she cared for her child. After discharge, Diane participated in weekly outpatient psychotherapy with a cognitive behavioral therapist who reinforced the gains she had made in ERP and who also addressed her depression using cognitive and behavioral strategies.

4

PANIC ATTACKS

Becca is a 25-year-old African American woman who had her first child 9 months ago. She reports a history of anxiety problems that began in high school. At that time, she had occasional panic attacks that would interfere with her participation in school-related activities, such as taking exams or participating in after-school sporting events. Her anxiety was managed successfully with psychotropic medication. After discontinuing medication in college, she had occasional panic attacks while she was studying for exams, but they were manageable. Becca reported a further decrease in her anxiety during pregnancy and noted that pregnancy was the "best time of my life." Her anxiety continued to be low following childbirth until the 6th month postpartum, when she began to wean her baby from breastfeeding. As she was weaning, she experienced a dramatic increase in her anxiety, such that she now has a panic attack approximately once every other day. These panic attacks leave her exhausted, and she often calls in sick to work or begs her husband to come home and take care of the baby because she is tired and shaken up.

Becca's case exemplifies the onset of postpartum panic disorder. She was vulnerable to developing this anxiety disorder, as she had been treated for panic attacks in high school (although at that time, she was not diagnosed with panic disorder per se because the panic attacks only occurred in response to a specific stressor, such as a test or sporting event, rather than coming out of the blue). Becca's clinical presentation followed a common course that we often observe in women who are vulnerable to developing panic disorder associated with childbirth. Specifically, she did not experience symptoms during pregnancy or in the postpartum period as she was breastfeeding. It was only after she began weaning her child that she began experiencing symptoms, and her symptoms occurred with a greater frequency and severity than she had experienced in the past. A biological mechanism to explain this clinical presentation is presented later in this chapter.

DEFINITION AND NATURE OF PANIC ATTACKS

A *panic attack* is a discrete episode of intense anxiety characterized by symptoms such as racing heart, difficulty breathing, sweating, trembling and shaking, and a belief that one is going crazy or is going to die. Panic attacks usually develop abruptly and peak within 10 to 15 min. A diagnosis of panic disorder is made when a person experiences recurrent panic attacks, and, for at least 1 month, either worries about having additional attacks, worries about the implications of the attacks, and/or changes her behavior because of the attacks (*Diagnostic and Statistical Manual of Mental Disorders*; 4th ed., text rev. [*DSM–IV–TR*]; American Psychiatric Association, 2000). Women with perinatal panic attacks seem to experience many of the same types of symptoms as women who experience panic attacks at other times in their lives (Guler et al., 2008; Wenzel, Gorman, O'Hara, & Stuart, 2001). However, C. T. Beck (1996) added that women with postpartum panic disorder often report hysterical crying, disorientation, and headaches. She also observed that these women (a) feel out of control, (b) become exhausted in their efforts to maintain composure, (c) experience lowered self-esteem and perceive that they are disappointing themselves and their families, and (d) are terrified by the prospect that their emotional distress will have adverse effects on themselves and their families (C. T. Beck, 1998).

As might be imagined, panic symptoms experienced during pregnancy and the postpartum period hold great meaning for women. Panic symptoms experienced during pregnancy are often interpreted as something being wrong with the baby (Ross & McLean, 2006; Weisberg & Paquette, 2002), and panic symptoms experienced during the postpartum period shake women's confidence in their ability to care for their newborn (C. T. Beck, 1998). The guilt, shame, and apprehension that are associated with these perceptions have the potential to cause further distress for the new mother.

More often than not, Becca's panic attacks come on suddenly when she is at home with the baby. Typical symptoms she experiences during panic attacks include racing heart, difficulty breathing, chest constriction, tingling and numbness in her extremities, and a foreboding sense that she is going crazy. After her attacks subside, she is exhausted, tearful, and shaky. Becca often asks her husband or her mother-in-law to take over the care of the baby after having a panic attack, as she is so disoriented that she feels she just needs to sleep. Over time, Becca has been choosing to stay at home more and more, as she is terrified of having a panic attack in public when she is with her baby. She also avoids driving alone with her baby in the car because she worries that a panic attack might make her run off the road and get into an accident. She is taking on fewer hours at work for fear that she might have a panic attack while on the job.

PREVALENCE

Much research on the prevalence of perinatal panic disorder has examined the frequency of panic attacks longitudinally in samples of women during pregnancy and through the postpartum period. Some of this research was conducted with women who were presenting for psychiatric treatment, which I regard as using a clinical sample. In contrast, other research was conducted with women who were receiving obstetric care or who were recruited from public records, which I regard as using a community sample. Accordingly, this section is divided into two parts: a summary of studies that examine the prevalence of perinatal panic symptoms and disorder in clinical samples and a summary of studies that examine the prevalence of perinatal panic symptoms and disorder in community samples.

Clinical Samples

A great deal of research has examined the expression of panic symptoms during pregnancy and the postpartum period in women who have preexisting panic disorder. Much research has suggested that panic symptoms remain the same or decrease in frequency and severity during pregnancy (e.g., Villeponteaux, Lydiard, Laraia, Stuart, & Ballenger, 1992) but that there is a resurgence of symptoms during the postpartum period. However, there is great variation in reported results from study to study, and there has yet to be a prospective study with a large sample size that accounts for relevant variables that could influence the course of panic symptoms throughout the transition to parenthood (e.g., type and dosage of medication, life stress).

In a series of studies often cited by scholars in this field, L. S. Cohen, Sichel, Dimmock, and Rosenbaum (1994a, 1994b) retrospectively examined the course of panic disorder during pregnancy through the 8th week postpartum in 49 women with panic disorder. During pregnancy, 57% of the women experienced no change in symptoms, 20% reported improvement, and 20% reported worsening (L. S. Cohen et al., 1994a). Eight weeks following childbirth, 35% of the women reported a worsening of symptoms. Interestingly, women with mild panic disorder were more likely to worsen in the postpartum period than were women with moderate to severe panic disorder, perhaps because most of the women with mild panic disorder were not taking medications (L. S. Cohen et al., 1994b). In a later study in which 10 women with preexisting panic disorder were followed prospectively throughout the 3 trimesters of pregnancy through the 9th month postpartum, seven women met criteria for panic disorder at every assessment throughout pregnancy, and all but one woman met criteria at the postpartum assessments. The majority of women in this sample increased their dosage of psychotropic medications soon after they gave birth (L. S. Cohen et al., 1996).

The studies by L. S. Cohen et al. (1994a, 1994b) have suggested that at least a subset of women experience an improvement in panic symptoms during pregnancy and that a subset of women experience an exacerbation of symptoms in the postpartum period. Several studies have demonstrated that symptoms can recur in the postpartum period several months following delivery, which may correspond to the time at which women are discontinuing breastfeeding (Cowley & Roy-Byrne, 1989; Curran, Nelson, & Rodgers, 1995; George, Ladenheim, & Nutt, 1987; Klein, 1994; Northcott & Stein, 1994; Wisner, Peindl, & Hanusa, 1996, for similar descriptions). As is seen later in this chapter, breastfeeding status has perhaps more significant implications for the expression of postpartum panic disorder than for any other anxiety disorder described in this volume.

A more recent study involved the retrospective analysis of the course of panic symptoms in women with preexisting panic disorder who had at least one pregnancy, compared with women with preexisting panic disorder who had never given birth (Bandelow et al., 2006). These researchers computed a "panic manifestation quotient," in which they identified the first appearance of panic symptoms or an exacerbation of at least moderate severity as a function of three observation periods—266 pregnancy days, 180 postpartum days, and the days without pregnancy or postpartum from ages 15 to 40. In line with the other studies reviewed in this section, they determined that panic manifestation quotients were lower during pregnancy in women who had been pregnant compared with women who had not been pregnant, and that panic manifestation quotients were higher in the postpartum period in women who had given birth compared with women who had not given birth. Notably, 10 of the 93 women in the sample who had been pregnant indicated that their symptoms were first observed in the postpartum period, which represents a

132-fold increase in risk compared with the nonpostpartum period. This finding replicated a statistic calculated over 15 years ago, which suggested that the postpartum period is a time of increased risk for the onset of new cases of panic disorder (Sholomskas et al., 1993). Contrary to expectation, panic manifestation quotients did not vary as a function of breastfeeding status.

Thus, there are conflicting findings regarding the course of panic symptoms throughout pregnancy and the postpartum period. In their comprehensive analysis on the course of symptoms in women with preexisting panic disorder, Hertzberg and Wahlbeck (1999) calculated that 41% of the pregnancies considered in eight studies were associated with an improvement in symptoms during pregnancy, and 38% were associated with a worsening of symptoms during pregnancy—a pattern of results that does not suggest a clear trend one way or the other. It also is important to note that studies assessing whether women experienced a worsening, improvement, or no change in their symptoms often find that "no change" is the most common response in pregnant women with preexisting panic disorder (Ross & McLean, 2006; Wisner et al., 1996). Clearly, women are at risk of experiencing a recurrence or increase in panic symptoms if they discontinue treatment during pregnancy and/or the postpartum period. Women with preexisting panic disorder who become pregnant should be carefully monitored so that the costs and benefits of treating (or not treating) panic symptoms can be weighed at multiple points during pregnancy In contrast, results from the studies reviewed in this section generally suggest that women with preexisting panic disorder will experience an increase in symptoms during the postpartum period, perhaps around the time they discontinue breastfeeding.

Community Samples

Research on the prevalence of perinatal panic disorder has suggested that it is less prevalent than many of the anxiety disorders described in this volume, but that it is at least as prevalent as rates of panic disorder in women representative of the general population. Throughout this section, the reader can compare the rates of panic disorder found in various samples of pregnant and postpartum women with the prevalence of panic disorder in women who participated in epidemiological research—1.3% (4-week rate; Jacobi et al., 2004).

Pregnancy

Three of the studies examining rates of generalized anxiety disorder (GAD) and/or obsessive–compulsive disorder (OCD) in pregnant women also investigated rates of panic disorder in this population. In their investigation of 175 pregnant and 172 nonpregnant women in their 3rd trimester of pregnancy in Africa, Adewuya, Ola, Aloba, and Mapayi (2006) found that 5.2% of the pregnant women met criteria for panic disorder, relative to only 1.7% of the nonpregnant women. This group difference was significant at only a statistical trend level ($p = .078$), although it is notable because the rate of panic disorder in the pregnant group was approximately 3 times the rate in the nonpregnant group. In contrast, Sutter-Dallay, Giaconne-Marcesche, Glatigny-Dallay, and Verdoux (2004) identified a smaller subset of pregnant women who met criteria for panic disorder (i.e., 1.4%). As was seen in the chapters on GAD and OCD, Mota, Cox, Enns, Calhoun, and Sareen's (2008) analysis of panic disorder in pregnant women in the National Epidemiologic Survey on Alcohol and Related Conditions yielded lower rates of panic disorder in pregnant women than in nonpregnant women. Specifically, they estimated rates of panic disorder in currently pregnant, pregnant in the past year, and nonpregnant women of 2.1%, 4.0%, and 3.7%, respectively.

Two additional studies focused specifically on panic disorder during pregnancy. Guler et al. (2008) interviewed 512 consecutive women in their 3rd trimester of pregnancy who received treatment in university obstetric clinics and found a 2.5% prevalence rate of panic disorder. Of these women, 46% had a history of panic disorder, whereas 54% reported that the onset of their panic symptoms occurred between the 6th and 28th week of gestation. The severity of their symptoms was similar to that in a matched sample of nonpregnant women who were also diagnosed with panic disorder. In addition, Meshberg-Cohen and Svikis (2007) reported a higher rate of panic disorder in their sample of pregnant women seeking care at a university OB/GYN clinic for the first time; the rate of panic disorder in this sample was 9.8%, relative to 3.4% in a sample of nonpregnant women. Collectively, results from these five studies suggest that the rate of panic disorder in community samples of pregnant women range from 1.4% to 9.8%, with four of the five studies identifying rates that are higher than the rate of a current diagnosis of panic disorder in women who participate in epidemiological research. This pattern of results does not support the notion that pregnancy "protects" women from panic disorder.

Postpartum Period

Investigations of panic disorder in the postpartum period in community samples paint a different picture than do studies that examine postpartum panic symptoms in clinical samples. In two of my own studies, I found rates of panic disorder of 1.4% in women who were approximately 8 weeks postpartum (Wenzel, Haugen, Jackson, & Brendle, 2005) and 1.5% in women who were between 4 and 7 months postpartum (Wenzel et al., 2001). Both of these rates are not much different from the rate of panic disorder in women representative of the general population. Navarro et al.'s (2008) large epidemiological study revealed a rate of 0.5% for diagnoses of panic disorder at 6 weeks postpartum. Matthey, Barnett, Howie, and Kavanagh (2003) identified rates of panic disorder of 2.7% and 0.5% in two samples of women who were recruited from antenatal clinics for participation in their program to prevent postpartum depression (Ns = 216, 192). It is difficult to explain the discrepancy in their rates, as the prevalence of panic disorder in their first sample points to an elevated rate of panic disorder in the postpartum period, and the prevalence of panic disorder in the second sample points to a diminished rate of panic disorder in the postpartum period. Finally, the rate of panic disorder in Rowe, Fisher, and Loh's (2008) high-risk sample of women enrolled in a residential parenting program was 2.9% at an average of 10.3 weeks postpartum, which is not appreciably different from the rate seen in Matthey et al.'s (2003) Sample 1, despite the fact that the sample was higher risk. In all, results from community studies suggest that the prevalence of panic disorder in women who are between 6 and 10 weeks postpartum ranges from 0.5% to 2.9%. My research also shows that rates drop even further at 6 and 12 months postpartum (Wenzel, 2005).

Results from epidemiological studies with community samples are at odds with results from studies using clinical samples of childbearing women with preexisting panic disorder. Although results are variable, there is a weak pattern in clinical studies, which suggests that pregnancy protects some women from panic symptoms but that there is an exacerbation in these symptoms in the postpartum period. In contrast, results from most studies using community samples indicate that the rate of panic disorder during pregnancy is higher than it is for women who are not necessarily pregnant or postpartum, but that during the postpartum period, rates fall to that which would be expected of women who are representative of the general population. Yet, two groups of researchers (Bandelow et al., 2006; Sholomskas et al., 1993) calculated that the postpartum period is a time when the risk of the onset of panic disorder is much greater than would be expected by chance. As is seen later in this chapter, there are distinct biological and psychological mechanisms to explain the onset and/or exacerbation of panic symptoms and panic disorder during the transition to parenthood, particularly in the postpartum period. It will be incumbent on future researchers to test prospectively the onset and exacerbation of panic symptoms during pregnancy and throughout the postpartum period to determine whether different mechanisms are at work in women who do and do not have preexisting panic disorder.

Agoraphobia

Agoraphobia is a condition that often accompanies panic disorder. Agoraphobic individuals experience anxiety when they go out in places from which escape might be difficult or in which help might not be available. As a result, those situations are either avoided or endured with a great deal of distress (*DSM–IV–TR*; American Psychiatric Association, 2000). According to data collected in the National Comorbidity Survey Replication, 0.8% of the population meets criteria for agoraphobia without panic disorder, and 1.1% of the population meets criteria for panic disorder with agoraphobia (Kessler et al., 2006).

Despite the accumulating research on panic symptoms and diagnoses associated with childbirth, there has been little research on the prevalence of associated agoraphobia during pregnancy and the postpartum period (March & Yonkers, 2001). The one study that identified the prevalence of agoraphobia during pregnancy (Sutter-Dallay et al., 2004) found an unexplainably high percentage of women who met diagnostic criteria for this anxiety disorder (i.e., 14%). In my longitudinal study of 147 postpartum women, not one reported clinically significant symptoms of agoraphobia (Wenzel, Haugen, Jackson, et al., 2005), and Navarro et al. (2008) found a prevalence of 0.6%. The rate of agoraphobia was slightly higher in Rowe et al.'s study (2.2%), but this rate could be elevated because these women were representative of a high-risk sample of people who often have poor mental and physical health. Thus, there are widely discrepant results in studies that identify agoraphobia in childbearing women. It will be important for future research to document the prevalence and course of agoraphobic anxiety and avoidance throughout pregnancy and the 1st year postpartum in women with and without histories of panic disorder.

> Although Becca has not been formally diagnosed with panic disorder with agoraphobia, she exhibits some agoraphobic symptoms. As stated previously, she often chooses to stay at home with the baby to avoid having panic attacks in public or while driving. She feels more comfortable going out in public when she is with her husband, whom she views as her "safety net." In addition, she is beginning to decline invitations to attend events with her mother's group or to get together with her girlfriends.

EFFECTS

An oft-cited case to illustrate the effects of panic disorder during pregnancy is described in a report by L. S. Cohen, Rosenbaum, and Heller (1989), who presented the case of a nulliparous, nonmedicated 29-year-old woman who had a history of panic attacks beginning at age 13. Although the frequency and severity of her panic attacks decreased during the 1st trimester, she experienced daily panic attacks and substantial anticipatory anxiety during the

2nd and 3rd trimesters. Near the end of her pregnancy, she had a panic attack that was followed by vaginal bleeding and placental abruption, which prompted a cesarean section. Fortunately, the baby was healthy and had Apgar scores within the normal range. The authors speculated that increased blood pressure and sympathetic arousal associated with her anxiety symptoms were responsible for the placental abruption, and they urged clinicians to balance the risks associated with taking and not taking medication for moderate to severe panic disorder during pregnancy, a topic that is discussed in greater length in Chapter 9.

Hirshfeld-Becker et al. (2004) retrospectively assessed pregnancy and delivery complications in parents with a history of maternal panic disorder compared with parents with major depression or no psychiatric disorder. In their analyses of pregnancy problems, a history of panic disorder was associated with a higher incidence of illness requiring medical attention during pregnancy, emotional problems requiring counseling, serious family problems, smoking at least a pack of cigarettes a day for at least 3 months, and taking medications of any type. Family problems, in turn, were associated with risk of offspring developing two or more childhood anxiety disorders. In contrast, a history of panic disorder was not associated with heavy bleeding, excessive nausea or vomiting, excessive weight loss or weight gain, infection requiring medical attention, high blood pressure or excessive fluid retention, convulsions, accidents requiring medical care, illnesses requiring medical care, or taking alcohol or drugs. In patients with a history of panic disorder, the number of pregnancy problems was associated with the occurrence of anxiety disorders in children. It is interesting that depression, but not panic disorder, was associated specifically with delivery complications. An important caveat to consider when interpreting these results is that the associations were between lifetime diagnoses of panic disorder and pregnancy problems; thus, it was unknown whether the mothers were experiencing acute symptoms of panic during pregnancy. In a recent study that did include patients who were currently diagnosed with panic disorder, Meshberg-Cohen and Svikis (2007) found that pregnant women who were diagnosed with panic disorder reported greater alcohol use than pregnant women without panic disorder.

Collectively, results from these studies raise the possibility that panic disorder during pregnancy is associated with behavioral and emotional maladjustment during pregnancy and the risk of complications nearing delivery. However, more research is needed before definitive conclusions can be drawn, as the L. S. Cohen et al. (1989) report is based on a single case study, and participants in the Hirshfeld-Becker et al. (2004) report had a history of panic disorder but were not necessarily having panic attacks during pregnancy. Moreover, there is no known investigation of the effects of panic symptoms and panic disorder that are observed in the postpartum period. However, we can speculate about the effects of postpartum panic disorder on the basis of studies that have examined impairment and disability in people with panic disorder who are not necessarily undergoing the transition to parenthood. Specifically, panic disorder is associated with impairment in social functioning (Carrera et al., 2006), marital distress (Markowitz, Weissman, Oullette, Lish, & Klerman, 1989), bodily pain and lower perceptions of general health (Carrera et al., 2006), increased health care utilization (Katon, 1996), impairment in occupational functioning (Edlund & Swann, 1987), and decreased time spent in hobbies (Markowitz et al., 1989). On the basis of this research, it would be reasonable to formulate the following hypotheses about women with perinatal panic disorder:

- Panic disorder is likely to be associated with impairments in close relationships during pregnancy and the postpartum period, particularly the marital or partner relationship.
- Panic disorder is likely to be associated with health concerns during pregnancy and the postpartum period (e.g., hypertension, gestational diabetes). A corollary of this hypothesis is that childbearing women with panic disorder would utilize more health care services than childbearing women without panic disorder.
- In women who work, panic disorder is likely to be associated with impairment in occupational functioning during pregnancy and difficulty adjusting to work following maternity leave.
- Panic disorder is likely to be associated with less time spent in hobbies and recreational pursuits outside of work and family responsibilities during pregnancy and the postpartum period.

Becca did not experience panic attacks during pregnancy and the period of time around delivery; she was surprised that her delivery went as smoothly as it did, and there were no complications or abnormalities in her baby daughter. Becca began to notice the effects of her panic attacks approximately 2 months after their onset at 6 months postpartum. As stated previously, she is taking on fewer hours at work for fear that she will have a panic attack, which is beginning to take a toll on the family's finances. Her husband has been disciplined twice at work for leaving early to come home after she had a panic attack. Becca and her husband had hoped to start trying to have another child when their daughter was a year old; recently, he indicated that he is no longer in favor of this plan because it is unclear that she would be able to handle two young children. Her husband's change of heart has prompted a great deal of shame and self-doubt in Becca.

COMORBIDITY WITH DEPRESSION

Little research has examined the overlap between perinatal panic and perinatal depression. In an exception, Bandelow et al. (2006) found that postpartum panic and depression overlapped in approximately 12% of their sample. In my longitudinal study of postpartum anxiety disorders, one of the two women in the sample of 147 women was diagnosed with major depressive disorder (Wenzel, Haugen, Jackson, et al., 2005). Obviously, these numbers are so small that definitive conclusions about the relation between postpartum panic disorder and postpartum depression cannot be drawn.

However, it can be speculated that perinatal panic disorder and depression would overlap on the basis of research conducted with samples of people representative of the general population. For example, Melartin et al. (2002) combined comorbidity estimates across several studies and determined that 16% of patients with major depression are diagnosed with comorbid panic disorder. Conversely, Starcevic et al. (2008) reported that approximately 52% of female patients with panic disorder with agoraphobia met criteria for major depression. Thus, we could speculate that rates of comorbidity between perinatal panic disorder and depression range from 16% to 52%. Because comorbidity is associated with poorer clinical course and outcome (Van Balkom et al., 2008), clinicians would be wise to be alert for both clusters of symptoms in childbearing women and to treat psychiatric symptoms especially aggressively in women who carry both diagnoses.

> Becca began to experience secondary symptoms of depression around the time her family noticed the decrease in her functioning because of panic disorder. The primary symptoms she experiences are a sense of worthlessness and excessive guilt. Becca is terribly embarrassed by her panic attacks, views herself as a bad mother and wife, and feels tremendous guilt at asking her husband and extended family members to come to the house and help her take care of her daughter when she has a panic attack. In addition, she cries frequently, lacks the motivation to engage in activities that had once brought her pleasure, and is constantly exhausted.

POSSIBLE ETIOLOGY

Although few studies have been conducted with the specific purpose of identifying variables that contribute to the etiology of perinatal panic disorder, several researchers have proposed mechanisms for the onset or exacerbation of perinatal panic on the basis of biological and psychological theories of panic disorder. In this section, I describe sociodemographic variables that have been found to be associated with postpartum panic symptoms. In addition, I outline biological and psychological explanations for the onset and exacerbation of panic symptoms in childbearing women.

Sociodemographic Factors

In one study that examined sociodemographic factors associated with panic symptoms during pregnancy, Guler et al. (2008) found no differences between pregnant women with and without panic disorder in age, marital status, education, and occupation, number of gestations, and parity. However, in my study on the longitudinal course of postpartum anxiety disorders (Wenzel, Haugen, Jackson, et al., 2005), I identified several sociodemographic variables that were associated with panic symptoms. In one analysis, I examined the degree to which four sociodemographic variables (i.e., mother's age, baby's age, number of children in the household, and socioeconomic status) predicted scores on the Beck Anxiety Inventory (BAI; A. T. Beck & Steer, 1990), which, as stated in Chapter 1, is a self-report inventory that assesses physical symptoms of anxiety such as racing heart, sweating, and difficulty breathing. Socioeconomic status was a negative predictor of BAI scores, meaning that women of lower socioeconomic status were more likely than women of higher socioeconomic status to report higher BAI scores.

In addition, BAI scores correlated negatively with mother's age, level of education attained by the mother, the baby's father's age, and income. Thus, younger women who had attained a lower level of education, who had their children with younger fathers, and who had lower incomes were more likely to report physical symptoms of anxiety. BAI scores correlated negatively with length of time in the relationship with the baby's father, suggesting that physical symptoms of anxiety are especially like to occur when women are in relationships with their baby's father for shorter periods of time. BAI scores were also associated with the couple's marital status, such that women who were not married to the baby's father reported higher BAI scores than women who were married to the father of their newborn. Furthermore, both a personal and family psychiatric history predicted scores on the BAI at 8 weeks postpartum, such that women who endorsed previous episodes of depression or anxiety disorders or indicated that a biological family member had experienced one or more of these disorders were more likely to report physical symptoms of anxiety on this inventory. In contrast, BAI scores were not associated with parity, mother or baby's father's ethnicity, the skill level of the mother and baby's father's jobs, and the level of education attained by the baby's father.

Unlike the pattern of associations that was found when women were assessed around 8 weeks postpartum, at the 6- and 12-month assessments the

BAI correlated with length of time that women were in a relationship with the baby's father but with no other sociodemographic variable. These results raise the possibility that sociodemographic variables play a role in the expression of anxiety in the early postpartum period, but that they play a lesser role as women adapt to their new life circumstances.

It is likely that the significant associations between BAI scores and these sociodemographic variables can be explained by the stress that they bring to new mothers. Retrospective research has found that childbearing women who experienced life stress had a 1.7-fold increase in risk of developing panic symptoms during their first pregnancy (Bandelow et al., 2006). For example, new mothers of low socioeconomic status who report a low income level might experience anxiety about the financial resources needed to provide for their newborn. Being in a relationship with the baby's father for only a short period of time or not being married to the baby's father could induce anxiety about issues such as whether the relationship will last and whether the baby's father will contribute time and resources to caring for the child. It is interesting that there were many more significant associations between scores on the BAI and sociodemographic factors than between these factors and symptoms of worry, as described in Chapter 2. One explanation for this pattern of results is that new mothers have little opportunity to engage in the conscious process of worry because of increased responsibilities and fatigue associated with sleep disturbance, so that much of their anxiety is expressed in physical symptoms such as racing heart and shallow breathing.

> Having given birth at age 25, Becca would not necessarily be considered a younger mother by many people. However, she and her husband are struggling financially. Because she is taking on fewer shifts at work because of her panic attacks, her husband is considering taking a second job. This possibility causes a great deal of anxiety for Becca, as she experiences a noticeable decrease in her symptoms when her husband is home with her. In addition, she and her husband had been dating for 6 months when she got pregnant, and they were married 6 months thereafter. Although the timing of the pregnancy was not optimal, Becca believes that her husband was "the one" and that they would have eventually married anyway. Nevertheless, they had not lived together until they were married, and there was a period of adjustment as they became acclimated to each other's habits. The current difficulties that they are experiencing because of Becca's panic attacks are the greatest challenge of their marriage to date. As Becca continues to become more anxious and depressed, she has started to wonder whether her husband will stay with her in the long run. Finally, Becca has a personal history of panic attacks that were cued during stressful situations, and she has a family history (i.e., mother and maternal grandmother) of anxiety and worry.

Biological Factors

Three main candidates for biological factors associated with the onset or exacerbation of perinatal panic disorder have been identified. Each of these variables is considered in this section.

Estrogen

There is evidence that premenstrual hormonal changes play a role in the expression of panic symptoms in some women, so it is logical to speculate that ovarian hormones may play a role in panic experienced in the postpartum period (Metz, Sichel, & Goff, 1988). As was stated previously, estrogen is elevated during pregnancy, and it drops dramatically in the first several days postpartum. Estrogen interacts with serotonin transporter sites, serotonin receptor sensitivity, and the metabolism of serotonin; it decreases monoamine oxidase activity; and it enhances the metabolism of norepinephrine transmission (Halbreich, 1997). Both serotonin and norepinephrine transmission are associated with panic disorder, so it is possible that changes in estrogen levels associated with pregnancy and childbirth affect the onset and exacerbation of panic symptoms. However, not all scholars agree that estrogen plays a role in the perinatal panic symptoms (e.g., Cowley & Roy-Byrne, 1989).

Progesterone

Progesterone might play the greatest role in the degree to which panic symptoms are expressed during pregnancy, as it exerts its anxiolytic effect by increasing the effect of adenosine, which is an inhibitory neurotransmitter than suppresses arousal (Cowley & Roy-Byrne, 1989). In addition, progesterone decreases the amount of plasma carbon dioxide (CO_2), which reduces the probability of hyperventilation (Klein, Skrobala, & Garfinkel, 1995). Hyperventilation is one physical symptom often experienced by people with panic disorder, so it is sensible that a reduction in hyperventilation would be associated with perceived improvement in panic symptoms. Moreover, there is evidence that progesterone metabolites work in much the same manner as anxiolytic medication at gamma-aminobutyric acid (GABA) receptor-binding sites (George et al., 1987).

Although progesterone seems to have anxiolytic effects, it is important to acknowledge that some of its actions may actually increase panic symptoms during pregnancy. Cowley and Roy-Byrne (1989) indicated that progesterone is responsible for the increased minute ventilation (i.e., the volume of air that can be inhaled in any one moment), increased tidal volume (i.e., air displaced between inhalation and exhalation), and hypoxia (i.e., body being deprived of oxygen). The phenotypic expression of increased minute ventilation, increased tidal volume, and hypoxia is hyperventilation. Thus, increased progesterone during pregnancy potentially contributes to two different mechanisms that affect the likelihood that a woman will experience hyperventilation during pregnancy—one that decreases the likelihood (i.e., by decreasing the amount of plasma CO_2) and one the increases the likelihood (i.e., by increasing minute ventilation and tidal volume). More research is needed to track the effects of increased levels of progesterone on the neurobiological functioning (i.e., adenosine, GABA binding sites) as well as on physiological functioning (i.e., breathing capacity).

Klein et al. (1995) hypothesized that panic symptoms would increase in the postpartum period because progesterone levels drop dramatically, and there is a corresponding increase in plasma CO_2 levels. They predicted that the first 3 weeks postpartum would be the time in which women would be at greatest risk of developing panic disorder. If women are breastfeeding, then they predicted that the first 3 weeks following weaning would be the time at which women would be at greatest risk of developing panic disorder. Retrospective research has found that weaning was associated with the onset or exacerbation of panic symptoms (Klein et al., 1995; Northcott & Stein, 1994; Villeponteaux et al., 1992), although in my longitudinal study (Wenzel, Haugen, Jackson, et al., 2005), breastfeeding status was not associated with BAI scores or diagnoses of panic disorder at any of the postpartum assessments.

Physiological Changes

In addition to the hormonal and neurochemical changes that women experience during pregnancy and the postpartum period, their bodies also go through tremendous physical changes that have the potential to exacerbate panic symptoms. For example, during pregnancy, women's reproductive organs impinge on their diaphragm, which causes them to take smaller breaths (March & Yonkers, 2001). Heart rate often increases to pump blood through the larger body and to the fetus. Nausea is common during the 1st trimester of pregnancy, and flutters of the baby kicking can resemble gastrointestinal symptoms of panic in later stages of pregnancy. Although these physical sensations are to be expected during pregnancy, some women who are vulnerable to panic disorder have the tendency to misinterpret these symptoms as catastrophic—a tendency that is described in the next section.

Psychological Factors

Two potential psychological candidates to explain the etiology of perinatal panic disorder have been proposed in the literature. For example, Klein et al. (1995) used cognitive theory to explain why there should be an increase in panic symptoms during pregnancy. As stated previously, pregnant women undergo many physiological changes, a number of which resemble panic symptoms. Panic disorder is associated with the tendency to misinterpret these symptoms as being more catastrophic than they really are (Clark et al., 1997), such that they are viewed as signals that something is terribly wrong with their or their baby's health or well-being. Thus, pregnancy provides many opportunities for these catastrophic misinterpretations to occur, which could in turn increase the likelihood of heightened anxiety.

A creative hypothesis about another psychological factor that contributes to the onset of postpartum panic disorder was proposed by Bybee (1989) in a brief letter to the editor in response to an article describing postpartum panic disorder. Specifically, he proposed that women are often taught to hyperventilate during labor as a strategy to manage their pain, and he reasoned that women may turn to this strategy during the postpartum period when they are experiencing profound sleep deprivation and emotional distress associated with a demanding infant. Thus, he suggested that hyperventilation is a learned behavior that can be treated with behavioral anxiety management strategies, such as diaphragmatic breathing.

Although these explanations for perinatal panic disorder are intriguing, they have yet to be subjected to empirical scrutiny. A large body of research has demonstrated that individuals with panic disorder indeed make catastrophic misinterpretations of their symptoms as signaling imminent physical and mental disaster, although there has yet to be published research that documents this phenomenon in childbearing women. Moreover, it will be important for empirical research to identify psychological mechanisms at work in vulnerable women whose symptoms improve during pregnancy versus vulnerable women whose symptoms worsen during pregnancy. It is possible that one's preexisting cognitive style can account for distinctions between these subsets of women, such that women who tend to catastrophize in other stressful situations in their lives would be particularly prone to misinterpret physical symptoms during pregnancy, and thus experience an increase in panic symptoms. In contrast, it is possible that women who do not demonstrate this tendency at other points in their lives would not necessarily make these misinterpretations and thus would experience no change or even a decrease in symptoms.

> Becca does not catastrophize the medical implications of her panic symptoms. In fact, each time she experiences a panic attack, she knows exactly what it is and knows that it will be over soon. However, she dwells on the implications of her symptoms for her abilities as a wife and mother. She often ruminates over the belief that her symptoms will never improve and that she is bound to be dependent on her husband and extended family forever for help with taking care of her child. Moreover, she

berates herself for not being a stronger person and focuses on the prediction that eventually her husband will leave her for someone who is "whole." Thus, Becca makes some catastrophic predictions about the implications of her symptoms for her emotional well-being and relationships with others, but these seem to be more of a consequence of her symptoms than a cause, and the predictions put her at risk of comorbid depression.

PRACTICAL IMPLICATIONS

Clinicians reading this book may find it difficult to make sense of the data that speak to the course of panic symptoms and disorder throughout pregnancy and the postpartum period. Is pregnancy associated with an increase or a decrease in panic symptoms? Does the postpartum period pose a substantial risk for the exacerbation of panic symptoms in women with preexisting panic disorder and the onset of new cases of panic disorder, or not? Does breastfeeding make a difference in the onset or exacerbation of panic symptoms during the postpartum period? The answer to all of these questions is that some data support these possibilities and some do not. My recommendation for clinicians is to identify possible risk factors for the onset and exacerbation of panic symptoms during pregnancy and the postpartum period and to carefully monitor for a worsening of symptoms. Young women who are of low socioeconomic status and/or who have been with the fathers of their babies for only a short period of time might be particularly vulnerable for panic symptoms during pregnancy and the postpartum period, perhaps because these variables create additional stress in an already stressful time in which they are transitioning to parenthood. In addition, women who have a personal or family history of anxiety or depression are at risk of experiencing panic symptoms during the postpartum period. It is possible that women's pregravid cognitive style plays a role in whether they develop panic symptoms during pregnancy and the postpartum period. Those who have the tendency to catastrophize when facing stress might be more likely to develop panic attacks, whereas those who maintain an especially positive attitude toward pregnancy and the transition to parenthood might be less likely to develop panic attacks.

It is important for mental health clinicians who work with postpartum women who experience panic attacks to understand that their symptoms hold great meaning to them. Many of these women experience shame and embarrassment and believe that their symptoms are indicative of incompetence as mothers or as wives. Cognitive behavioral therapy (CBT) would be a logical choice of intervention to address these beliefs. However, even if clinicians do not choose to treat women with postpartum panic disorder from a cognitive behavioral standpoint, it is still important to be mindful of these powerful beliefs so that the new mother can develop a healthy view of herself in this new role.

Becca sought help for panic disorder when she was 10 months postpartum, at the insistence of her husband, who indicated that her symptoms were causing significant strain on the family. She first saw her gynecologist, who prescribed a selective serotonin reuptake inhibitor (SSRI) and referred her to a psychologist for CBT. Becca was terrified to attend regular psychotherapy sessions, predicting that her therapist could declare her incurable and that she would have to face the fact that she would be impaired forever. Her therapist recognized that her difficulties with panic disorder were weighing substantially on her sense of self-worth. Thus, the first few sessions were spent educating Becca about panic disorder and placing it in the context of the events associated with the transition to parenthood. In addition, the therapist educated her about the efficacy of SSRIs and CBT in the treatment of panic disorder. Becca began to have some hope that her symptoms could be managed, and she became much more motivated to attend sessions and practice implementing the anxiety management skills in her life.

5

SOCIAL ANXIETY

Lily is a 32-year-old Asian American woman who gave birth to her first child 3 months ago. She is currently on maternity leave from her job as an attorney at a high-profile law firm. She is one of the few women in the office who opted to have children, and she is the first of her female friends, all of whom hold similar professional positions, to have children. Since the birth of her baby, Lily has felt increasingly distant from her circle of friends. She is worried that she will bore her friends with talk about late-night feedings and diapers and that she is not caught up on the latest professional gossip. Recently, she accompanied her husband to his office holiday party, and she worried about not being able to hold "an intelligent conversation" and about others' negative judgments about her appearance. Lately, she has avoided opportunities to interact with others whom she views as "professional and together," such as by avoiding her friends' phone calls and delaying a planned office visit with her baby.

Lily is experiencing social anxiety with a postpartum onset. This case of social anxiety is different from many other cases that clinicians typically come across. Social anxiety is one form of anxiety that often has an onset in the teenage years and runs a chronic course (Reich, Goldenberg, Vasile, Goisman, & Keller, 1994; Stein & Stein, 2008). Nevertheless, this case illustrates a form of postpartum social anxiety that characterized many of the women in my community sample (Wenzel, Haugen, Jackson, & Brendle, 2005), and it is hoped that this chapter will demonstrate that perinatal social anxiety deserves attention from clinicians because it can interfere with postpartum adjustment and has the potential to put women at risk for depression.

The *Diagnostic and Statistical Manual of Mental Disorders* (4th ed., text revision [*DSM–IV–TR*]; American Psychiatric Association, 2000) does not specify a time period for which an adult must experience social anxiety to qualify for a diagnosis of social anxiety disorder. Nevertheless, it would be clinically wise to refrain from making a diagnosis of social anxiety disorder until the individual has experienced clinically significant social anxiety that persists over at least a few months. Thus, Lily would not yet meet diagnostic criteria for social anxiety disorder because the onset occurred a couple of weeks after her daughter was born. Nevertheless, her symptoms would be worth monitoring to assign a diagnosis if they persist, to determine the degree to which they are interfering with her life and causing her distress, and to identify other emotional disturbances that might stem from them.

DEFINITION AND NATURE OF SOCIAL ANXIETY

Social anxiety is defined as excessive fear of embarrassment or negative evaluation that is associated with avoidance of and distress in social and evaluative activities. A diagnosis of social anxiety disorder is made when a person meets five criteria: (a) there is marked or persistent fear of interactions with or evaluation by others that is excessive and cued by the feared situation; (b) exposure to the feared situation almost always provokes anxiety; (c) the person recognizes that the fear is excessive; (d) the feared situation is avoided or endured with extreme distress; and (e) the avoidance, anxious anticipation, or distress causes life interference, or the person has marked distress about having the fear (*DSM–IV–TR*; American Psychiatric Association, 2000). I should note here that the "official" term for social anxiety at this level is *social phobia* in the *DSM–IV–TR*. However, many leading scholars in the field instead refer to the condition as *social anxiety disorder* because this name better captures the degree to which the disorder is pervasive and impairing (Liebowitz, Heimberg, Fresco, Travers, & Stein, 2000). I adopt the term *social anxiety disorder* to be consistent with this standard in the field.

The literature on social anxiety associated with childbirth is virtually nonexistent. A few of the epidemiological studies of psychiatric disorders during pregnancy and the postpartum period assessed the prevalence of social anxiety disorder in these samples, although they included little, if any, commentary about the implications of their findings. Much of my knowledge of social anxiety associated with childbirth comes from my longitudinal study of community women who were followed throughout the 1st year postpartum (Wenzel, Haugen, Jackson, et al., 2005), which suggests that some cases of clinically significant social anxiety have their onset soon after childbirth. Socially anxious women in this sample identified many adverse effects from their symptoms, including avoidance of social situations, allowance of others to initiate and direct conversations, a perceived inability to participate in deep and meaningful conversations, and a failure to find common ground with others, particularly with others who do not have children. Some of these women reported a belief that they were unable to talk about anything other than child rearing. In addition, body image concerns often fueled social anxiety that occurred in the postpartum period, as many of these women expressed concern that others would judge their appearance negatively. Consequently, they avoided social contact with others, which could have deleterious effects on their relationships.

PREVALENCE

Only a few investigations have examined the prevalence of social anxiety disorder in pregnant and postpartum samples. Rates found in these studies can be compared with rates of social anxiety disorder in women who are not necessarily pregnant or postpartum—1-month prevalence rates of social anxiety disorder in women range from 1.4% (Lampe, Slade, Issakidis, & Andrews, 2003) to 5.2% (W. J. Magee, Eaton, Wittchen, McGonagle, & Kessler, 1996).

Pregnancy

Adewuya, Ola, Aloba, and Mapayi (2006) found statistically significant differences in the prevalence of social anxiety disorder in 175 pregnant women in their 3rd trimester and 172 nonpregnant women, such that this disorder was diagnosed in 6.4% and 1.7% of the pregnant and nonpregnant women, respectively. In contrast, Sutter-Dallay, Giaconne-Marcesche, Glatigny-Dallay, and Verdoux (2004) found a smaller prevalence rate of only 2% in their sample of pregnant women in their 3rd trimester of pregnancy. In their analysis of the National Epidemiologic Survey on Alcohol and Related Conditions, Mota, Cox, Enns, Calhoun, and Sareen (2008) found that rates of social anxiety disorder in currently pregnant, pregnant in the past year, and nonpregnant women were 3.3%, 2.5%, and 3.4%, respectively. Women who had been pregnant in the past year had significantly lower rates of social anxiety disorder than did women who were not pregnant, a pattern that the authors had difficulty explaining. Collectively, research conducted to date suggests that rates of social anxiety disorder in pregnant women range from 2.0% to 6.4%, with two of the three studies indicating that the rate of social anxiety disorder in this population falls within the expected range for women who are not necessarily pregnant or postpartum.

Postpartum Period

In my longitudinal study of postpartum anxiety disorders in 147 community women, my students and I found that 4.1% of the sample met diagnostic criteria for social anxiety disorder and that another 15% were regarded as having subsyndromal expressions of social anxiety disorder at 8 weeks postpartum (Wenzel, Haugen, Jackson, et al., 2005). The 4.1% rate is not particularly noteworthy, as it is consistent with the 1-month prevalence of social anxiety disorder in women who are not necessarily pregnant or postpartum. However, what was striking was that the majority of the women who were diagnosed with social anxiety disorder stated that their symptoms had a postpartum onset, similar to what I present in the case description of Lily.

The percentages of women who met diagnostic criteria for social anxiety disorder at the follow-up assessments in my study continued to decline, with 2.3% of the sample meeting criteria at the 6-month assessment (which included a mixture of cases that had been diagnosed at 8 weeks postpartum and cases that had been subsyndromal at 8 weeks postpartum), and 1.7% meeting criteria at the 12-month assessment (Wenzel, 2005). These rates are in the lower end of the range of 1-month prevalence rates of women who are representative of the general population. Only one woman who had a postpartum onset of social anxiety disorder continued to meet diagnostic criteria at the 6- and 12-month assessments; the rest of the women who endorsed social anxiety disorder with a postpartum onset were either subsyndromal for a diagnosis or did not meet criteria at all by the 6- and 12-month assessments. This finding is heartening, as it suggests that childbearing women can be assured that most cases of clinically significant social anxiety with a postpartum onset are relatively transient.

Only two other studies have reported rates of postpartum social anxiety disorder. Navarro et al. (2008) reported a much lower rate of social anxiety disorder at 6 weeks postpartum (i.e., 0.2%) than I found in my study at 8 weeks postpartum. It is unclear why the rate they obtained is so much different from rates obtained in samples of women representative of the general population who participate in epidemiological research, although it is consistent with the observation described in previous chapters that Navarro et al. (2008) generally obtained lower rates of pathology than other studies. The rate of social anxiety disorder in Rowe, Fisher, and Loh's (2008) study of high-risk women enrolled in a residential parenting program was 6.5% in women who were approximately

10.3 weeks postpartum. Thus, at 6 to 10 weeks postpartum, rates of social anxiety disorder range from 0.2% to 6.5%, and results from epidemiological research indicate that rates drop to 2.3% at 6 months postpartum and 1.7% at 12 months postpartum.

EFFECTS

In my longitudinal study on postpartum anxiety disorders, my students and I uncovered the interesting finding that symptoms of social anxiety, symptoms of depression, and number of children in the household predicted distress in the partner relationship at 8 weeks postpartum (Wenzel, Haugen, Jackson, et al., 2005). What made this finding particularly compelling was that the influence of social anxiety was detected after all of the variance in relationship distress that could be explained by the sociodemographic factors and depressive symptoms was controlled. In contrast, scores on a measure of worry symptoms and on a measure of physical anxiety symptoms did not predict levels of relationship distress. This means that there is something unique about social anxiety that has a deleterious effect on the quality of the partner relationship. My research also showed that socially anxious women perceived that their partners were less caring than women who did not report symptoms of social anxiety (Haugen, Brendle, Schmutzer, & Wenzel, 2003).

It is important to recognize that most partner relationships suffer, to some degree, in the early postpartum period (cf. Haugen, Schmutzer, & Wenzel, 2004). On a measure of relationship distress (i.e., the Dyadic Adjustment Scale; Spanier, 1976), the average woman in my longitudinal study reported that the quality of her relationship was in the mildly distressed range at 8 weeks postpartum. However, at 6 months postpartum, the relationships of women who reported few, if any, symptoms of social anxiety rose well into the functional range. In contrast, women who reported many symptoms of social anxiety continued to score below the cutoff between functional and dysfunctional relationships (Schmutzer, Brendle, Haugen, Jackson, & Wenzel, 2002). Because problems in the partner relationship predict depression in postpartum women (C. T. Beck & Driscoll, 2006) and in women at other times in their lives (O'Mahen, Beach, & Banawan, 2001), we can speculate that socially anxious women are at risk of problems with emotional adjustment as the postpartum period continues.

In addition, the larger literature on social anxiety disorder presents some hints about other areas of impairment in childbearing women with this type of psychiatric disturbance. For example, research has suggested that social anxiety disorder is associated with impairment in occupational functioning (Ruscio et al., 2008), impairment in home management (Ruscio et al., 2008), and decreased satisfaction in many life domains (e.g., family, social relations, work, finances; Fehm, Beesdo, Jacobi, & Fiedler, 2008). On the basis of this research, it would be reasonable to formulate the following hypotheses about women with perinatal social anxiety disorder:

- In women who work, social anxiety disorder is likely to be associated with impaired occupational functioning during pregnancy and difficulty adjusting to work following maternity leave.
- Social anxiety disorder is likely to be associated with impairment in household responsibilities during pregnancy and the postpartum period.
- Social anxiety is likely to be associated with decreased life satisfaction during pregnancy and the postpartum period.

The most obvious area of Lily's impairment is in her close relationships. Before having her daughter, she had strong friendships with several friends from law school as well as several coworkers. However, she worries that many of these individuals judge her negatively for putting her family before her career, and as a result, she has had little contact with them. Her coworkers continue to invite her to go to happy hour after work, but Lily does not respond to the messages. Her friends from law school get together for dinner once a month, and she has not attended those outings, either. Lily attempted to join a mothers' group to make new friends, but she felt equally awkward with these women, perceiving that they were judging her negatively for not leaving her professional position and devoting herself to full-time motherhood. In addition to these concerns, Lily views herself as not losing her baby weight quickly enough and is having difficulty finding clothes that fit her, which has prompted worries that others will view her as overweight and unworthy of attention. As a result of these socially anxious concerns, Lily feels isolated from the world, but at the same time she is dreading going back to work.

COMORBIDITY WITH DEPRESSION

As might be expected, there is substantial overlap between social anxiety and depression. For example, Lecrubier and Weiller (1997) reported that 48% of their clinical sample of patients with social anxiety disorder also met criteria for major depressive disorder. Conversely, Pini et al. (1997) indicated that 11.1% of their patients diagnosed with major depression carried secondary diagnoses of social anxiety disorder. My longitudinal research confirmed that there was a high overlap between social anxiety and depression, as approximately half of the women who were diagnosed with social anxiety disorder reported clinically significant symptoms of depression at 8 weeks postpartum (Wenzel, Haugen, Jackson, et al., 2005).

> Although she does not meet criteria for major depressive disorder, Lily experiences some depressive symptoms and views them as bothersome. Her mood is clearly more depressed than she has ever experienced in her life. She gets little pleasure out of engaging in activities that she used to enjoy, whether or not the activities involve social interaction. Furthermore, she reports that she is eating a great deal less than what is normal for her, although she cannot pinpoint whether this is due to depression or to the fact that she is trying to eat less so that she loses the baby weight. In contrast, Lily does not believe that her sleep and energy are lower than what would be expected for a mother of a 3-month-old child.

POSSIBLE ETIOLOGY

As might be expected from such a small literature on the phenomenology of perinatal social anxiety disorder, little work has been done to identify candidates that could explain the etiology of social anxiety during the transition to parenthood. Nevertheless, results from my longitudinal study point to sociodemographic characteristics that are especially prevalent in women who experience postpartum social anxiety. In addition, my research raises the possibility that breastfeeding status could affect the expression of postpartum social anxiety. I describe these results in the following section, along with research on people with social anxiety disorder who are not necessarily undergoing the transition to parenthood, in order to generate hypotheses about variables that contribute to the etiology of perinatal social anxiety that can be tested in future research.

Sociodemographic Factors

My research suggests that there are a number of sociodemographic variables associated with postpartum social anxiety. In an analysis that was nearly identical to that described in Chapter 4 on panic disorder, I examined the degree to which mother's age, baby's age, number of children in the household, and socioeconomic status predicted scores on the Social Interaction Anxiety Scale (SIAS; Mattick & Clarke, 1998). Both mother's age and socioeconomic status were negative predictors associated with SIAS scores at 8 weeks postpartum, meaning that younger age and lower socioeconomic status predicted higher levels of social anxiety (Wenzel, Haugen, Jackson, et al., 2005). In addition, SIAS scores correlated negatively with the level of education attained by the mother, age of the baby's father, the skill level of the baby's father's job, the level of education attained by the baby's father, and income level. SIAS scores were also associated with the women's marital status, such that women who were not married to the father of their newborn scored higher on the SIAS than women who were married to the father of their newborn. In contrast, SIAS scores were not associated with parity, the ethnicity of the mother or the baby's father, or the length of time the woman was in a relationship with the baby's father. Unlike the case of many of the other types of anxiety that are considered in this volume, a personal and family psychiatric history did not predict symptoms of social anxiety at 8 weeks postpartum.

Similar to the pattern that was observed with BAI scores described in Chapter 4 on panic disorder, there were only three significant associations between SIAS scores and sociodemographic variables at 6 or 12 months postpartum. Specifically, women who were not married to the father of their newborn scored higher on the SIAS at 6 months postpartum than women who were married to the father of their newborn. In addition, younger women scored higher on the SIAS at 6 months postpartum, as did women with lower levels of educational attainment. There were no significant associations between background variables and SIAS scores at the 12-month postpartum assessment. As stated previously, it seems that anxiety symptoms are much more reactive to circumstances that might be stressful for women early in the postpartum period, and that these variables play a lesser role in exacerbating anxiety as the postpartum period progresses.

> Lily is not characterized by the sociodemographic variables that I found to be related to postpartum social anxiety symptoms—she is not particularly young to be starting her family, she is married to the father of her baby, she and her husband both have graduate degrees, and their professions allow them the luxury of having no financial concerns. Thus, Lily is not experiencing much life stress generated by sociodemographic factors. On the other hand, Lily is experiencing stress associated with other aspects of her life. She and her husband are financing a home for her aging parents, and she is finding that they are able to take on fewer and fewer household responsibilities. In addition, she and her husband are beginning the process of putting their current home on the market and looking for a larger home. It is possible that the stress caused by these factors has weakened her psychological resources to cope with the transition to parenthood.

Biological Factors

To date, there has been no speculation into the biological factors that make women vulnerable to social anxiety during pregnancy and the postpartum period. However, research on biological factors associated with social anxiety in people representative of the general population is quickly accumulating.

For example, there is evidence that a behaviorally inhibited temperament, which is characterized by socially anxious behavior, is associated with the corticotropin-releasing hormone (CRH) gene (Smoller et al., 2005). CRH levels are high during pregnancy, and CRH plays a role in determining the length of pregnancy and the timing of labor and delivery. It is possible that elevations in CRH levels during pregnancy make some women vulnerable to symptoms of social anxiety. Moreover, if CRH levels are elevated in socially anxious pregnant women, it is possible that they could affect the length of gestation. In addition, Stein and Stein (2008) concluded that serotonergic dysfunction is at work in social anxiety disorder, and we have seen that dramatic changes in estrogen have the potential to disrupt the serotonin system. Finally, oxytocin levels affect the neural circuitry associated with fear during social functioning (Kirsch et al., 2005), so it is possible that the high level of oxytocin that is present near delivery and while lactating could affect the expression of social anxiety.

In my longitudinal study, I found that breastfeeding status predicted scores on the SIAS and beyond the background variables indicated previously (Wenzel, Haugen, Jackson, et al., 2005). Nonbreastfeeding women were more likely than breastfeeding women to endorse higher scores on the SIAS at 8 weeks postpartum. In addition, women who were diagnosed with social anxiety disorder or who were subthreshold for social anxiety disorder at 6 months postpartum were less likely than women without social anxiety disorder to be breastfeeding. One explanation for this pattern of results is that women who do not breastfeed experience a more dramatic change in hormone levels soon after they give birth than women who do breastfeed, which could in turn prompt on onset of postpartum social anxiety. However, I also believe that the significant association between breastfeeding status and symptoms of social anxiety could be explained by psychological mechanisms. It is not uncommon for women to report that they are uncomfortable with breastfeeding, particularly when they are called on to do so in public (Ledley, 2009). It is reasonable to speculate that the decision not to breastfeed is associated with variables indicative of social anxiety, such as discomfort with public exposure or lack of self-confidence. In other words, the decision not to breastfeed could be another consequence of social anxiety, rather than a cause of it.

Psychological Factors

Scholars have yet to speculate about the psychological processes that make women vulnerable to developing perinatal social anxiety disorder. Fortunately, there is a rich literature on the psychological processes associated with social anxiety disorder in general from which we can draw and apply to pregnant and postpartum women. For example, socially anxious people lack confidence in themselves, and as a result, they judge themselves harshly and believe that they performed poorly in their interactions with others (Wenzel & Kashdan, 2008). The transition to parenthood is a time of great uncertainty, which makes it especially likely that their doubts about themselves will be salient. It is possible that the stress of caring for a newborn and adjusting to a new role, as well as exhaustion and sleep deprivation, will exacerbate the tendency of some women to focus on their shortcomings at the expense of their successes because they have available fewer cognitive resources to evaluate their negative appraisals.

In addition, people with social anxiety disorder are characterized by several biases in the manner in which they allocate their attention (Schultz & Heimberg, 2008). First, socially anxious individuals are characterized by *self-focused attention*, defined as "an awareness of self-referent, internally generated information that stands in contrast to an awareness of externally generated information derived through sensory receptors" (Ingram, 1990, p. 156). When socially anxious people perceive that they are being watched, they begin to monitor themselves for signs of anxiety, which in turn provokes physiological, cognitive, and emotional indicators of perceived threat. They then take those signs as facts that they are indeed performing poorly. Anxiety is exacerbated when socially anxious people focus their attention on these anxiety reactions, which precludes them from garnering any external positive feedback and distracts them from the interactional task at hand (Clark & Wells, 1995). Second, socially anxious people scan their environment for signs that others do not approve of them (Rapee & Heimberg, 1997). This information processing style could make some women vulnerable to social anxiety, particularly in the postpartum period, when they could perceive that others are judging their parenting style or their ability to "fit in" after this profound transition.

Following social interactions, socially anxious people have the tendency to engage in *post-event processing*, which occurs when they engage in extensive review and analysis of their performance after a social interaction (Brozovich & Heimberg, 2008). Rather than learning from mistakes they might have made during the interaction, socially anxious people who engage in post-event processing ruminate over perceived social errors and their implications, which only exacerbates emotional disturbance. One could speculate that after interacting socially with others, pregnant and postpartum women with this cognitive style would ruminate over whether they talked too much about the baby, whether they had anything meaningful to contribute to conversation, and whether others will be less interested in them now that they have a new focus in their life. Thus, post-event processing is another cognitive style that could contribute to the development of social anxiety disorder during the transition to parenthood.

Many people engage in one or more of these processes from time to time, and in times of low stress they can bring perspective and balance to the conclusions that they draw as a result of these tendencies. However, the transition to parenthood is characterized by a great deal of stress, and new mothers often do not have the opportunity to systematically evaluate their negative beliefs or get reassurance and balance from others. The postpartum period, then, might be a time when women who are characterized by one or more of these styles to develop clinically significant difficulties with social anxiety.

> Even before she became pregnant, Lily had engaged in a number of these cognitive processes when she interacted with others. She views herself a shy person who is more comfortable allowing others to be in the spotlight. Although she has an extensive circle of friends and enjoys socializing with them, she has had difficulty interacting with people whom she meets for the first time, such as the new boyfriend of one of her friends or a new coworker who joined the group for a social outing. During these interactions, she often has the perception that others will be upset that they were "stuck" sitting next to her because she is boring. As a result, she is hyperaware of any indication that a new person with whom she is interacting does not like her. On a few occasions, she has chosen to leave social gatherings early, believing that her departure would allow others to have more fun. Moreover, Lily has a history of analyzing social interactions with others whom she perceived as more attractive or more accomplished than her. However, she usually had the opportunity to discuss her fears with her husband, and he was able to help her put them in perspective.

PRACTICAL IMPLICATIONS

Perinatal social anxiety has rarely been considered in the research literature. However, it is clear that a small percentage of women develop clinically significant expressions of social anxiety disorder following childbirth. It would be helpful for physicians and mental health professionals to be aware that social anxiety can intensify in the postpartum period so that they can help their patients understand the nature and expected course of their symptoms. These women can be assured by health care providers that, in most cases, their symptoms will decrease over the first 6 months postpartum. However, women whose symptoms persist across the 1st year postpartum should be monitored; not only are these women likely experiencing more severe instances of social anxiety disorder that could be associated with life interference, but they are also more likely to have interpersonal difficulties that put them at risk of continued maladjustment and depression.

Clinicians who work with women who become pregnant should be cognizant of warning signs that might be associated with the onset or exacerbation of social anxiety. Such warning signs could be sociodemographic variables that have the potential to cause stress in a new mother's life (e.g., younger age, low income) as well as cognitive styles that lead women to interpret their social performance as deficient. During pregnancy, women who are characterized by these warning signs should do what they can to ensure that a strong social support network is available for them as they transition to the new role as mother. By continuing to engage in social interaction, postpartum women with social anxiety disorder can ensure that they are continuing to connect with their social support system and actively engage in their environment.

> Lily opted not to seek treatment for her social anxiety because she regarded it as something she has always dealt with to some degree and that she must accept as part of her character. However, she agreed to purchase a self-help book on cognitive behavioral strategies for managing social anxiety. Lily responded well to bibliotherapy and actively made attempts to implement the strategies in her daily life. Over time, Lily's confidence improved, and she began to realize that her new role in life could bring added depth to some of her relationships.

Most of the focus of this chapter has been on new cases of social anxiety disorder that develop in the postpartum period. However, it is feasible that women with preexisting social anxiety disorder would have a particularly difficult transition to parenthood. For example, relative to people without social anxiety disorder, people with social anxiety disorder have smaller social support networks and are less satisfied with those networks (Torgrud et al., 2004). The implication of this is that socially anxious women might have little support as they experience the stress of pregnancy and the postpartum period. Moreover, the cognitive processes associated with social anxiety disorder that were outlined earlier in the chapter could interfere with socially anxious women's ability to utilize the health care system, as their insecurity might inhibit them from asking questions at medical appointments or calling their obstetrician in the event of a problem. It also is feasible that socially anxious women would be hesitant to take advantage of other ways to obtain support and information, such as attending childbirth preparation classes and breastfeeding classes or joining a mother's group. Thus, clinicians who work with women with preexisting social anxiety are encouraged to be cognizant of instances in which their symptoms interfere with a healthy transition to parenthood and recommend intervention when necessary.

6

CHILDBIRTH-RELATED FEAR AND TRAUMA

Samantha is a 26-year-old single Caucasian woman who unexpectedly became pregnant by her boyfriend of 5 years. She has always told her friends that she would never have children because she is petrified of labor and delivery. She has a low pain threshold and experiences great distress when she goes through routine procedures, such as getting a flu shot. Thus, she predicts that labor and delivery will be excruciating for her and that she will simply not be able to take it. In addition, 2 years ago Samantha's older sister had problems during labor and hemorrhaged, almost resulting in her death. Her sister has vowed not to have any more children as a result of this incident. Now that she is pregnant, Samantha predicts that the same thing will happen to her. As a result, she avoids most reminders of the baby—she does not talk about the pregnancy with others, she has not read books or gathered other information to educate herself about pregnancy and child rearing, and she has even skipped several of her prenatal appointments.

Kellie is a 30-year-old separated American Indian woman who gave birth at a small hospital on a reservation 2 hr away from her home. She does not have contact with her husband at present because she took out a restraining order against him for domestic violence. When she went into labor, one of her aunts was recruited to drive her to the hospital. Her aunt complained about the inconvenience along the way and made it known to Kellie that she would not stay with her in the delivery room. Kellie worried about who would take care of her other two children and whether her estranged husband would use this opportunity to take them away. When she and her aunt were still a half hour away from the hospital, the frequency and intensity of her labor pains increased substantially, and Kellie was terrified that they would not make it to the hospital. Fortunately, they did make it to the hospital before the baby was born, and she was rushed to the delivery room. The pain continued to be excruciating, but there was no time to administer an analgesic. As the baby was being born, she heard the doctor shout, "It's not breathing!" Kellie screamed and panicked, pleading to know what was going on. The doctor and nurse ignored her, rushing around. She was sure that her baby would not make it. Although the baby lived, he was put into the neonatal intensive care unit, and Kellie had difficulty obtaining information about what was wrong with him. Throughout the childbirth experience, she viewed the medical staff at the hospital as being cold and uncaring of the ordeal she had endured. When Kellie was finally able to take the baby home, although he was healthy, she felt strangely numb and disconnected.

Although more than 75% of women report some degree of fear associated with childbirth (Melender, 2002), a minority of women experience fears of phobic proportions, and they are vulnerable to the development of childbirth-related posttraumatic stress symptoms as a result (Fairbrother & Woody, 2007; Söderquist, Wijma, & Wijma, 2004; Wijma, 2003). One focus of this chapter is on clinically significant childbirth-related fears and the manner in which they affect labor and delivery, as well as birth outcomes and child development. In addition, several situational variables increase the likelihood of posttraumatic stress symptoms following childbirth, including painful labor, complications during labor, and perceptions of medical staff as being unhelpful (Allen, 1998; Czarnocka & Slade, 2000). A second focus of this chapter is on the phenomenology and consequences of perinatal posttraumatic stress disorder (PTSD). Most of the discussion of PTSD focuses on posttraumatic stress resulting from a difficult labor and delivery; however, this chapter also considers instances in which women report clinically significant instances of posttraumatic stress during pregnancy.

FEAR OF CHILDBIRTH

Although some degree of fear surrounding labor and delivery is to be expected in pregnant women, excessive fears of childbirth have the potential to affect prenatal care and cause significant distress. This section describes research on fears of childbirth and their psychiatric sequelae.

Definition and Nature of Childbirth-Related Fears

Women typically report a number of fears of childbirth, including pain during labor, their own health complications or death, health complications or death of the fetus, painful injections, and losing control during labor (Areskog, Kjessler, & Uddenberg, 1982; Areskog, Uddenberg, & Kjessler, 1981; Geissbuehler & Eberhard, 2002). It is normal for women to have some degree of fear or apprehension about pregnancy, labor, delivery, and postpartum adjustment, and it is normal for women to report that their childbirth-related fears are more severe than other fears that they might have. However, a small percentage of women experience such extensive fear that they meet diagnostic criteria for specific phobia.

According to the *Diagnostic and Statistical Manual of Mental Disorders* (4th ed., text revision [*DSM–IV–TR*]; American Psychiatric Association, 2000), there are five criteria for specific phobia: (a) a marked or persistent fear that is excessive and cued by the feared stimulus; (b) exposure to the feared stimulus almost always provokes anxiety; (c) the person recognizes that the fear is excessive; (d) the feared stimulus is avoided or endured with extreme distress; and (e) the avoidance, anxious anticipation, or distress causes life interference, or the person has marked distress about having the fear. In this chapter, I use the term *fear of childbirth* when describing studies in which the authors did not specifically assign diagnoses of specific phobia, and I use the term *specific phobia* only in cases in which women met *DSM–IV–TR* criteria for this anxiety disorder. The vast majority of the research to date focuses on women who report high levels of fear but who may or may not meet diagnostic criteria for a specific phobia.

Aspects of specific phobia of childbirth are unique among the pool of phobic disorders in general. Wijma (2003) noted that specific phobia of childbirth can differ from other specific phobias in that it only reaches clinically significant proportions after a woman has become pregnant. At that point, she is unable to fully avoid or escape the fact that she will have to face childbirth, so the amount of fear continually increases as she approaches her delivery date. Subtle avoidance behavior is manifested by not acknowledging the pregnancy, not thinking about childbirth, and not planning for delivery and beyond.

> Samantha meets criteria for specific phobia. She endorses fear in excess of that which nearly all pregnant women report. She has experienced anxiety about the impending childbirth every day since she learned that she was pregnant. Whenever someone mentions the pregnancy, the blood drains from her face, and she begins to shake. She indicates that she pictures herself lying on the bed in the delivery room in a pool of blood and with the heart-rate monitor flatlining. As stated previously,

she avoids exposure to aspects of childbirth and her pregnancy by not talking about the pregnancy, not preparing for delivery and beyond, and missing her scheduled prenatal appointments. She refuses to buy maternity clothes and wears the baggiest clothes that she already owns (e.g., oversized sweatshirts, sweatpants) so that she does not see her belly and can pretend that her life is back to normal. Her phobic behavior has the potential to cause life interference because she is not engaging in healthy behavior to care for her unborn child.

Prevalence

Specific phobias are the most common anxiety disorder, with a 12-month prevalence rate of 8.7% (Kessler, Chiu, Demler, & Walters, 2005). That rate includes all specific phobias, so it is not appropriate to compare rates of childbirth-related specific phobia with rates of specific phobias in the general population. Nevertheless, some work has been done with childbearing women to identify the prevalence of fears associated with childbirth. Nearly all of this research has been conducted with women who are currently pregnant. For example, Melender (2002) administered a questionnaire to 329 pregnant women and found that 78% endorsed fears of pregnancy, childbirth, or both. In their analysis of more than 8,000 pregnant women, Geissbuehler and Eberhard (2002) found that 57.5% reported "some fear" and that 5.3% reported "intense fear." An early, exploratory study of fear of childbirth found that 6% of pregnant women reported a severe fear of childbirth, with severe defined as instances in which it interfered with their daily functioning or emotional well-being. It is possible that these women would have been diagnosed with specific phobia. This study identified another 17% of women who reported a moderate fear of childbirth, with moderate defined as instances in which women clearly endorsed such fears, but that the fears did not cause life interference (Areskog et al., 1981). Thus, the majority of pregnant women (i.e., 57.5%–78.0%) admitted to some fear of childbirth, and a noticeable minority of pregnant women (i.e., 5.3%–6.0%) reported fears of childbirth that were persistent and/or associated with life interference and distress.

Effects

Correlational research suggests that fear of childbirth is associated with aversive experiences during labor. For example, fear of delivery assessed in the first phase of labor is associated with the amount of pain relief used and the duration of labor (Alehagen, Wijma, & Wijma, 2001), although it is unclear whether this association can be explained by the fact that women with childbirth fears actually experience more pain or whether women with childbirth fears find pain more aversive and have a diminished ability to tolerate it. Other research has suggested that both explanations could be at work. In an elegant experimental study, Saisto, Kaaja, Ylikorkala, and Halmesmäki (2001) found that not only did women with a fear of labor perceive labor as more painful than women without such a fear, they also tolerated much less pain on a cold presser task conducted before delivery. Additional research has suggested that fear of childbirth is associated with the type of delivery that women have when they give birth. Ryding (1993) identified a subset of fearful women who scheduled elective cesarean sections in order to avoid labor, and she later determined that fear of childbirth increases women's risk of undergoing an emergency cesarean section (Ryding, Wijma, Wijma, & Rydhström, 1998). Finally, relative to women who report a low fear of delivery, those with a high fear of delivery also endorse more intrusive memories of the delivery experience, raising the possibility that they are at particular risk of developing PTSD (see the next section). Also, the likelihood is increased that these women will admit that they are hesitant about having additional children and report a lack of confidence in their parenting and breastfeeding abilities (Areskog, Uddenberg, & Kjessler, 1983b).

Many mental health professionals assume that fear of childbirth dissipates following delivery, as delivery would serve as an intense, prolonged exposure to the feared stimulus. This assumption is only partially correct. For example, Wijma and Wijma (1992) reported that postdelivery, women who had endorsed a high fear of childbirth during pregnancy continued to report higher levels than women who had endorsed a low fear of childbirth. However, their level of fear dropped significantly compared with their level predelivery, and a follow-up study (Zar, Wijma, & Wijma, 2001) found that fear level continued to drop through the 5th week postpartum. In other words, fear of childbirth decreases significantly following the childbirth experience, but women who report pronounced fears of childbirth during pregnancy continue to report a higher level of fear in the postpartum period, relative to women who reported a low fear of childbirth during pregnancy. Although this research has shown that fear of childbirth usually decreases substantially after a woman gives birth to her first child, a small proportion of women who have previously given birth report "intense fear" of childbirth, usually in instances in which they had a difficult labor and delivery (Geissbuehler & Eberhard, 2002).

> Samantha went into labor 6 days after her projected due date. In the
> month preceding delivery, she begged her obstetrician to arrange for an
> elective cesarean section so that she could be under anesthesia when she
> had the child. However, her insurance company would not cover the pro-
> cedure because it was not medically necessary, and she could not afford
> to pay for the procedure out-of-pocket. Although Samantha's labor was
> quite short for a first child, she screamed in pain and pleaded with the

medical staff to do something, saying she couldn't take it anymore. An epidural was administered despite the fact that her labor was not prolonged. Two days after Samantha gave birth to her healthy baby girl, she described labor and delivery as the worst experiences of her life and vowed not to have another child. However, as she bonded with her baby over time, her view on this issue softened, and on her baby's first birthday she told her family that she would consider having another child if she could afford an elective cesarean section.

Comorbidity With Depression

There is not much research on comorbid fear of childbirth and depression. In one descriptive study, Hofberg and Brockington (2000) presented four cases of women who developed a phobia of childbirth, which they viewed as secondary to depression during pregnancy. Epidemiological research conducted with people who are not necessarily pregnant or postpartum has suggested that rates of comorbidity between specific phobias and depression are higher than would be expected by chance, although less than rates of comorbidity between depression and other anxiety disorders such as generalized anxiety disorder and social anxiety disorder (McGlinchey & Zimmerman, 2007). In the National Comorbidity Survey, more than 40% of people diagnosed with specific phobia had a lifetime history of depression, relative to 14% of people who were not diagnosed with specific phobia (Choy, Fyer, & Goodwin, 2007). It is interesting that people who reported more than one specific fear were more likely to report a history of depression than people who endorsed only one fear. This finding suggests that it would be worthwhile to assess for the presence of other specific phobias in women who endorse fears associated with childbirth, as women who have another phobia in addition to their fear of childbirth would be more likely to experience depression, which would in turn be associated with greater impairment.

> Samantha does indeed have a history of other phobias—when she was younger, she exhibited symptoms of school phobia. She also reports fears of insects, snakes, and vermin, although she does not believe that these fears cause life interference. During the second half of her pregnancy, she endorsed some symptoms of depression. Her mood was much lower than was normal for her, and she had difficulty concentrating on professional and personal activities, in part because she was preoccupied with the impending labor and delivery. She rarely slept through the night, and when she was able to fall asleep, she slept restlessly. Moreover, she was consumed with guilt, as she began to wonder if she was a bad person for not being more excited about the pregnancy. After giving birth to her baby girl, she experienced the blues during the 1st week and a half postpartum. However, her depressive symptoms

subsided as the postpartum period progressed and as she developed a bond with her baby.

Possible Etiology

The following sections describe correlates of childbirth fears that have the potential to explain their etiology, including sociodemographic factors (e.g., parity), biological factors (e.g., reactivity to perceived threat), and psychological factors (e.g., learning).

Sociodemographic Factors

With the other anxiety disorders described in this volume, there is only mixed evidence that nulliparous women are more likely to report higher anxiety than parous women. This is not the case with childbirth fears. There is clear evidence that women who have never given birth usually score much higher than women who have had previous children on self-report inventories that measure fears of childbirth (e.g., Alehagen et al., 2001; Areskog et al., 1981; Wijma, Wijma, & Zar, 1998; Zar et al., 2001). As stated previously, if parous women endorse a significant fear of childbirth, it is usually because they had a previous delivery that they viewed as traumatic (Areskog et al., 1981). It is possible that parity exerts its effects on fear of childbirth through cognitive mechanisms, as women who have not yet had a childbirth experience are likely to overestimate the pain and adversity they will experience and catastrophize about the possibility of unlikely complications.

In addition, women with a previous psychiatric history or who endorsed psychiatric problems during pregnancy are more likely than those without psychiatric problems to endorse a fear of childbirth (Areskog, Uddenberg, & Kjessler, 1983a). In contrast, many other sociodemographic variables are not associated with fear of childbirth, including age and educational attainment (Areskog et al., 1981). Unlike some of the other anxiety disorders described in this volume, there is no evidence that sociodemographic variables that increase the stress in the lives of pregnant women increase the likelihood of a fear of childbirth.

Biological Factors

No research has considered the mechanism by which hormonal changes associated with pregnancy would increase the likelihood that women would experience a fear of childbirth. One general model for the etiology of specific phobias suggests that people with specific phobias have a nonspecific genetic predisposition to experience anxiety or alarm reactions, which interacts with specific life experiences that teach them to be fearful of a particular object or situation (Antony & Barlow, 2002). This means that people who have a biological predisposition to be reactive to perceived threat, as evidenced by heightened arousal and alertness, are particularly likely to develop phobias when they have an adverse experience with a phobic stimulus. For example, an overly aroused woman who hears "horror stories" from others about childbirth is more likely to develop a specific phobia of childbirth than a woman who does not exhibit overarousal.

Psychological Factors

In a seminal paper that is still widely cited today, Rachman (1977) described three psychological pathways to development of a phobia. The first pathway involves *classical conditioning,* which is evidenced when a person has a negative experience with a previously neutral stimulus and subsequently associates the fear response with that stimulus. This pathway explains fear of childbirth in pregnant women who are fearful because a previous childbirth had been traumatic. The second pathway involves *vicarious learning,* which occurs when a person learns to be fearful of a stimulus by observing the reactions of others. This pathway explains fear of childbirth in pregnant women like Samantha who have witnessed others exhibiting fear behavior, such as her sister's unwillingness to have more children after she experienced a significant delivery complication. Finally, the third pathway involves *instruction,* which occurs when a person is given information about the danger associated with the stimulus. This pathway explains fear of childbirth in pregnant women when they are told by others how painful labor is, or when they are given information by their health care provider about serious complications that can occur during labor and delivery. This pathway also pertains to Samantha, as she developed a fear of childbirth only after she had acquired the knowledge that labor and delivery are painful. All three of these mechanisms are behavioral in nature, in that they involve learning.

Practical Implications

Many women have some degree of fear of childbirth, which can be normalized by clinicians when pregnant women overtly express concern about the fear that they are experiencing. When a pregnant woman admits to fear of childbirth, clinicians would be wise to assess the degree to which this fear is associated with avoidance behavior and life interference. Avoidance behavior could manifest in not acknowledging the pregnancy, which could be associated with engagement in unhealthy behaviors such as smoking or drinking, as well as in missing important appointments to ensure that the pregnancy is progressing normally. Intervention should be swift in instances in which the woman is not engaging in adequate prenatal care. In addition, clinicians should assess for fear of childbirth in women who do not spontaneously express such fears for the same reasons.

> Samantha's nurse–midwife noticed that she had inconsistent attendance at her prenatal care visits and that she missed her 20-week ultrasound. When she questioned her about this, Samantha was reluctant to disclose the reason for her absence, partly because she was fearful that she would be somehow forced to attend all subsequent appointments and partly because she was embarrassed. At first, the nurse–midwife asked questions about her partner relationship and whether there was anything her boyfriend was doing to her that she did not want others to see. Samantha realized that her nurse–midwife wondered whether she was being abused, which could not have been further from the truth—her boyfriend was thrilled that they were going to have a child together and was talking about proposing. To ensure that her nurse–midwife did not think that her boyfriend was abusing her, Samantha reluctantly admitted that she was very uncomfortable with being pregnant and that she did not know how she was going to face labor. Her nurse–midwife discussed her concerns with empathy and sensitivity and strongly encouraged her to seek help through psychotherapy.

TRAUMATIC STRESS

As stated earlier in this chapter, women who have clinically significant fears of childbirth have an increased likelihood of having a traumatic birth experience. In some instances, a traumatic birth experience can result in PTSD. This section describes the research on traumatic childbirths and their psychiatric sequelae. It also includes research on the prevalence and effects of preexisting posttraumatic stress symptoms whose onset occurred well before or during pregnancy.

Definition and Nature of Traumatic Stress

A trauma that can precipitate a diagnosis of PTSD is one in which a person experiences or witnesses an event associated with actual or threatened death or injury, and the person responds with fear, horror, or helplessness (American Psychiatric Association, 2000). Nearly all of the cases of childbirth-related PTSD that have been described in the literature stem from stressful experiences during labor and delivery. Some women believe that their bodies are being torn apart during childbirth and wonder whether they and their babies will survive (Boyce & Condon, 2000). Moreover, many women experience a sense of helplessness in response to the physical pain and to a perceived lack of support and information provided by medical staff. A few women develop traumatic stress symptoms that stem from threatened abortion and threatened premature delivery (Ichida, 1996) or after a history of infertility or complicated pregnancies (Moleman, van der Hart, & van der Kolk, 1992). The investigation of childbirth-related PTSD is a relatively new phenomenon, as the third version of the *DSM* (i.e., *DSM–III–R;* American Psychiatric Association, 1987) indicated that the traumatic experience was to be outside the range of usual experience. At that time, childbirth would not have qualified as an event outside the usual range of experience, as about half the population goes through childbirth at some point (Bailham & Joseph, 2003; Crompton, 1996a; Olde, van der Hart, Kleber, & van Son, 2006).

In addition, the person must report symptoms in three different clusters to qualify for a *DSM–IV–TR* diagnosis of PTSD. First, the trauma must be persistently reexperienced in at least one way. *Reexperiencing* can take the form of nightmares, flashbacks, intrusive memories, or distress and/or physiological reactivity to reminders of the trauma. Second, the person must report three symptoms of avoidance of stimuli associated with the trauma and/or a general numbing of responsiveness. *Avoidance* takes the form of avoiding thoughts, feelings, activities, places, or people associated with the trauma. Extreme avoidance can manifest in an inability to recall important aspects of the trauma. *Numbing* includes symptoms such as decreased interest or participation in significant activities, a sense of estrangement from others, restricted range of affect, and a sense of a foreshortened future. Third, the individual must report two symptoms of *increased arousal,* such as sleep disturbance, irritability, concentration difficulties, hypervigilance, and exaggerated startle response. Traumatic stress symptoms that last between 1 and 3 months are regarded as acute, and traumatic stress symptoms that last more than 3 months are regarded as chronic (American Psychiatric Association, 2000). In this chapter, I refer to posttraumatic stress symptoms to capture subsyndromal manifestations of PTSD, usually as measured by responses to self-report inventories of posttraumatic stress. In some instances, scholars regard women as meeting criteria if they score above a certain threshold on self-report inventories that assess diagnostic criteria for PTSD; I point out these definitions of PTSD diagnoses when relevant. I use the term *PTSD* without qualification in instances in which women were diagnosed with PTSD through the use of an established clinical interview.

> At 2 months postpartum, Kellie has been diagnosed with acute PTSD. Whenever she is able to grab a couple hours of sleep, she sleeps fitfully because she has nightmares about the traumatic birth experience, particularly the instance in which her doctor said that the baby was not breathing. Often, she is unable to get to sleep even though all of her children, including her newborn, are sleeping. In addition, she is often "jolted" when she is nursing her baby and has a flashback of the traumatic

childbirth. Kellie tries to avoid intrusive memories of the traumatic childbirth, but she is constantly bombarded with them when she is caring for her baby. Not only does she feel detached from her newborn, she also feels disconnected from her other children and her extended family. Moreover, she exhibits a restricted range in affect, having difficulty showing love toward her children, especially her newborn. Despite the fact that she is extremely fatigued, Kellie is hyperalert to any signs of danger and is easily startled when her older children burst into the room to talk to her.

Prevalence

As was seen earlier in the chapter when I described the prevalence of childbirth-related specific phobia, we cannot compare rates of PTSD that is due to a traumatic childbirth with rates of PTSD in women who are not necessarily pregnant or postpartum because in epidemiological studies, PTSD is diagnosed in response to any number of traumatic events (e.g., a car accident, a sexual assault). However, research with childbearing women has suggested that approximately one third of women experience a stressful labor and delivery that they view as traumatic (Creedy, Shochet, & Horsfall, 2000; Soet, Brack, & Dilorio, 2003). In a sample of first-time mothers, Lyons (1998) indicated that 10% of 42 women interviewed on postnatal wards reported fear that they might die during childbirth and that 14% reported fear that their baby might die. It should also be noted that some cases of childbirth-related PTSD have been diagnosed in women who do not describe their labor and delivery as traumatic, perhaps because they are reluctant to admit a negative birth experience or are motivated to avoid talking about it (Soet et al., 2003).

It is not uncommon for women to ruminate over negative experiences during labor and delivery during the postpartum period, which often causes more distress than the apprehension that they experienced about labor and delivery during pregnancy (Arizmendi & Affonso, 1987). Rates of PTSD at 3 to 6 weeks postpartum diagnosed via self-report inventories of symptoms that correspond to *DSM–IV–TR* criteria range from 0.8% (Ford, Ayers, & Bradley, 2010) to 4.6% (Creedy et al., 2000). Another 18.5% (Onoye, Goebert, Morland, Matsu, & Wright, 2009) to 30.0% (Soet et al., 2003) endorse subsyndromal posttraumatic stress symptoms during this time period. The percentage of women who meet criteria for PTSD later in the postpartum period ranges from 0.9% at 3 months (Ford et al., 2010) to between 1.5% and 6.4% at 6 months postpartum (Ayers & Pickering, 2001; Zaers, Waschke, & Ehlert, 2008) and 0.9% at 11 months postpartum (Söderquist, Wijma, & Wijma, 2006). Zaers et al. (2008) reported that 10.6% of women continue to report subsyndromal posttraumatic stress symptoms at 6 months postpartum. In contrast, I obtained a different pattern of results in my longitudinal study of postpartum anxiety disorders, as no women met criteria for childbirth-related PTSD at 8 weeks, 6 months, or 12 months postpartum (Wenzel, Haugen, Jackson, & Brendle, 2005).

All of the studies described previously reported the prevalence of PTSD in women who had live births. It is equally important to consider instances of PTSD in women who experience pregnancy loss. For example, Engelhard, van den Hout, and Arntz (2001) reported prevalence rates of 25% and 7% for PTSD diagnosed via a self-report inventory of symptoms that correspond to *DSM–IV–TR* criteria at 1 month and 4 months, respectively, following a pregnancy loss. When women are forced to deliver a fetus that has not or will not survive, approximately 25% experience intrusive memories of the delivery (Hunfeld, Wladimiroff, & Passchier, 1997). Moreover, women who terminate a pregnancy in the 2nd or early 3rd trimester report significantly more symptoms of intrusive memories, avoidance, and hyperarousal 14 days following the event than women who deliver premature infants and women who deliver healthy babies, with 64% of these women being regarded as "cases" of PTSD on the basis of their scores on a self-report inventory (Kersting et al., 2009). Although posttraumatic stress symptoms associated with a late pregnancy termination decreased significantly over the 1st year following the event, they remained elevated compared with symptoms in the other two groups.

Finally, although the studies described in this section reveal a great deal about the prevalence of PTSD associated with childbirth-related events, they do not account for women who meet diagnostic criteria for PTSD during pregnancy, usually because of an unrelated traumatic event. Results from epidemiological studies described in previous chapters indicate that few, if any, women who are interviewed in obstetric care clinics meet criteria for PTSD (0%, Sutter-Dallay et al., 2004; 0.6%, Adewuya, Ola, Aloba, & Mapayi, 2006). However, rates are much higher in studies designed specifically to assess aspects of perinatal PTSD; for example, Ford et al. (2010) reported that approximately 38% of 136 women in their sample of women between 33 and 37 weeks pregnant had experienced a previous traumatic event and endorsed posttraumatic stress symptoms and that 7.2% met criteria for PTSD according to a self-report inventory that assessed the presence of *DSM–IV–TR* symptoms. Morland et al. (2007) found a 16% rate of PTSD in their sample of 101 women in their 1st trimester of pregnancy and reported that an additional 23% of their sample reported subsyndromal posttraumatic stress symptoms. Interestingly, there is documentation of some women who would be regarded as having PTSD during pregnancy on the basis of fear of their impending childbirth (i.e., pretraumatic stress). For example, Söderquist et al. (2004) found that 2.3% of 940 women at 32 weeks' gestation met criteria for PTSD for this reason as determined by their score on a self-report inventory that corresponded to *DSM–IV–TR* criteria, and an additional 5.8% were subsyndromal for PTSD.

Rates of PTSD are even higher in high-risk samples of pregnant women, such as those enrolled in perinatal drug treatment programs (26%; Eggleston et al., 2009). Research has shown that rates of PTSD during pregnancy vary as a function of type of trauma; for example, Seng, Sperlich, and Low (2008) reported that, in a sample of 1,259 nulliparous women who were at no more than 28 weeks' gestation, 4.1% had PTSD attributable to a nonabuse trauma exposure, 11.4% had PTSD attributable to physical or sexual abuse in adulthood, 16.0% had PTSD attributable to physical or sexual abuse in childhood, and 39.2% had PTSD attributable to physical or sexual abuse in both periods.

As a whole, results from these studies indicate that posttraumatic stress symptoms are quite common in pregnant and postpartum women. Up to a third of postpartum women view labor and delivery as traumatic, with between 10% and 15% of these women reporting a belief during labor and delivery that they or their baby might die. Rates of PTSD (as diagnosed according to responses on a self-report inventory that corresponds to *DSM–IV–TR* criteria) in the first several weeks following childbirth are as high as 5%, and an additional 30% of women report subsyndromal posttraumatic stress symptoms. Rates of PTSD remain fairly consistent with these values at 6 months postpartum and drop significantly in the second half of the 1st year postpartum. Rates of postpartum PTSD have the potential to be even higher in women who experience a 2nd or 3rd trimester pregnancy loss. Lest we fall into the trap of believing that PTSD is only a problem after a traumatic labor and delivery experience, we must acknowledge that up to 16% of pregnant women may suffer from PTSD from other traumatic stressors and even may experience pretraumatic stress that is due to fear of their impending childbirth.

Effects

There is a paucity of research on the manner in which preexisting posttraumatic stress symptoms affect pregnancy, labor, delivery, and postpartum adjustment. However, some studies show that women who have experienced previous traumatic events are at increased risk of pregnancy and delivery complications (e.g., Chang, Chang, Lin, & Kuo, 2002; Glynn, Wadhwa, Dunkel-Schetter, Chicz-Demet, & Sandman, 2001). Pregnant women with preexisting PTSD are at risk of specific pregnancy complications, such as spontaneous abortion and preterm contractions (Seng et al., 2001). In addition, posttraumatic stress symptoms of intrusion and avoidance predict the likelihood of being classified as a high-risk pregnancy and the subjective amount of pain and distress experienced during delivery (Lev-Wiesel, Chen, Daphna-Tekoah, & Hod, 2009). Research has also shown that a history of abuse is associated with poor self-care during pregnancy, such as use of tobacco, alcohol, or illicit drugs and gaining too much weight (Morland et al., 2007; Seng et al., 2008).

The potential effects of an aversive childbirth experience are many. Women who experience a difficult childbirth are at an increased likelihood of experiencing symptoms of postpartum depression, state anxiety, and perceived stress and of engaging in binge drinking (Onoye et al., 2009). In addition, research has shown that women who report negative birth experiences are at more likely to describe their infants as ill-tempered, lack self-confidence, have difficulties coping with life problems, and endorse depressive symptoms (Quine, Rutter, & Gowen, 1993). Women who have posttraumatic stress symptoms following childbirth avoid reminders of childbirth, such as their own babies or other mothers (Ballard, Stanley, & Brockington, 1995; C. T. Beck, 2004). As a result, these women are at high risk of impairment in their relationships with their infants, which could in turn foster insecure attachment style in the baby (Bailham & Joseph, 2003; Ross & McLean, 2006). Many studies have shown than women with posttraumatic stress symptoms decide not to have any more children or do so only if they are guaranteed to have a cesarean section (Allen, 1998; Czarnocka & Slade, 2000; Ryding, Wijma, & Wijma, 1997; Ryding, Wijma, & Wijma, 1998b). Some women who have had traumatic childbirths go so far as to terminate unplanned pregnancies (Goldbeck-Wood, 1996) or undergo voluntary sterilization (Fones, 1996). In other instances, posttraumatic stress symptoms resurface during gynecological procedures and sexual intercourse (Fones, 1996; Goldbeck-Wood, 1996), consequences of which could be avoidance of regular gynecological care and sexual relations with one's partner. In severe cases, these symptoms and associated dysfunction can last for several years (Ballard et al., 1995). Other research has suggested that postpartum PTSD is associated with adverse interpersonal consequences, such as a lowered perception of social support (Ford et al., 2010; Söderquist, Wijma, & Wijma, 2006), which in turn exacerbates psychiatric symptoms.

It is difficult to extrapolate hypotheses about other areas of disability in postpartum women with PTSD, as much of the literature that examines disability associated with PTSD does so with distinct samples of trauma survivors, such as veterans, people who have experienced sexual assault, or people who have been in a motor vehicle accident. The degree to which research with these specific samples applies to women who develop PTSD associated with childbirth is unclear. Several areas of disability associated with PTSD have been documented in a large general population mental health survey (i.e., the Canadian Community Health Survey Cycle; $N = 36,984$), in which respondents indicated whether they had been diagnosed with PTSD by a health care professional (Sareen et al., 2007). This study is less rigorous than the studies examining consequences of anxiety disorders described in previous chapters because it relies on participants' self-reports of PTSD diagnoses; however, the advantage of applying results of this study to childbirth-related

PTSD is that respondents who were diagnosed with PTSD could have experienced any number of traumatic events. Thus, results from this analysis are relevant to people in general who are diagnosed with PTSD, rather than a specific subsample. The authors found that diagnoses of PTSD were associated with increased odds of many chronic physical health conditions; low psychological well-being; and impairment in activities at home, work, school, or leisure. These results raise the possibility that women with PTSD following childbirth will experience a range of negative effects in their lives that extend beyond the relationship with their infant and difficulty handling subsequent obstetric and gynecological procedures.

> Kellie has had a great deal of difficulty caring for her children and managing the household since she brought her baby home from the hospital. She is apathetic about caring for her baby boy and often asks her oldest child to soothe the baby when he screams. Whenever she can, she leaves her baby with her aunt or a neighbor, and she goes on long drives with the reasoning that she "just needs to get away." She lives in close proximity to her neighbors, and she can't stand it when she hears one of their young children screaming or crying. Because she feels detached from her other children as well, she is less diligent about her usual parenting activities, such as preparing meals and making sure that they are wearing clean clothes. Her older children are beginning to get in trouble at school and in the neighborhood because they are not supervised. Her extended family members have noticed this change in her behavior, but rather than providing help and support, they criticize her for having children with "the bum" in the first place. Kellie views herself as being all alone and struggles each day to provide minimum care for her children.

Comorbidity With Depression

Research has shown that there is significant comorbidity between posttraumatic stress symptoms and depression throughout the 1st year postpartum. White, Matthey, Boyd, and Barnett (2006) examined traumatic stress and depressive symptoms in a sample of 400 women who gave birth in a public hospital. Of the nine women who met criteria for PTSD or acute stress reaction at 6 weeks postpartum, six scored above the cutoff for major depression on a self-report inventory. Moreover, 42% of women with subsyndromal levels of traumatic stress symptoms scored above the cutoff on this inventory for minor depression. At 6 months postpartum, seven women met criteria for PTSD, six of whom scored above the cutoff for major depression, and the other of whom scored in the minor depressive range. Similarly, at 12 months postpartum, six women met criteria for PTSD, four of whom scored above the cutoff for major depression, and the remaining two scored in the range indicating minor depression. Zaers et al. (2008) obtained a lower but still elevated rate of depression in women with posttraumatic stress symptoms—12% of women with syndromal or subsyndromal posttraumatic stress symptoms reported at least subsyndromal depression 6 weeks following childbirth, and this rate of overlap increased to approximately 16% at 6 months postpartum. Using a different approach to analyses, Söderquist et al. (2006) found that 65% of their sample who reported clinically significant posttraumatic stress symptoms at some point within the first 11 months postpartum also reported clinically significant depressive symptoms at some point within the same time period.

This pattern of results is in line with findings from large epidemiological studies, which suggest that people with PTSD have elevated rates of depression. For example, Sareen et al. (2007) found that 37% of their sample of people who reported they had been diagnosed with PTSD indicated that they had been diagnosed with major depression during the previous year, which is more than a 10-fold increase over people who did not report that they had been diagnosed with PTSD. Even higher rates of comorbidity have been reported in samples of people who experienced a specific trauma, such as those who experienced a flood (53%; Green, Lindy, Grace, & Leonard, 1992) and those who survived a motor vehicle accident (45%; Shalev et al., 1998). Although diagnoses of PTSD and depression share three diagnostic criteria—sleep disturbance, anhedonia, and concentration difficulties—research has demon-strated that this overlap does not account for the high rate of comorbidity (Elhai, Grubaugh, Kashdan, & Frueh, 2008; Franklin & Zimmerman, 2001). Instead, depression can be regarded as a logical response to a trauma (Franklin & Zimmerman, 2001), given that trauma often is associated with a real, perceived, or threatened loss. Many women who experienced a traumatic childbirth have been threatened with the loss of their own lives and/or their babies' lives, and it is likely that in the aftermath they are coping with other perceived losses, such as the loss of the hope for a strong mother–infant bond. When clinicians identify women who present with comorbid posttraumatic stress and depressive symptoms, intervention should be especially aggressive, as comorbidity is associated with more impairment and greater distress (Blanchard, Buckley, Hickling, & Taylor, 1998).

> Kellie had experienced postpartum depression with her other two children, so she expected that she would experience some depressive symptoms with her newborn as well. Perhaps her most significant depressive symptom is fatigue—she has very little energy to take care of her household respon-sibilities and views herself as living her life as if she were in a fog. She has little appetite and usually only eats a few bites of whatever she fixes for the kids. Furthermore, she struggles with significant guilt over her difficulty bonding with her newborn. Kellie worries that her avoidance of her baby girl is going to set the stage for a troubled relationship in the future, and she wonders if she has already created irreversible damage. She admits

that she often thinks that her family would be better off without her, although she claims that she would never do anything to hurt herself because she hopes to protect her children from their abusive father.

Possible Etiology

The following sections describe correlates of childbirth-related PTSD that have the potential to explain its etiology, including sociodemographic factors (e.g., socioeconomic status), stressors (e.g., preterm labor), biological factors (e.g., changes in the hypothalamic–pituitary–adrenal [HPA] axis), and psychological factors (e.g., lack of coping resources).

Sociodemographic Factors

In my longitudinal study of postpartum anxiety disorders (Wenzel, Haugen, Jackson, et al., 2005), I examined the degree to which postpartum traumatic stress symptoms as measured by the Impact of Events Scale (IES; Horowitz, Wilner, & Alvarez, 1979) were associated with the sociodemographic variables discussed in the previous chapters on the other anxiety disorders. At 8 weeks postpartum, IES scores correlated negatively with the skill level of the mother's job and the level of education attained by the mother. Interestingly, IES scores were significantly associated with both the mother's and the baby's father's ethnicity, such that Hispanic women or women whose infants were fathered by Hispanic men scored highest on this measure. It is unclear why this pattern of results emerged, although Hispanic ethnicity has been associated with PTSD in other samples (Schnurr, Lunney, & Sengupta, 2004). In contrast, IES scores were not associated with parity, mother's or baby's father's age, the baby's father's skill level of his job or level of educational attainment, length of time the mother was in the relationship with the baby's father, whether the woman was married to the baby's father, socioeconomic status, or income level. Other researchers have replicated the lack of association between parity and posttraumatic stress symptoms (Creedy et al., 2000; Czarnocka & Slade, 2000; Söderquist et al., 2006; but see Wijma, Söderquist, & Wijma, 1997, for an exception), and one study (Czarnocka & Slade, 2000) identified unplanned pregnancy and a previous psychiatric history as additional variables associated with posttraumatic stress symptoms.

Although I did not find an association between posttraumatic stress symptoms and socioeconomic status, other research has found that lower socioeconomic status is indeed associated with more severe postpartum stress symptoms in the postpartum period (Lyons, 1998). As is discussed in the section on psychological factors associated with postpartum posttraumatic stress symptoms, a strong predictor of PTSD is a perception of incompetence or unhelpfulness of medical staff assigned to labor and delivery. It is possible that women of lower socioeconomic status receive care in lower quality settings, which could reinforce this perception and increase the likelihood of delivery complications. Moreover, women of higher socioeconomic background receive more support from their family and peers, feel better prepared for labor, and are more satisfied with the information that is provided to them during pregnancy (Quine et al., 1993); all of these variables could affect women's satisfaction with their birth experience.

Very little has been written about cultural variables and their relation to perinatal anxiety disorders. The one exception is in the literature on post-partum posttraumatic stress. Matthey, Silove, Barnett, Fitzgerald, and Mitchell (1999) examined traumatic stress symptoms following childbirth in a sample of 31 Cambodian refugees who had given birth in Australia. They found that a history of previous trauma was associated with higher levels of traumatic stress symptoms following childbirth, whereas having a difficult birth experience was less related to endorsement of these symptoms in this sample. There were some surprising instances in which expected variables were not associated with traumatic stress symptoms following childbirth, such as whether women had been in a refugee camp, the length of time they had been in Australia, and the extent of their social support network. Many refugees have gone through traumatic experiences in their homeland, a circumstance that, along with uncertain relocation experiences, disrupts their sense of controllability and predictability. It is sensible that women who have fled violence and persecution would be at particular risk of reporting high levels of traumatic stress symptoms during this time of great transition and uncertainty, a notion that will be important to test in a design that includes a matched sample of nonrefugee women.

Other research using nonrefugee samples has confirmed that a history of exposure to trauma, especially interpersonal violence, is associated with increased risk of traumatic stress symptoms during pregnancy (Harris-Britt, Martin, Li, Casanueva, & Kupper, 2004; Loveland Cook et al., 2004; Morland et al., 2007; Rodriguez et al., 2008) and the postpartum period (M. M. Cohen, Ansara, Shei, Stuckless, & Stewart, 2004; Onoye et al., 2009). In addition, research has shown that women who have a history of childhood sexual abuse may be at a particularly high risk of developing traumatic stress symptoms associated with childbirth (Lev-Wiesel, Daphna-Tekoah, & Hallak, 2009; Soet et al., 2003). According to Boyce and Condon (2000), many of these women reexperience the sexual trauma during childbirth, either because the pain reminds them of the pain that they experienced during the assault or because they perceive that they are tied down and unable to escape. Menage (1993) noted that many women feel powerless during obstetric and gynecological procedures, much like they felt during their sexual assault. In contrast, it has been suggested that women who suffer from PTSD as a result of other events, such as natural disasters, are less likely to experience traumatic stress symptoms in response to a stressful childbirth experience (Crompton, 1996a). Thus, clinicians should take care to assess for a history of exposure to traumatic events, as such a history could make women vulnerable to have a difficult childbirth and childbirth-related posttraumatic stress symptoms.

> Kellie fits the sociodemographic profile of a woman at risk of childbirth-related PTSD. She graduated from high school but sought no additional postsecondary education. She is not currently working and receives government assistance; thus, she is of very low socioeconomic status. Most important, she has a history of previous trauma, although her posttraumatic stress symptoms did not qualify for a diagnosis of PTSD until now. Specifically, her estranged husband beat her on many occasions when he was intoxicated, and on three occasions the beatings were severe enough that she needed medical attention. One beating took place when she was 4 months pregnant, and she was convinced that the baby would not make it. On another occasion, she blacked out after the beating, and when she came to she realized that her husband had left with her children. He did not bring the children home for 3 days, and during that time she was terrified that she would never see them again.

Additional Stressors

Unlike the other anxiety disorders covered in this volume, postpartum posttraumatic stress symptoms have been studied extensively in relation to stressful events that characterize labor and delivery experiences. For example, several studies have found an association between maternal and infant complications and later posttraumatic stress symptoms. Specifically, elevated rates of posttraumatic stress symptoms have been documented in mothers of premature infants (Holditch-Davis, Bartlett, Blickman, & Miles, 2003), women with preeclampsia (Engelhard et al., 2002; van Pampus, Wolf, Schultz, Weijmar, & Aarnoudse, 2004), women who underwent emergency cesarean section (Callahan & Hynan, 2002; Creedy et al., 2000; Ryding et al., 1998b), and women whose physicians used forceps during the delivery (Creedy et al., 2000). In addition, Czarnocka and Slade (2000) found that women whose partners were not present during delivery reported more severe posttraumatic stress symptoms than women whose partners were present. Collectively, these studies indicate that medical occurrences that threaten the life of the mother or baby, as well as the lack of a supportive other's presence, contribute to a negative birth experience that in turn puts postpartum women at risk of posttraumatic stress symptoms. Kellie indeed perceived that the baby was not going to live when the doctor exclaimed that he was not breathing and when the medical staff were too rushed to answer her questions. She also did not have a supportive person in the delivery room with her.

Biological Factors

No research has been conducted to identify biological factors that have the potential to increase postpartum women's risk of experiencing post-traumatic stress symptoms. However, research with people with PTSD who are not neither necessarily pregnant nor postpartum has suggested that changes in the HPA axis, particularly in levels of cortisol, might be associated with posttraumatic stress symptoms. Usually, increased stress is associated with an increase in cortisol levels, as the function of cortisol is to manage the body's defensive reaction when it becomes activated in the face of stress. Contrary to what might be expected, people with PTSD are characterized by low cortisol levels, which Yehuda (2001) suggested is indicative of a suppressed HPA axis caused by the adaptation to chronic stress. This neurobiological alteration occurs after the person has experienced a traumatic event, which makes it unlikely that it functions as an etiological factor for the development of PTSD. However, it is possible that altered HPA axis functioning in women who have already experienced trauma would increase the likelihood that they would develop PTSD following a difficult childbirth. Because pregnancy and childbirth are associated with significant changes in cortisol levels, it is important for future research to measure cortisol levels before childbirth and examine the degree to which they predict posttraumatic stress symptoms and comorbid psychiatric disturbance following childbirth.

Psychological Factors

Allen (1998) advanced a psychological theory of the development of traumatic stress symptoms following childbirth on the basis of a qualitative analysis of 20 women who had experienced a traumatic childbirth. She viewed the main precipitant of posttraumatic stress symptoms as a perception of being out of control, which is prompted by intense pain and the prediction that the baby will be harmed during labor in some way. Women often attempt to reduce perceived threat by seeking information and reassurance from medical staff and their partners. Unfortunately, in many instances they do not get the help and support that they need, which reinforces their sense of helplessness. Much research on this topic has verified aspects of this theory, including perceptions of being out of control (Ballard et al., 1995), expectations that the baby will be harmed (Ballard et al., 1995), and a lack of support provided by medical staff (Creedy et al., 2000; Wijma et al., 1997). One area in which women report especially high perceptions of being out of control is in the pain that they experience during labor (Ballard et al., 1995; Soet et al., 2003), and research has shown that control over analgesics correlates negatively with traumatic stress symptoms (Keogh, Ayers, & Francis, 2002). These findings raise the possibility that restoring a sense of control over one aspect of the delivery process protects women from developing posttraumatic stress symptoms in the postpartum period.

In addition to the psychological factors described in Allen's (1998) model, other research has suggested that the strength of a woman's coping resources is associated with the development of postpartum posttraumatic stress symptoms. For example, Czarnocka and Slade (2000) found that women who develop traumatic stress are less confident in their ability to cope with labor and delivery than women who do not develop traumatic stress symptoms. Lyons (1998) speculated that women who have a pattern of difficulty coping with adversity are more likely to associate negative emotions with their memories of childbirth, which would lead them to interpret their labor and delivery experience in a negative manner. This suggestion is provocative, as it indicates that the perception of the birth experience is more important than the actual events that take place during delivery (cf. Ford et al., 2010; Olde et al., 2006). A recent investigation testing a cognitive model of postpartum posttraumatic stress symptoms confirmed that posttraumatic cognitions of the birth experience, including negative appraisals of the self, negative appraisals of the world, and self-blame, explained the association between women's prior dysfunctional beliefs and coping skills and posttraumatic stress symptoms 3 weeks and 3 months following childbirth (Ford et al., 2010). It follows that cognitive behavioral therapy could be useful in helping women to acquire coping skills and strategies to view adversity with as much balance and accuracy as is possible. Moreover, Ford et al. (2010) found that social support predicted posttraumatic stress symptoms at 3 months postpartum, suggesting that an intervention for these symptoms as the postpartum period progresses should include the utilization of one's support network.

Results from two studies indicated that anxiety sensitivity predicts posttraumatic stress symptoms (Keogh et al., 2002; Fairbrother & Woody, 2007). *Anxiety sensitivity* is defined as the "tendency to respond fearfully to anxiety symptoms," which "is based on beliefs that these symptoms have undesirable consequences" (McNally, 1989, p. 193). Most women experience anxiety during labor and delivery, as well as many physical symptoms that could be interpreted as catastrophic. It is possible that women who are high in anxiety sensitivity react especially adversely during labor and delivery, which could contribute to a perception of a negative birth experience. In the larger literature, anxiety sensitivity has been linked most directly with panic disorder (Olatunji & Wolitzky-Taylor, 2009); thus, it will be important for future research to investigate the relevance of this construct in other perinatal anxiety disorders, particularly perinatal panic disorder.

Collectively, this research points to psychological factors that have the potential to predispose women to develop childbirth-related PTSD. Women who demonstrate a lack of coping resources to deal with stressful life problems may also have difficulty coping with the pain and uncertainty of labor. It is possible that these women are especially likely to develop a sense of uncontrollability and unpredictability during labor and delivery. In addition, women who are high in anxiety sensitivity may be particularly reactive to emotional and physical symptoms that they interpret as being dangerous. During the course of labor and delivery, they might react with especially great alarm if they indeed experience a delivery complication or if the medical staff who work with them are unresponsive or unsupportive. Negative appraisals about the labor and delivery experience facilitate the onset of posttraumatic stress symptoms.

> Kellie has a history of failing to cope effectively with life stressors. At times, she does not pay her bills when she is short on funds, allowing her utilities to be cut off. She becomes easily overwhelmed with parenting her two older children. Her neighbors stay up until late hours listening to loud music, but she does not say anything to them about it, claiming that she would just say something stupid. Thus, Kellie has little confidence in her own abilities and gives up rather than figuring out a solution to the problems that she is experiencing.

Practical Implications

Perceptions of inadequate medical care were reported in several studies examining childbirth-related PTSD. The key features that health care professionals should attend to in order to minimize the degree of traumatic stress associated with labor and delivery include (a) the woman's perception of control, (b) the attitude of the medical staff (e.g., caring, supportive, listening), and (c) the amount of information given during the birth experience (Menage, 1993). Unfortunately, in many instances, when women express their concerns about previous experiences with inadequate medical care, a rupture arises in the doctor–patient relationship, and these women are given psychiatric referrals without the medical staff truly understanding the basis of their claims (Beech & Robinson, 1985). Thus, it is important to listen carefully to women's concerns about the responsivity of medical staff during their labor and delivery experiences, provide validation and understanding, investigate any specific complaints, and identify medical staff behaviors that might be addressed to prevent future damage.

The literature on psychological factors associated with the development of childbirth-related PTSD is more developed than that of the other anxiety disorders considered in this volume other than obsessive–compulsive disorder. It clearly indicates that perceptions of uncontrollability and poor coping contribute significantly to the appraisal of the childbirth experience, and negative appraisals of the childbirth experience contribute significantly to the development of childbirth-related PTSD. Pregnant women, especially those with a history of trauma or current posttraumatic stress symptoms, would benefit from cognitive behavioral therapy so that they can develop strategies for constructing accurate and balanced appraisals and for tolerating the stress associated with childbirth. This approach to treatment also has the potential to be efficacious in postpartum women who have developed posttraumatic stress symptoms, as it would assist them in viewing the childbirth experience in perspective and developing strategies to manage symptoms such as the reexperiencing of the traumatic event. In addition, because research has shown that a strong social support network buffers people from the effects of trauma (e.g., Hyman, Gold, & Cott, 2003) and that women with childbirth-related posttraumatic stress symptoms view their support networks in a negative light, it is important to target the utilization of one's support network in treatment.

> Kellie did not attend any follow-up appointments after she gave birth, claiming that the hospital was too far away and she could not find transportation to get there. However, she had a case manager who visited the home every 2 weeks. This case worker noticed many of Kellie's symptoms, and she referred her to a clinical social worker. Although this social worker was not trained to conduct evidence-based treatment for PTSD, she worked with Kellie to develop concrete mood management and problem-solving strategies. Kellie continues to struggle with intrusive memories of her childbirth experience, but she has become more proactive in taking care of her household responsibilities and in asking people to help her take care of her newborn when she is overwhelmed.

7

A BIOPSYCHOSOCIAL MODEL
OF PERINATAL ANXIETY

As research on perinatal anxiety accumulates, it is important to integrate and evaluate it in light of a coherent conceptualization of anxiety that occurs during the transition to parenthood. Having such a model will allow clinicians to explain perinatal anxiety to their patients and identify women who are vulnerable to its development. It will also allow scholars to generate targeted hypotheses and carry out subsequent research to uncover specific mechanisms at work in the etiology of perinatal anxiety. Chapters 2 through 6 highlighted three main sources of variables that could account for the onset and exacerbation of anxiety during pregnancy and the postpartum period: (a) sociodemographic factors, (b) biological factors, and (c) psychological factors. In this chapter, I incorporate these into the beginnings of a biopsychosocial model of perinatal anxiety.

This is not the first time that a biopsychosocial model involving perinatal anxiety has been developed. Ross, Sellers, Gilbert Evans, and Romach (2004) theorized that biological risk factors (i.e., personal and family psychiatric history, history of premenstrual mood symptoms, high plasma cortisol, and high plasma progesterone) would have a direct effect on the expression of perinatal anxiety and depression as well as an indirect effect on these emotional disturbances by exacerbating reactivity to life stress. They conceptualized life stress in much the same way as I have throughout this volume, including socio-demographic variables such as low household income and a lack of social support. Using structural equation modeling, they determined that a personal and family psychiatric history and high plasma progesterone levels influenced anxiety and life stress. The relation between these biological variables and depression was mediated by anxiety and life stress, which suggests that anxiety had a closer relation with these variables than did depression in their study. Thus, their model implicates anxiety as a key construct in understanding mood associated with the transition to parenthood.

It is interesting that their model fit well for data collected during the 3rd trimester of pregnancy, but it did not fit well for data collected at the 6th week postpartum. To explain this unexpected finding, Ross et al. (2004) speculated that different types of life stress that were not measured in their study might be operative in the postpartum period, such as the aftermath of obstetric complications, child care stress, and infant temperament. An important conclusion from their study is that different etiological factors may be at work in prenatal emotional disturbance and in postpartum emotional disturbance.

The theoretical model I present in this chapter expands on that described by Ross et al. (2004). As in Ross et al., biological factors and life stress are cornerstones of the model. However, I divide biological factors into two separate categories: those that pertain to genetic vulnerability for perinatal anxiety disorders and those that pertain to the neurochemical variability that is endured during pregnancy and in the postpartum period. In addition, I include a third domain of factors that make women vulnerable to the development of perinatal anxiety disorders: those that are psychological in nature, such as cognitive styles that can predispose some women to respond to stress and transition with anxiety. I have not collected data in support of this model, so I will not speculate about the magnitude of relations among the variables. Nevertheless, this model should provide a useful starting point for conceptualizing the onset and exacerbation of perinatal anxiety, which can serve as a basis for future researchers to generate specific hypotheses for empirical research that will contribute to the refinement of our understanding of this emotional disturbance.

THE GENERAL BIOPSYCHOSOCIAL MODEL

Figure 7.1 displays the general biopsychosocial model of perinatal anxiety, which is based in a diathesis-stress framework. The circles on the left side of the figure represent three domains of vulnerability: (a) genetic vulnerability, (b) neurochemical variability, and (c) psychological vulnerability.

Genetic vulnerability is determined by a personal or family history of anxiety and/or depression. A woman who has had chronic difficulties with

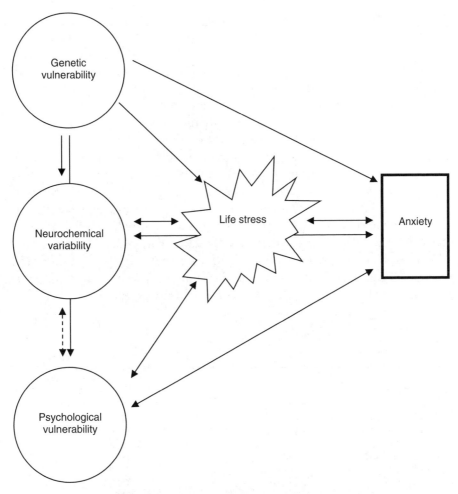

Figure 7.1. Biopsychosocial model of anxiety in childbearing women. Solid lines represent associations that have been demonstrated with empirical data in either childbearing or nonchildbearing samples. The dotted line represents a proposed association that has not yet been subject to empirical scrutiny.

anxiety or depression or who has many family members who have been diagnosed with anxiety disorders or depression would be characterized by a high level of genetic vulnerability; conversely, a woman who does not have a personal or family history of anxiety or depression would be characterized by a low level of genetic vulnerability.

Neurochemical variability reflects the dramatic changes in hormone levels associated with pregnancy, labor and delivery, and lactation and their influence on neurotransmitters associated with mood (e.g., catecholamines, serotonin). It is likely that no increase or decrease in any one hormone is related to the expression of perinatal anxiety disorders, but rather that some women are particularly sensitive to the rapid changes in hormone levels (Altemus, 2001; Glover & Kammerer, 2004; Nonacs, 2005), which could in turn affect neurotransmission that plays a role in the regulation of mood. However, it is likely that changes in levels of some hormones are particularly important at certain points during pregnancy and the postpartum period. For example, oxytocin levels rise substantially right before delivery and remain elevated during lactation. Changes in levels of oxytocin, then, might be more important to explain an increase in anxiety observed around the time of delivery or in the postpartum period than earlier in pregnancy.

Psychological vulnerability includes the cognitive styles that characterize people with various anxiety disorders as well as the ability to implement effective coping in times of stress. Psychological vulnerability has the potential to have the most specificity with regard to the particular type of anxiety disorder that is expressed in pregnant and postpartum women. Table 7.1 displays the psychological vulnerabilities described in Chapters 2 through 6 and their association with specific anxiety disorders. With the exception of the psycho-

TABLE 7.1
Psychological Vulnerability Factors for Perinatal Anxiety Disorders

Psychological variable	Associated anxiety disorder
Intolerance of uncertainty	GAD, OCD
Inaccurate beliefs about worry	GAD
Poor problem orientation	GAD
Cognitive avoidance	GAD
Probability bias	OCD
Morality bias	OCD
Overestimation of responsibility	OCD
Inaccurate beliefs about the need to control intrusive thoughts	OCD
Catastrophic misinterpretations of bodily symptoms	Panic disorder
Hyperventilation as learned behavior	Panic disorder
Negative self-talk about one's social skills	Social anxiety disorder
Self-focused attention	Social anxiety disorder
Tendency to scan environment for indications of rejection	Social anxiety disorder
Post-event processing	Social anxiety disorder
Classical conditioning of childbirth fear	Specific phobia
Vicarious learning of childbirth fear	Specific phobia
Instruction of childbirth fear	Specific phobia
Perceptions of being out of control during labor and delivery	PTSD
Inadequate coping resources	PTSD
Negative appraisals of the self or world	PTSD
Anxiety sensitivity	PTSD

Note. GAD = generalized anxiety disorder; OCD = obsessive–compulsive disorder; PTSD = posttraumatic stress disorder.

logical variables associated with perinatal obsessive–compulsive disorder (OCD) and three of the variables associated with posttraumatic stress disorder (i.e., perception of being out of control, negative appraisals, and anxiety sensitivity), empirical research has yet to be conducted that demonstrates that these factors indeed characterize pregnant and postpartum women with these anxiety disorders. It is possible that empirical research will show that some of these variables, such as poor problem orientation, cognitive avoidance, and inadequate coping resources, are nonspecific and characteristic of several types of perinatal anxiety disorders. Nevertheless, this list is grounded in the state of the literature at the time this volume was written, and it provides a starting point for understanding the psychological mechanisms by which each perinatal anxiety might be expressed.

These three domains of vulnerability are interrelated, as can be seen from the arrows that connect them in Figure 7.1. Genetic vulnerability for anxiety and depression influences the neurochemical variability experienced during pregnancy and the postpartum period as well as the psychological vulnerabilities associated with various anxiety disorders. This pathway supports the contention I proposed earlier in the book, in that genetic vulnerability has the potential to prompt perinatal anxiety disorders through both biological and psychological mechanisms. I also include a bidirectional arrow between neurochemical variability and psychological vulnerability. I speculate that hormonal changes associated with childbirth and their effects on neurotransmission would affect the manner in which psychological vulnerability is expressed, and conversely, I speculate that maladaptive psychological tendencies influence the neurochemistry associated with mood, with which hormones associated with childbirth are closely involved. However, research has not been designed to investigate this possibility; thus, the arrow is represented by a dotted line.

In Ross et al.'s (2004) model, biological vulnerability was directly related to life stress as well as anxiety, and life stress also mediated the relation between biological vulnerability and anxiety. I adopt a similar approach in the biopsychosocial model presented in this chapter. In this model, each of the three domains of vulnerability is directly associated with life stress and directly associated with anxiety. However, they are also indirectly associated with anxiety through reactivity to life stress. Women who are characterized by few vulnerability factors will likely experience perinatal anxiety only in the context of significant life stress above and beyond the demands of pregnancy and childbirth, whereas women who are characterized by many vulnerability factors will likely experience perinatal anxiety even when there is very little life stress above and beyond the demands of pregnancy and childbirth.

This general biopsychosocial model can be applied to both prenatal and postpartum anxiety, as it indicates broad domains of vulnerability and does not define specific types of life stress that are most likely to exacerbate anxiety during the transition to parenthood. However, Ross et al.'s (2004) data raise the possibility that different variables are at work in prenatal versus postpartum mood disturbance. In the next section, I propose some specific variables that have the potential to be more relevant to one time period or the other.

SPECIFIC BIOPSYCHOSOCIAL MODELS

Regardless of whether a woman develops anxiety during pregnancy or in the postpartum period, I believe that biological vulnerabilities, psychological vulnerabilities, and life stress can account for its etiology. Some factors are likely to be equally relevant to both pregnancy and the postpartum period, such as a woman's genetic vulnerability. However, in this section, I identify specific variables that have the potential to put women at particularly high risk of anxiety disorders during pregnancy and during the postpartum period. Each of the specific variables described in these sections can be inserted into the general categories of vulnerability illustrated in Figure 7.1.

A Biopsychosocial Model of Prenatal Anxiety

Although there are many avenues by which the elevated level of progesterone during pregnancy might reduce anxiety, Cowley and Roy-Byrne (1989) raised the possibility that progesterone is associated with increases in aspects of respiratory functioning associated with hyperventilation, which is a common physical symptom in panic disorder. Some women whose respiratory systems are reactive to such changes could be at risk of developing panic disorder during pregnancy. In addition, cortisol levels rise steadily throughout pregnancy until they are 3 times higher than normal in the 3rd trimester (Sichel & Driscoll, 1999). As has been mentioned previously in this volume, cortisol is the stress hormone that is secreted in situations in which a person is faced with threat or danger. However, in most circumstances cortisol decreases when the threat has passed. A chronically high level of cortisol during pregnancy could create a neurochemical context for overarousal, which could exacerbate symptoms associated with any one of the anxiety disorders discussed in this book. Moreover, prolactin also increases steadily during pregnancy. Although an elevated level of prolactin has been associated with anger and irritability in women (Sichel & Driscoll, 1999), it also decreases the responsivity of the hypothalamic–pituitary–adrenal (HPA) axis, which could alter neurotransmission associated with many expressions of anxiety. Thus, it is possible that progesterone, cortisol, and prolactin are three neurochemical variables that are especially relevant in understanding prenatal anxiety.

In addition, it is possible that certain psychological vulnerabilities are more likely to trigger anxiety during pregnancy than in the postpartum period.

As was stated in the Introduction to this volume, pregnancy is a time of great uncertainty, and most women worry about issues such as their baby's health and their own health. Women who have difficulty tolerating uncertainty might be particularly vulnerable to the development of generalized anxiety disorder during pregnancy. In addition, pregnancy is a time in which women go through tremendous physical changes, and they experience many odd physical sensations that they do not typically notice when they are not pregnant. Women who have the tendency to catastrophize about the implications of these symptoms might be particularly vulnerable to panic disorder during pregnancy. Finally, I reference the same life stress variables that Ross et al. (2004) found to be associated with anxiety and depression in their biopsychosocial model of prenatal mood disturbance: sociodemographic variables such as low income and low socioeconomic status, as well as an inadequate social support network.

A Biopsychosocial Model of Postpartum Anxiety

It is possible that the postpartum period is a time of increased risk of anxiety disorders because of the dramatic drop in estrogen and progesterone, both of which could have exerted protective effects during pregnancy (Sichel & Driscoll, 1999). Specifically, estrogen stimulates neurotransmission in the HPA axis (Halbreich, 1997), which could improve mood and decrease many expressions of anxiety, whereas progesterone stimulates gamma-aminobutyric acid receptors and lowers plasma CO_2 levels (Klein, Skrobala, & Garfinkel, 1995), which could decrease the chance that a woman experiences panic-like anxiety. If elevations in the level of these hormones are indeed protective factors that buffer women from experiencing an increase in anxiety during pregnancy, then the loss of these factors during a time that requires tremendous adjustment could be particularly devastating. In addition, the inflammatory response system is activated in late pregnancy and the early postpartum period, which disrupts HPA axis functioning and increases cortisol (Kendall-Tackett, 2008; Maes et al., 2000), thereby altering neurochemicals that are important for mood regulation. Moreover, oxytocin levels increase around the time of delivery and remain elevated as women breastfeed. Oxytocin promotes maternal bonding, so it is possible that women with some of the psychological vulnerability factors would be especially sensitive to an elevated level of this hormone and would attach great meaning to thoughts of harm coming to their babies, with whom they are intimately bonded. As a result, it is possible that they would develop obsessive–compulsive symptoms at this time, rather than at other times, in their lives (C. T. Beck & Driscoll, 2006).

The postpartum period provides a context that is especially likely for some of the psychological vulnerabilities to become activated. For example, many of the cognitive biases described by Abramowitz and his colleagues would be particularly salient in the postpartum period, when new mothers come face to face with the reality of new parenthood (Abramowitz, Schwartz, Moore, & Luenzmann, 2003). As was stated in Chapter 3 on OCD, most new mothers experience bizarre, intrusive thoughts of harming their children after they have given birth. However, it is only those people who have the tendency to believe that having those thoughts increases the likelihood that they will act on them (i.e., probability bias) or that having those thoughts is equivalent to actually engaging in the behavior (i.e., morality bias) who are vulnerable to the development of postpartum OCD. In addition, Bybee's (1989) theory that hyperventilation is a learned behavior that generalizes from its use as a way to manage pain during labor, by definition, can only operate during the postpartum period, rather than in pregnancy. Moreover, I propose that the cognitive biases and styles associated with social anxiety disorder (i.e., negative self-talk about one's social skills, self-focused attention, scanning the environment for signs of rejection, and post-event processing) would be heightened in the postpartum period as women's life circumstances have changed dramatically—they are consumed with caring for their newborn and likely not as actively engaged in other areas of their life (e.g., socializing regularly with friends), and they are no longer pregnant but still carrying baby weight.

Ross et al.'s (2004) analyses raised the possibility that sociodemographic variables like low socioeconomic status and low social support are more relevant to understanding the etiology of prenatal anxiety than postpartum anxiety. This conclusion is at odds with my research suggesting that at 8 weeks postpartum several domains of anxiety (e.g., physical symptoms as measured by the Beck Anxiety Inventory [A. T. Beck & Steer, 1990], social anxiety as measured by the Social Interaction Anxiety Scale [Mattick & Clarke, 1998], and traumatic stress symptoms as measured by the Impact of Events Scale [Horowitz, Wilner, & Alvarez, 1979]) correlate with sociodemographic variables that have the potential to be stressful. I continue to theorize that these variables contribute to life stress and the etiology of postpartum anxiety, but it will be important for future research to replicate these findings. In addition, my former student's work suggests that it is not the size of or satisfaction with one's social support network that accounts for anxiety at 8 weeks postpartum, but rather the frequency of negative social support, which is defined as unhelpful interactions with others (Haugen, 2003). It is possible that this very specific aspect of social support is most relevant to the life stress that makes women vulnerable to develop postpartum anxiety disorders, rather than prenatal anxiety disorders. Finally, the alternative possibilities identified by Ross et al., including the aftermath of obstetric complications, child care stress, and infant temperament, would be reasonable candidates for life stress that make women vulnerable to develop anxiety disorders particularly in the postpartum period.

PRACTICAL IMPLICATIONS

The key point from this chapter is that genetic vulnerability, neuro-chemical variability, psychological vulnerability, and life stress interact to prompt the onset or exacerbation of anxiety during pregnancy and/or the postpartum period. Although I speculated about the degree to which some of the neurochemical variables, psychological vulnerabilities, and life stressors might be differentially associated with the expression and anxiety during pregnancy versus the postpartum period, it is likely that most of these variables interact with one another in a unique and complex way that is not fully understood and have some relevance to the expression of anxiety in both time periods. This model was developed on the basis of the current state of the literature with pregnant and postpartum women as well as the literature on anxiety disorders in people in general who are not necessarily pregnant and postpartum. Not only must the domains in this model be tested in empirical research, but the specific components of each domain must be identified. The identification of tangible biological, psychological, and life stress variables that increase a woman's vulnerability to a perinatal anxiety disorder can then lead to more targeted interventions.

Women cannot change their personal and family psychiatric histories or the fact that their bodies undergo tremendous physical changes associated with childbirth. However, they can be cognizant of these vulnerabilities and prepare themselves for the stress that occurs during the transition to parenthood. Pregnant women who know they are vulnerable to anxiety and depression during times of change can ensure that other areas of their lives are in order, that their social support network is intact, and that they have clear and accurate expectations for the upcoming change in their lives. Moreover, there is evidence that omega-3 fatty acids, exercise, and St. John's wort can reduce the inflammatory response system, which could in turn regulate HPA axis functioning (Kendall-Tackett, 2008). In other words, these interventions can modify the intensity of the body's reaction to biological changes associated with childbirth.

The psychological vulnerabilities that predispose women to have difficulty with the transition to parenthood can also be modified. Clinicians who are aware of the manner in which these vulnerabilities contribute to perinatal anxiety disorders can be alert for them as they work with child-bearing women and refer them for treatment that will address them. Although psychotropic medications are efficacious in reducing symptoms of anxiety disorders, they do not directly provide women with strategies for recognizing when they are engaging in an unhelpful cognitive style and modifying it. Chapter 10 describes some psychotherapeutic approaches that can achieve this goal.

II

CLINICAL MANAGEMENT OF ANXIETY IN CHILDBEARING WOMEN

8

ASSESSMENT OF PERINATAL ANXIETY

At present, only 20% of obstetricians and gynecologists routinely screen for anxiety disorders in their practice (Coleman, Carter, Morgan, & Schulkin, 2008). Because perinatal anxiety disorders are clearly associated with life interference, risk of adverse effects to the fetus or infant, and substantial distress, it is crucial that clinicians be aware of signs that a child-bearing woman might be experiencing clinically significant difficulties with anxiety and conduct a systematic assessment. The course of perinatal anxiety can fluctuate, so it is important to screen for anxiety symptoms at repeated assessments throughout pregnancy and the 1st year postpartum (C. T. Beck & Driscoll, 2006). This chapter describes warning signs that indicate that clinicians should conduct a more thorough assessment for perinatal anxiety disorders, measures designed specifically to detect anxiety symptoms in pregnant and postpartum women, measures that assess anxiety disorders that were not developed specifically with samples of pregnant and postpartum women but that might have relevance to this population, and guidelines for arriving at a diagnosis.

WARNING SIGNS

Most childbearing women will not overtly verbalize that they are struggling with anxiety; in fact, many women know that something does not seem right but are unable to put a name to their emotional experiences. There are several warning signs that signal the need to conduct a more systematic assessment for perinatal anxiety disorders. For example, agitation or restlessness (e.g., hand wringing, leg tapping, pacing) is indicative of a high level of arousal, which could underlie any one of the anxiety disorders discussed in this volume. When clinicians notice indicators of agitation, they might ask their patient if she is especially nervous or anxious about any aspect of pregnancy or childbirth. Although tearfulness is also an indicator of depression, it may serve as a marker for perinatal anxiety, as worries about their own or their baby's health are frightening and hold great meaning for women. Frequent "what if" questions about the possibility of catastrophes, an excessive number of calls in between sessions, and excessive reassurance seeking are verbal indicators that a childbearing woman is struggling with symptoms of generalized anxiety disorder (GAD).

Clinicians should also be alert for indicators of avoidance, such as missed appointments, lack of eye contact, and submissive posture, as these nonverbal behaviors may also point to an underlying problem with anxiety. Women with significant fears of childbirth might miss appointments so that they can avoid reminders of the pregnancy; socially anxious women might miss appointments because they are nervous about interacting with health care providers, whom they view as authorities, or fear that they will be judged negatively; women with panic disorder might miss appointments because they are too fearful to leave their home; and women with intrusive thoughts of harming their infant might miss appointments because they fear that their child will be taken away from them if they disclose these thoughts to a health care provider. Lack of eye contact and submissive posture could also signify social anxiety or shame about the contents of intrusive thoughts.

On the basis of her clinical observation, Crompton (1996b) identified several warning signs for women who may be at risk of having traumatic childbirth experiences. These signs include obvious indicators of injury; a need for control, a detailed birth plan, and/or insistence on home birth; failure to keep antenatal appointments; extreme fear of needles; and severe agitation. Signs that a woman is actively experiencing a traumatic labor and delivery include lack of trust; an indication that she perceives that she cannot escape; signals of reexperiencing, such as flashbacks; and extreme agitation, screaming, and/or crying. However, Crompton noted that other women experiencing traumatic childbirth present very differently—rather than displaying externalizing behavior, they exhibit signs that suggest that they are internalizing the trauma (e.g., silence, submissiveness, extreme modesty). The most important point is that clinicians involved in labor and delivery must recognize that many women experience childbirth as traumatic and that they can alleviate the psychiatric sequelae by proceeding with sensitivity and competence.

MEASURES SPECIFIC TO PERINATAL ANXIETY

Edinburgh Postnatal Depression Scale

Perhaps the most frequently used inventory to assess postpartum psychiatric symptoms is the Edinburgh Postnatal Depression Scale (EPDS; Cox, Holden, & Sagovksy, 1987). The EPDS is a 10-item self-report inventory that was originally designed to assess symptoms of depression following childbirth. For each item, women are asked to select one of four choices that best represents the severity of the symptom in question. Items are scored on a scale of 0 to 3, and responses to each item are summed to obtain a total score. A score of 12 on this inventory or a nonzero response to the item assessing suicidal thoughts indicates that a more thorough evaluation for perinatal depression is warranted (Nonacs, 2005). This scale is widely available in its entirety on multiple Internet sites.

During the past decade, it has been recognized that the EPDS is also a useful screening tool for anxiety. Several groups of researchers have identified an anxiety subscale of the EPDS that consists of three items: one that pertains to unnecessary self-blame, one that pertains to anxiety or worry for no good reason, and one that pertains to feeling scared or panicky for no good reason (Brouwers, van Baar, & Pop, 2001a; Kabir, Sheeder, & Kelly, 2008; Ross, Gilbert Evans, Sellers, & Romach, 2003; Rowe, Fisher, & Loh, 2008; Tuohy & McVey, 2008). This subscale can be used to measure anxiety during pregnancy (Brouwers et al., 2001a) as well as in the postpartum period (Ross et al., 2003; Tuohy & McVey, 2008). The scale ranges from 0 to 9, and the cutoff score that indicates a probable anxiety disorder is 6 (Matthey, 2008). The internal consistency of this scale ranges from .60 (Brouwers et al., 2001a) to .80 (Tuohy & McVey, 2008).

Although the three-item anxiety scale is effective in identifying women with postpartum depression (Kabir et al., 2008), more research needs to be done to determine whether scoring at or above the cutoff on this scale predicts a *Diagnostic and Statistical Manual of Mental Disorders* (4th ed., text revision [*DSM–IV–TR*]; American Psychiatric Association, 2000) diagnosis of one or more of the anxiety disorders. In fact, results from one study (Rowe et al. 2008) indicated that neither the EPDS total score nor the score on the three-item anxiety scale distinguish postpartum women with an anxiety disorder from those with depression. Nevertheless, clinicians who use the EPDS in their practice can use responses to Items 3, 4, and 5 as a first step in screening for perinatal anxiety. However, they should also be aware that these items do not cover the full range of anxiety disorders covered in this volume. The item on self-blame is nonspecific and does not readily correspond to one particular anxiety disorder, the item on worry and anxiousness roughly corresponds to generally anxious symptoms, and the item on feeling scared and panicky roughly corresponds to panic symptoms. Clinicians should recognize that women who score below the cutoff on this subscale may still be struggling with clinically significant symptoms of anxiety, particularly in the realms of obsessive–compulsive disorder (OCD), social anxiety disorder, specific phobia, and posttraumatic stress disorder (PTSD).

Cambridge Worry Scale

The Cambridge Worry Scale (CWS; Green, Kafetsios, Statham, & Snowdon, 2003) is a 16-item self-report measure that assesses various domains of women's worries (e.g., something being wrong with the baby, giving birth, unemployment) during pregnancy. Items are rated on a 6-point Likert-type scale (0 = *not a worry*; 5 = *extremely worried*). Coefficient alphas range from .76 (Green et al., 2003) to .81 (Öhman, Grunewald, & Waldenström, 2003), and test–retest correlations between various administrations of the measure throughout the course of pregnancy range from .69 to .72 (Green et al., 2003). The scale can be divided into four factors: (a) sociomedical (e.g., worry about going to the hospital and having examinations), (b) socioeconomic (e.g., worry about money and employment), (c) health (e.g., worry about miscarriage, something being wrong with the baby, one's own health), and (d) relationships (e.g., worry about the partner, family, and friends; cf. Jomeen & Martin, 2005). Each of these factors correlates with scores on the State–Trait Anxiety Inventory (STAI), and the total score on this measure predicts scores on the EPDS above and beyond scores on the STAI. This scale in its entirety can be found in Green et al.'s (2003) Figure 1.

The CWS appears to be a sound measure of worry during pregnancy and captures some unique variance of the anxiety experience of pregnant women beyond what is accounted for by standard measures of anxiety. However, there are no data that speak to the clinical utility of this measure in identifying women who are at risk of GAD. In fact, the developers of this measure clearly stated that they constructed the measure to capture the range of normal worry during pregnancy, rather than pathology. Thus, this measure has the potential to be a useful tool for scholars who wish to conduct research on worry across the course of pregnancy, but at present there is no justification for its use in clinical settings.

Pregnancy Anxiety Scale

The Pregnancy Anxiety Scale (Levin, 1991) is a 10-item self-report measure that assesses three dimensions of pregnancy-specific anxiety: (a) anxiety about being pregnant, (b) anxiety about childbirth, and (c) anxiety about hospitalization. Scores on each of these dimensions add up to an overall score of pregnancy anxiety. Levin constructed this measure by selecting items from a larger 53-item inventory of the same name designed by Pleshette, Asch, and Chase (1956), with the intention of establishing adequate psychometric properties on an existing measure that had already been used in the literature. Items that were judged as having adequate face validity and yielded a relatively normal distribution of responses were chosen for the current version. Examples of items include "Did you read anything that frightened you about having a baby?"; "Were you afraid the pain of childbirth would be bad?"; and "Were you afraid you would be alone in the hospital?" Respondents indicate whether each item is true or false. Items are worded in a manner that measures the retrospective assessment of anxiety during pregnancy by postpartum women, although Levin emphasized that they could easily be reworded so that they were relevant to pregnant women who have not yet given birth. This scale can be found in its entirety in Levin's (1991) Table 1.

Levin (1991) reported an internal consistency of .63 (Kuder-Richardson formula) for this scale, which is a value that is somewhat low but minimally acceptable. Although this measure is valuable because it is specific to anxiety experienced during pregnancy, its limitations include a lack of clinical cutpoints and a lack of correspondence with a diagnosable anxiety disorder. Moreover, it does not appear to have been used in any scholarly investigation since its publication. In fact, another researcher developed her own measure, titled the Pregnancy Anxiety Scale (Côté-Arsenault, 2003), but it is entirely different from the one Levin (1991) described. Although Levin is to be applauded for conducting careful research to validate an existing instrument on anxiety experienced during pregnancy, it seems that this measure would be useful only in circumstances in which a researcher aims to measure anxiety during pregnancy retrospectively in samples of postpartum women.

Delivery Fear Scale

The Delivery Fear Scale (Alehagen, Wijma, & Wijma, 2001; Wijma, Alehagen, & Wijma, 2002) is a 10-item self-report inventory in which women rate items pertaining to fears of delivery on a 10-point Likert-type scale when they are in labor (1 = do not agree at all; 10 = agree totally). Items are read orally by another person and consist of statements such as "I can stand the pain" and

"I don't want to go on anymore." Items are summed to obtain a total score, with higher scores being indicative of a greater fear of labor. The internal consistency of this scale (coefficient alpha) is .87 (Alehagen et al., 2001) to .88 (Wijma et al., 2002), and scores on this measure correlate positively with the STAI and other measures of childbirth-related fears. This scale in its entirety can be found in Alehagan et al.'s (2001) Table 2.

This measure would be useful for researchers who wish to investigate the manner in which fear experienced during labor is associated with the course of labor and delivery. However, it is unlikely that this measure would have clinical utility in diagnosing perinatal anxiety disorders, as most childbearing women are fearful during labor. It would be more clinically useful to diagnose women with a specific phobia of childbirth well before they are in labor. If the measure were to be administered earlier in pregnancy, items would need to be reworded, which would necessitate that researchers reestablish adequate psychometric properties.

Perinatal Posttraumatic Stress Disorder Questionnaire

The Perinatal Posttraumatic Stress Disorder Questionnaire (DeMier, Hynan, Harris, & Manniello, 1996) is a 14-item self-report inventory that assesses symptoms in the three symptom clusters associated with PTSD: reexperiencing, avoidance and numbing, and increased arousal. Although this scale had sound psychometric properties (Callahan & Hynan, 2002; DeMier et al.,1996; Quinnell & Hynan, 1999), it was recently modified so that items are now rated on a 0 (*not at all*) to 4 (*often, for more than a month*) Likert-type scale (Callahan, Borja, & Hynan, 2006). The coefficient alpha of this modified scale is .90, and it has good convergent validity with a standard measure of posttraumatic distress and correlates less strongly or not at all with divergent measures. A principal components analysis confirmed that the modified scale yielded three factors corresponding to the *DSM–IV–TR* symptom clusters. Moreover, a clinical cutpoint of 19 identifies women who would be appropriate for referrals for mental health services.

This scale can be found in its entirety in Callahan et al.'s (2006) Appendix A. Empirical data have suggested that it reliably identifies women who are experiencing distress and would benefit from mental health services. In addition, it could serve as a screening instrument for PTSD associated with childbirth, as clinicians could quickly assess whether women endorse enough symptoms associated with each symptom cluster to warrant a diagnosis of PTSD. Women who endorse one reexperiencing symptom, three avoidance or numbing symptoms, and two symptoms of arousal or increased startle should be assessed more thoroughly for PTSD.

Wijma Delivery Experiences Questionnaire

The Wijma Delivery Expectancies Questionnaire (W-DEQ; Wijma, Wijma, & Zar, 1998) is a 33-item self-report inventory that assesses the cognitive and emotional aspects of fear of childbirth. It includes items such as "fantastic" and "frightful," which women rate on a 7-point Likert-type scale (0 = *not at all;* 6 = *extremely*). Version A assesses women's expectancies before delivery, and Version B assesses their perception of their delivery following childbirth. Wijma et al. (1998) reported that both versions have good internal consistency (coefficient α = .93 for Version A and .94 for Version B). The overlap between the W-DEQ and the STAI is approximately 30%, suggesting that there is a substantial amount of variance in fear of childbirth that cannot be accounted for by general anxiety. The scale in its entirety can be found in Wijma et al.'s Table 1.

The W-DEQ is the most widely studied measured of anxiety associated with childbirth, so researchers who wish to compare their results with others in the literature should consider administering this inventory to their samples of pregnant and postpartum women. On the other hand, many of the items pertain more to general distress (e.g., "lonely") than specifically to fear of childbirth. Moreover, the degree to which high scores on the W-DEQ identify women who meet diagnostic criteria for a specific phobia is unclear.

Comment

It is a true testament to the degree to which the study of perinatal anxiety is growing that so many measures specific to anxiety associated with childbirth have been developed. The researchers who created them have taken care to ensure that these measures have strong psychometric properties and have specific relevance to the experience of childbirth. However, the limitation of these instruments is that they are used primarily in research settings and will likely not be a part of a standard assessment battery that is administered in clinical settings. At this point, we have only one instrument that yields a clinical cutpoint to identify distressed women in need of mental health services (i.e., the Perinatal Posttraumatic Stress Disorder Questionnaire) and no instruments that yield clinical cutpoints that designate women who are likely to meet diagnostic criteria for a perinatal anxiety disorder. Although such a cutpoint exists for the EPDS, it is questionable whether it will identify women who meet criteria for anxiety disorders in domains that are not assessed on that measure, such as social anxiety disorder or PTSD. Clearly, the next step in advancing a system for identifying perinatal anxiety disorder is to develop a new inventory or adapt an existing inventory that covers the full spectrum of perinatal anxiety disorders and that determines cutpoints that predict specific anxiety disorder diagnoses.

ADAPTATION OF EXISTING INSTRUMENTS

On the one hand, it can be argued that it is preferable to assess perinatal anxiety with measures specifically designed for that purpose because they were validated on samples of women who were pregnant or had recently given birth. On the other hand, as was stated previously, the manner in which scores on these inventories relate to *DSM–IV–TR* diagnoses of anxiety disorders is unclear. This section describes several measures that are used to assess symptoms of anxiety disorders in the general population and that clinicians could use to aid in the diagnoses of anxiety disorders in pregnant and postpartum women. Nearly all of these measures are reproduced in Antony, Orsillo, and Roemer's (2002) *Practitioner's Guide to Empirically Based Measures of Anxiety*, which is an excellent compilation of anxiety measures that would be beneficial to administer in clinical and research settings alike. Unless otherwise specified, the reader can assume that the measures described in this section can be found in this resource. Measures that are not found in this resource are free and readily attainable, and I specify the source where they are located.

Generalized Anxiety Disorder

The Penn State Worry Questionnaire (PSWQ; Meyer, Miller, Metzger, & Borkovec, 1990) is a widely used 16-item measure to assess the intensity and excessiveness of a person's worry. Items are rated on a 5-point Likert-type scale (1 = *not at all typical;* 5 = *very typical*), and ratings assigned to each item are summed to obtain a total score, with higher scores being indicative of a more severe level of worry. This measure has excellent psychometric properties and takes only 3 min to complete (Roemer, 2002). The items on this measure are general enough that they are relevant to the worries of childbearing women, as well as worries that people experience at other times in their lives. Although this measure yields quality information about the severity of a person's worry, it does not assess the full range of *DSM–IV–TR* criteria. Newman et al. (2002) suggested that the PSWQ is best used as a screening measure; empirical research has suggested that a score of 65 is the optimal cutpoint that distinguishes between those who meet diagnostic criteria for GAD and those who meet diagnostic criteria for other anxiety disorders (Fresco, Mennin, Heimberg, & Turk, 2003). Thus, clinicians who identify high scorers on this measure should follow up with a careful assessment to determine whether they meet diagnostic criteria for GAD.

The Generalized Anxiety Disorder Questionnaire–IV (GAD-Q-IV; Newman et al., 2002) was constructed to assess symptoms consistent with a *DSM–IV–TR* diagnosis of GAD. The item format varies depending on the particular *DSM–IV–TR* criterion being assessed—some items require *yes* or *no* responses (e.g., "Do you experience excessive worry?"), whereas others assessing life interference and distress require ratings on 9-point Likert-type scales (0 = *none/no distress*; 8 = *very severely/very severe distress*). It has a .67 agreement (κ coefficient) with a structured clinical interview to diagnose GAD. Responses to this measure predict diagnoses of GAD with 83% sensitivity and 89% specificity, meaning that 83% of people who are diagnosed with GAD via clinical interview are identified as such on this inventory, and 89% of people who are not diagnosed with GAD via clinical interview are also not identified as such on this inventory. Of all measures that assess worry and other symptoms associated with GAD, this measure is the most straightforward in identifying people who are likely to meet diagnostic criteria for GAD. The full version of the scale can be found in Newman et al. (2002).

Finally, the Brief Measure of Worry Severity (Gladstone et al., 2005) is an eight-item inventory that assesses the degree to which worry interferes with life functioning. Items are rated on a 4-point Likert-type scale (0 = *not true at all*; 3 = *definitely true*) and are summed to obtain a total score, with higher scores being indicative of a greater severity of worry. The items on this measure are general enough that they are relevant to the consequences of worry in child-bearing women, as well as the consequences of worry that people endure at other times in their lives. This inventory has excellent psychometric properties, although it does not differentiate people with GAD from people who are diagnosed with other anxiety disorders. However, I recommend this measure because (a) it can be used as a brief screening tool, as it only takes 1 to 2 min to complete, and (b) it has been used with childbearing women to determine the degree to which worry severity predicts postpartum depression (Austin, Tully, & Parker, 2007). The full set of items on this measure is included in Gladstone et al. (2005).

Obsessive–Compulsive Disorder

C. T. Beck and Driscoll (2006) recommended the Yale-Brown Obsessive Compulsive Scale (Y-BOCS; Goodman, Price, Rasmussen, Mazure, Fleischman, et al., 1989; Goodman, Price, Rasmussen, Mazure, Delgado, et al., 1989), a 10-item clinician-administered semistructured interview, to assess the severity of obsessions and compulsions in women endorsing perinatal OCD. Items are rated on a 5-point Likert-type scale, with each item containing different descriptors depending on the specific symptom being assessed. Half of the items pertain to obsessions, and the other items pertain to compulsions. Responses to each item are summed to obtain a total score, with higher scores being indicative of a greater severity of obsessive compulsive symptoms. Many clinicians administer a 64-item checklist prior to conducting the interview to identify the most significant domains of obsessive–compulsive symptoms. Although this interview has excellent psychometric properties, it takes around 30 min to administer (Antony, 2002a), which may preclude its use by clinicians who have a finite amount of time to meet with their patients.

Many commonly used self-report inventories assess obsessive–compulsive symptoms. The Maudsley Obsessional Compulsive Inventory (Hodgson & Rachman, 1977) is a 30-item measure that yields scores on four subscales: (a) checking, (b) cleaning, (c) slowness, and (d) doubting. Items are rated in a true–false format, and responses to items are summed to obtain subscale and total scores. The Obsessive Compulsive Inventory–Revised (OCI-R; Foa et al., 2002) is an 18-item measure in which patients rate the distress caused by a range of obsessive–compulsive symptoms. Items are rated on a 5-point Likert-type scale (0 = *not at all;* 4 = *extremely*) and are summed to obtain a total score. The OCI-R yields six subscales: (a) washing, (b) obsessing, (c) hoarding, (d) ordering, (e) checking, and (f) neutralizing. The optimal cutpoint to distinguish between those who meet criteria for OCD and those who do not meet criteria for any anxiety disorder is 21. The full version of this scale can be found in Foa et al. (2002). Finally, the Padua Inventory–Washington State University Revision (Burns, Keortge, Formea, & Sternberger, 1996) is a 39-item inventory that assesses the severity of obsessive–compulsive symptoms. Items are rated on a 5-point Likert-type scale (0 = *not at all;* 4 = *very much*). The measure yields five subscales: (a) contamination obsessions/washing compulsions, (b) dressing/grooming compulsions, (c) checking compulsions, (d) obsessive thoughts of harm to self or others, and (e) obsessive impulses to harm self or others. All of these measures have excellent psychometric properties (Antony, 2002a).

The advantage of administering one or more of these self-report inventories to pregnant or postpartum women is that they can complete the measure in the waiting room before the appointment, which can provide useful information in which the clinician can follow up during the appointment. In addition, their scores can quickly be compared with normative values. However, it is possible that the contents of these measures are not relevant to the clinical presentation of the obsessive–compulsive childbearing woman, as many of the items in these measures tap into specific content areas (e.g., distress while handling money), and there are no questions that pertain specifically to harm coming to the infant. In contrast, the clinician can tailor the focus of Y-BOCS questions to pertain to the specific obsessions and compulsions that the woman reports. If a clinician chooses to administer a self-report inventory of obsessive–compulsive symptoms, it will be imperative that he or she follow up and ask whether the woman is experiencing other obsessions or compulsions that were not captured on the measure.

Panic Disorder

The Panic and Agoraphobia Scale (Bandelow, 1999) is a 13-item self-report inventory that assesses the severity of panic attacks, agoraphobic avoidance, anticipatory anxiety, disability and functional impairment, and worries about health. Its items are formatted in different ways depending on the nature of the specific symptom; for example, symptoms of panic attacks are indicated on a checklist, whereas impairment is rated on a 5-point Likert-type scale (0 = no impairment; 4 = extreme impairment). Items rated on the Likert-type scales are summed to obtain a total score, which places patients in categories of borderline or remission, mild, moderate, severe, and very severe. This measure has sound psychometric properties (Antony, 2002b). Because the nature of panic attacks in childbearing women does not seem to be different from the nature of panic attacks that women experience at other times in their lives (Wenzel, Gorman, O'Hara, & Stuart, 2001), this measure should be relevant for use with pregnant and postpartum women. The one caveat is that pregnant women might endorse some symptoms of panic attacks that are a consequence of the pregnancy, such as difficulty breathing, nausea, and hot flushes. Thus, clinicians should follow up in instances in which pregnant women endorse these symptoms and assess the degree to which they are experienced only in the context of a panic attack or in excess of that which would be expected in most pregnant women.

Recently, Newman, Holmes, Zuellig, Kachin, and Behar (2006) published the Panic Disorder Self-Report, a measure that provides information consistent with the DSM–IV–TR diagnostic criteria for panic disorder in the same manner as the GAD-Q-IV, discussed previously. The DSM–IV–TR criteria are phrased as questions, and respondents circle yes or no to each one. In addition, respondents rate the degree to which their symptoms cause life interference and distress on 5-point Likert-type scales (0 = not at all; 4 = very severely/disabling). This measure has a .93 agreement (κ coefficient) with a structured clinical interview to diagnose panic disorder. Responses to this measure predict diagnoses of panic disorder with 100% sensitivity and 89% specificity, meaning that 100% of people who are diagnosed with panic disorder via clinical interview are identified as such on this inventory, and 89% of people who are not diagnosed with panic disorder via clinical interview are also not identified as such on this inventory. Thus, this measure has the potential to be efficient and accurate in identifying instances of panic disorder in pregnant and postpartum women. However, as on the Panic and Agoraphobia Scale, pregnant women might endorse symptoms of anxiety that are actually part of the physical changes they experience during pregnancy, so the clinician should take care to ensure that they are in excess of what would normally be experienced by pregnant women. The full scale in its entirety can be found in Newman et al. (2006).

Social Anxiety Disorder

The Liebowitz Social Anxiety Scale (Liebowitz, 1987) is a widely used clinician-administered scale to assess fear or anxiety and avoidance in various social and evaluative situations. Its 24 items are rated on two 4-point Likert scales: (a) fear or anxiety (0 = none; 3 = severe) and (b) avoidance (0 = never [0%]; 3 = usually [67–100%]). Several subscales can be derived from the measure, including total fear, fear of social interaction, fear of performance, total avoidance, avoidance of social interaction, and avoidance of performance. Total and subscale scores are obtained by summing the items, with higher scores being indicative of more severe social anxiety. This measure has excellent psychometric properties and takes 20 to 30 min to administer (Orsillo, 2002b). A cutpoint of 30 is optimal in differentiating those who meet criteria for social anxiety disorder and those who do not meet criteria for any anxiety disorder (Mennin et al., 2002). This is a very common measure in the field that yields valuable information about social anxiety, but like the Y-BOCS, it might not be feasible for many clinicians to take the time to administer it.

The Social Interaction Anxiety Scale (Mattick & Clarke, 1998) is a 20-item self-report inventory that assesses cognitive, behavioral, and affective reactions to interpersonal interaction. Items are rated on a 5-point Likert-type scale (0 = not at all; 4 = extremely), and responses to items are summed to obtain a total score, with higher scores being indicative of more severe social anxiety. The measure has excellent psychometric properties (Orsillo, 2002b). Limitations of this measure include the fact that items pertain only to social interaction, rather than a broad array of social and evaluative situations, and that items do not correspond to a diagnosis of social anxiety disorder. Nevertheless, I include it here because postpartum women often specifically report increased concerns about social interaction with others, and it has been an effective measure of social anxiety in my research with postpartum women (Wenzel, Haugen, Jackson, & Brendle, 2005). Because this inventory takes no more than 5 min to complete, it has the potential to be useful in screening for symptoms of social anxiety in the postpartum period that otherwise would be missed.

Newman, Kachin, Zuellig, Constantino, and Cashman-McGrath (2003) developed a self-report inventory that corresponds to the diagnostic criteria for social anxiety disorder—the Social Phobia Diagnostic Questionnaire. Some of the items are rated using a yes/no format (e.g., "Do you try to avoid social situations?"), whereas others require respondents to make ratings on a Likert-type scale of 0 to 4 (e.g., life interference; 0 = no interference; 4 = very severe/disabling). This measure has a .66 agreement (κ coefficient) with a structured clinical interview to diagnose social anxiety disorder. It shows an 85% sensitivity and an 82% specificity, meaning that 85% of people who are diagnosed with panic disorder via clinical interview are identified as such on this inventory, and 82% of people who are not diagnosed with panic disorder via clinical interview are also not identified as such on this inventory. Thus, this measure has the potential to be efficient and accurate in identify instances of social anxiety disorder in childbearing women. The measure can be found in its entirety in Newman, Kachin, et al. (2003).

PTSD

The Clinician Administered PTSD Scale (CAPS; Blake et al., 1995) is a structured clinical interview to determine whether the respondent meets *DSM–IV–TR* criteria for PTSD. After establishing that the respondent meets Criterion A of the PTSD diagnosis (i.e., that she experienced an event in which there was real or perceived threat to her or someone close's health or well-being, and that she responded with fear, horror, or helplessness), the clinician assesses the frequency (0 = *never*; 4 = *daily or almost every day*) and the intensity (0 = *none*; 4 = *extreme*) of the 17 symptoms in the reexperiencing, avoidance/numbing, and increased arousal clusters. The scale can be used in two ways: the frequency and intensity of the 17 items can be summed for a total score, or clinicians can examine responses from each item to make a decision regarding whether the respondent meets diagnostic criteria for PTSD. The CAPS has been used to establish diagnoses of PTSD in a wide range of trauma survivors and has excellent psychometric properties (Orsillo, 2002a). Thus, there is no reason to believe that this interview would be problematic in the assessment of PTSD associated with a traumatic childbirth experience. The limitation of the CAPS is that it takes 45 to 60 min to administer, which might be difficult for clinicians who have limited time to see a large caseload of patients. It can be obtained at no cost by contacting the National Center for PTSD.

Clinicians whose time will not allow them to administer a structured interview like the CAPS might consider using the PTSD Checklist (Blanchard, Jones-Alexander, Buckley, & Forneris, 1996), a 17-item inventory that assesses the specific symptoms of PTSD. Items are rated on a 5-point Likert-type scale, indicating the degree to which each symptom bothers the respondent (1 = *not at all*; 5 = *extremely*). Responses to each item are summed to obtain a total score, with higher scores being indicative of more severe posttraumatic stress symptoms. This measure has good psychometric properties (Orsillo, 2002a). A cutoff of 44 predicts diagnoses of PTSD with a sensitivity of .94 and a specificity of .86, meaning that the measure correctly identifies 94% of people who are diagnosed with PTSD using a clinical interview, and that 86% of people who are not diagnosed with PTSD via clinical interview are also not identified as such on this inventory (Blanchard et al., 1996). Because this measure simply lists the 17 reexperiencing, avoidance/numbing, and increased arousal symptoms associated with PTSD without referencing specific traumatic events, it should be relevant to assess posttraumatic stress symptoms in women who experienced a traumatic childbirth.

PRACTICAL IMPLICATIONS

Ideally, clinicians would have the time and resources to administer screening inventories to pregnant and postpartum women, such as the self-report inventories described earlier in this chapter, and then use well-established structured or semistructured clinical interviews to determine whether child-bearing women who score high on screening inventories meet diagnostic criteria for an anxiety disorder. If clinicians have the time and resources to complete thorough assessments, then I would recommend that childbearing women complete measures of worry, obsessions and compulsions, panic attacks, social anxiety, childbirth fears (for pregnant women), and posttraumatic stress symptoms. This can even be done through an automated system, in which women respond to standard screening questions using a touch tone phone, and the responses are then forwarded to their provider (Kim, Bracha, & Tipnis, 2007). However, most mental health clinicians do not have the time and resources to administer screening instruments and clinical interviews when they are first assigned patients, and health care professionals who are not psychologists, psychiatrists, or clinical social workers generally will not have the training to administer or interpret them.

When clinicians do not use established inventories to assess for anxiety disorders, some basic questions can be posed to childbearing women that will begin to identify those who are at an increased likelihood of being diagnosed with a perinatal anxiety disorder (see Table 8.1). If women respond positively to these questions, then they should be assessed more thoroughly to determine whether they meet diagnostic criteria for an anxiety disorder. Throughout the assessment, clinicians should take care to use language that indicates that anxiety associated with pregnancy and the postpartum period is to be expected, but that it is also important to seek treatment if it is causing problems in their lives. It is also important for perinatal women to visit their obstetrician or family doctor to rule out medical causes of their anxiety symptoms. For example, thyroid dysfunction and anemia are common in perinatal women and are associated with symptoms often seen in GAD and panic disorder. Preeclampsia is also characterized by panic-like symptoms (Ross & McLean, 2006).

This volume has identified six distinct domains of anxiety symptoms in childbearing women: worry, obsessions and compulsions, panic attacks, social anxiety, fear of childbirth, and posttraumatic stress. In clinical practice,

TABLE 8.1

Screening Questions to Identify Anxiety Disorders in Childbearing Women

Disorder	Screening question
Generalized anxiety disorder	Have you found yourself worrying more of the time than not?
	Do you have difficulty controlling your worry?
	What kinds of problems has worrying caused for you?
Obsessive–compulsive disorder	Do you have any thoughts that don't make sense to you and that keep coming back even though you try not to think about them?
	Have you been engaging in any behaviors that you do over and over again?
	What kinds of problems have these thoughts and/or behaviors caused for you?
Panic disorder	Have you had any panic attacks that seem to come out of nowhere?
	Have you done anything differently because of these attacks?
	What kinds of problems have these panic attacks caused for you?
Social anxiety disorder	Have you been especially nervous or anxious when interacting with others?
	What kinds of problems has nervousness when interacting with others caused for you?
Specific phobia	Are you especially anxious or fearful about labor, delivery, or parenthood?
	Are there things that you have avoided because of this fear?
Posttraumatic stress disorder	What was your birth experience like? Was it difficult or traumatic? Have you experienced any other events in your life that you would view as traumatic?
	Do you experience unwanted reminders of the parts of childbirth (or trauma) that were difficult?
	Do you go out of your way to avoid reminders of the parts of childbirth (or trauma) that were difficult for you?
	Have you been more easily startled since you gave birth to your child (or experienced the trauma)?
	What kinds of problems have these symptoms caused for you?

the boundaries between these domains are not as clear, and in fact there is substantial comorbidity among the anxiety disorders (e.g., Sanderson, DiNardo, Rapee, & Barlow, 1990). The following are guidelines to differentiate among anxiety disorder diagnoses in childbearing women:

- *GAD versus OCD.* Does the patient report worry about everyday things, or are the thoughts experienced as bizarre or out of character? The former clinical presentation is more likely to be associated with a diagnosis of GAD, whereas the latter clinical presentation is more likely to be associated with a diagnosis of OCD. As was stated in Chapter 3, checking behavior is more strongly associated with GAD than with OCD, so the presence of this ritual should not sway a clinician to assign a diagnosis of OCD rather than GAD.

- *GAD versus panic disorder.* Some people with GAD engage in such a degree of catastrophic thinking that they experience panic attacks (cf. Barlow et al., 1985). A diagnosis of panic disorder should only be assigned when women experience panic attacks that come out of the blue, in situations in which they do not expect to be nervous or anxious.

- *GAD versus adjustment disorder with anxious mood.* In Chapter 2, I presented several pieces of information to justify assigning a diagnosis of GAD in instances in which women endorse clinically significant worry for less than 6 months. I would follow this recommendation when conducting research with child-bearing women, as the clinical characteristics of people who report worry for less than 6 months are similar to the clinical characteristics of people who report worry for 6 or more months (Kessler, Brandenburg, et al., 2005). Moreover, my experience is that some childbearing women have a rather sudden onset of clinically significant worry. Researchers who follow this practice can simply report this in the description of their sample. However, most facilities require that clinicians record diagnoses according to *DSM–IV–TR* criteria in patients' charts. Thus, I recommend that clinicians assign a diagnosis of GAD when excessive worry has persisted for at least 6 months and adjustment disorder with anxiety mood when excessive worry has persisted for less than 6 months to ensure that the chart is as consistent with practice guidelines as possible. In most instances, the treatment plan will be similar for women with either of these diagnoses.

- *Panic disorder versus specific phobia.* Many people have panic attacks when they are confronted with a phobic stimulus. Women should be diagnosed with specific phobia if they only have panic attacks when they are confronted with something that reminds them of childbirth. In contrast, women should be diagnosed with panic disorder if their panic attacks come out of the blue, in situations in which they do not expect to be nervous or uncomfortable.

Because anxiety disorders in childbearing women are only now beginning to be recognized, it is imperative for clinicians to be alert for warning signs that their patients may be experiencing clinically significant symptoms of anxiety and to have a working knowledge of questions that they can ask to assess for anxiety disorders. It is equally as important for clinicians to keep in mind that some degree of anxiety during pregnancy and the postpartum period is normal and should not be overpathologized (Oates, 2002). Anxiety disorders are only diagnosed when the symptoms cause noticeable life interference or personal distress.

9

PHARMACOTHERAPY
FOR PERINATAL ANXIETY

The use of psychotropic medication for women experiencing emotional disturbances during pregnancy and/or the postpartum period has been the subject of extensive discussion. Although clinical guidelines suggest that medications for anxiety disorders are relatively safe for pregnant and lactating women, some reports have identified specific abnormalities in the fetus or infant of women taking these medications. Furthermore, these medications are not designated by the U.S. Food and Drug Administration (FDA) as safe to take during pregnancy or while breastfeeding. Thus, the decision to medicate a pregnant or lactating woman is made on the basis of a number of factors—many of which are unsupported by data—and evaluated collaboratively by the woman and her prescribing physician.

In this chapter, we outline the factors that women and their clinician typically consider when deciding whether to initiate a course of pharmacotherapy for a perinatal anxiety disorder. In addition, we discuss findings from research that examined the effects of taking these medications on the fetus, newborn, and developing child. We comment briefly on data (or the lack

This chapter was coauthored with Scott Stuart, MD, University of Iowa, Iowa City.

thereof) that speak to the efficacy of these medications in reducing symptoms of perinatal anxiety disorders. Finally, we describe the recommendations made by experts in the field and provide our own evaluation of this issue on the basis of empirical research and clinical wisdom.

FACTORS AFFECTING THE DECISION TO MEDICATE

The decision to medicate a pregnant or lactating woman is complex. First, there is concern that psychotropic medication use has deleterious effects on the developing fetus and that small amounts of these medications are passed to the infant through breast milk. Currently, the FDA provides guidelines for clinicians by assigning all medications to one of five risk categories during pregnancy: (a) *Category A* indicates that well-designed research with humans has failed to demonstrate that there is risk to the fetus if the medication is taken during pregnancy; (b) *Category B* indicates that well-designed animal studies have failed to demonstrate that there is risk to the fetus if the medication is taken during pregnancy, but there are no well-designed studies in humans; (c) *Category C* indicates that animal studies have demonstrated that there may be adverse risk to the fetus if the medication is taken during pregnancy, but there are no well-designed studies in humans, and the benefit of taking the medication might outweigh the risk; (d) *Category D* indicates that there is evidence from research with humans that there is risk to the fetus if the medication is taken during pregnancy, but the benefit of taking the medication might outweigh the risk; and (e) *Category X* indicates that animal and/or human research has demonstrated that there is risk to the fetus if the medication is taken during pregnancy and that the risk of taking the medication outweighs the benefits. Most of the medications that are commonly prescribed to treat anxiety disorders fall into Categories C and D. Although it would be logical to conclude that Category B medications are safer than Category C medications, it has been noted that Category C medications may be preferable because the existing knowledge on these drugs is based, in part, on research with human subjects, whereas the existing knowledge on Category B drugs is based on animal subjects (Birndorf & Sacks, 2008).

Although at present many clinicians use these FDA guidelines to assist them in deciding whether to medicate pregnant patients, it should be acknowledged that there are many criticisms of this classification scheme. Critics have raised concern that the categories (a) are confusing and overly simplistic; (b) incorrectly give the impression that risk increases systematically from Category A to Category X; (c) incorrectly give the impression that all medications in the same category are associated with a similar level of toxicity; (d) fail to identify adverse effects as a function of severity, incidence, or type of effect, or dose, duration, frequency, route of administration, or gestational time of exposure; and (e) focus only on effects of planned prescribing, not inadvertent exposure (Public Affairs Committee of the Teratology Society, 2007). Moreover, these categories apply only to pregnancy and say nothing about safety for use in lactating women.

In response to these concerns, the FDA developed a Proposed Rule that contains a new set of guidelines for labeling risk associated with medication use in both pregnant and lactating women. Categories A through X will be eliminated, and pregnancy and lactation subsections of labels will include descriptive information including a risk summary, clinical considerations, and discussion of available data. At the time of this writing, the Proposed Rule is in the development stage and will likely be revised on the basis of comments from experts in the field. Until the Proposed Rule is published in its final form, the existing categories of pregnancy risk will be used.

Currently, then, there are no "official" FDA guidelines for risk of medication use in lactating women. However, Dr. Thomas Hale, a renowned professor of pediatrics, has developed a categorical scheme for lactation risk that is well-regarded by scholars and clinicians alike. As in the FDA guidelines, he has developed five categories of risk: (a) *L1, Safest* designates medications that have been taken by a large number of breastfeeding women with no adverse effects to the infant, and results from controlled studies suggest that there is little, if any, risk to the nursing infant; (b) *L2, Safer* indicates that limited studies have found no adverse effects in breastfeeding infants, and/or evidence suggests that risk to the nursing infant is remote; (c) *L3, Moderately Safe* indicates that there are either no controlled studies examining risk in nursing infants, or results from controlled studies document only minimal, nonthreatening adverse effects, and the medication should only be given when the potential benefit outweighs the risk; (d) *L4, Possibly Hazardous* indicates that there is possibly risk to the nursing infant, but the benefit of using the drug may outweigh the risk to the infant in serious situations; and (e) *L5, Contraindicated* indicates that there is a high risk of significant adverse effects to the infant, and the risk of using the drug outweighs the benefits of breastfeeding. As we discuss the various medications for anxiety disorders in this chapter, we identify the FDA risk category for pregnant women and Hale's (2008) risk category for lactating women.

In addition to concerns about effects on the fetus and newborn, the physiological and hormonal changes that childbearing women experience make finding the optimal dosage of medications a formidable task. Pregnant women may need higher dosages than they would otherwise because of an increase in total body water, which has the potential to lower drug serum concentrations (Birndorf & Sacks 2008). Antidepressant levels decrease during pregnancy, perhaps because of increases in plasma volume and hepatic microsomal enzyme activity and/or in renal clearance rates (Altshuler & Hendrick, 1996; Jeffries & Bochner, 1988). This means that there might be a recurrence of symptoms that is commensurate with the fall in serum antidepressant levels. In addition, drug binding decreases because women's total protein content is lower during pregnancy. It is recommended that clinicians carefully monitor drug levels, side effects, therapeutic response, and toxicity throughout pregnancy because women's bodies are continually changing during this time (Birndorf & Sacks, 2008). Such monitoring should continue in the early postpartum period because the rapid physiological and hormonal changes could render what was once a therapeutic dose now toxic to the new mother.

Clinicians who are deciding whether to medicate a pregnant or postpartum woman for clinically significant symptoms of anxiety must weigh the degree to which the medication might harm the fetus in utero or the nursing infant against the costs of not medicating, as it is possible that an anxiety disorder might interfere with adequate self-care, compliance with prenatal care, and/or care of the newborn (cf. Goldstein & Sundell, 1999). According to Nonacs, Cohen, Viguera, and Mogielnicki (2005), clinicians must keep in mind four types of risk as they make the decision of whether to medicate a pregnant or postpartum woman:

> 1) risk of pregnancy loss or miscarriage, 2) risk of organ malformation or teratogenesis (i.e., the risk of major organ malformation that occurs within the first 12 weeks of gestation; L. S. Cohen & Rosenbaum, 1998), 3) risk of neonatal toxicity or withdrawal symptoms during the acute neonatal period, and 4) risk of long-term neurobehavioral sequelae. (p. 25)

These groups of risk are considered in the following section on specific medications for perinatal anxiety disorders.

MEDICATIONS FOR PERINATAL ANXIETY DISORDERS

Table 9.1 summarizes the first-line medications that are efficacious in treating the anxiety disorders described in this volume. Medications included in this table are either those that are approved by the FDA for the treatment of one or more particular anxiety disorders or those that have been subjected to randomized, placebo-controlled studies and have been found to be efficacious. Medications that are regarded as adjunctive or second-line treatments are not included in this table. In addition, none of the medications has been designated as efficacious in the treatment of specific phobia related to childbirth, as exposure-based psychotherapy is widely regarded as the first-line treatment for specific phobias (Van Ameringen, Mancini, & Patterson, 2009). Although a few studies have demonstrated the efficacy of medications for certain types

TABLE 9.1
Common Medications for Anxiety Disorders

Medication	Anxiety disorders treated	FDA pregnancy risk category	Hale's lactation risk category
Benzodiazepines			
Alprazolam (Xanax)	GAD Panic disorder Social anxiety disorder	D	L3
Clonazepam (Klonopin)	Panic disorder Social anxiety disorder	D	L3
Diazepam (Valium)	GAD Panic disorder	D	L3
Lorazepam (Ativan)	GAD Panic disorder	D	L3
Azapirones			
Buspirone (BuSpar)	GAD	B	L3
Serotonin reuptake inhibitors			
Fluoxetine (Prozac)	OCD Panic disorder	C	L2
Sertraline (Zoloft)	OCD Panic disorder PTSD Social anxiety disorder	C	L2
Paroxetine (Paxil)	GAD OCD Panic disorder PTSD Social anxiety disorder	D	L2
Citalopram (Celexa)	OCD Panic disorder	C	L2
Escitalopram (Lexapro)	GAD OCD Panic disorder Social anxiety disorder	C	L2
Fluvoxamine (Luvox)	OCD Panic disorder Social anxiety disorder	C	L2
Venlafaxine (Effexor)	GAD Panic disorder PTSD Social anxiety disorder	C	L3

(*continues*)

TABLE 9.1
Common Medications for Anxiety Disorders *(Continued)*

Medication	Anxiety disorders treated	FDA pregnancy risk category	Hale's lactation risk category
Tricyclic antidepressants			
Imipramine (Tofranil)	Panic disorder	D	L2
Clomipramine (Anafranil)	OCD Panic disorder	C	L2
Monoamine oxidase inhibitors			
Phenelzine (Nardil)	Panic disorder Social anxiety disorder	C	—

Note. Data from Dent and Bremner (2009); Hale (2008); Mathew and Hoffman (2009); Pollack and Simon (2009); Stewart, Jenike, and Jenike (2009); Van Amaringen, Mancini, and Patterson (2009). FDA = U.S. Food and Drug Administration; GAD = generalized anxiety disorder; OCD = obsessive–compulsive disorder; PTSD = posttraumatic stress disorder.

of specific phobias, such as flying phobia, we know of no randomized, placebo-controlled studies that have examined the efficacy of medications in the treatment of specific phobia of childbirth. The following sections describe the safety profile of five main classes of medications used to treat anxiety disorders during pregnancy and the postpartum period: (a) benzodiazepines, (b) azapirones, (c) serotonin reuptake inhibitors, (d) tricyclic antidepressants, and (e) monoamine oxidase inhibitors.

Benzodiazepines

Benzodiazepines are medications that have sedative, anxiolytic effects and that exert their action on the inhibitory neurotransmitter, gamma-aminobutyric acid. They are the most frequently prescribed medications for some anxiety disorders, such as panic disorder (Bruce et al., 2003), in spite of the fact that the American Psychiatric Association (1998) recommends antidepressants as the first-line treatment. Prolonged use may be associated with the development of tolerance and dependence, and withdrawal symptoms may occur when these medications are discontinued. Benzodiazepine use may be associated with side effects such as drowsiness and cognitive/memory impairments.

As is evident in Table 9.1, all of the benzodiazepines recommended for the treatment of the anxiety disorders described in this volume are in the FDA's Category D, meaning that well-designed studies have determined that benzodiazepine use during pregnancy is associated with risk to the fetus. Benzodiazepine use during the 1st trimester of pregnancy has been associated with the development of oral cleft (i.e., cleft lip and/or cleft palate) as well as skeletal abnormalities and central nervous system dysfunction. Specifically, the risk of oral cleft in infants of mothers on benzodiazepines is 0.6%, which is a 10-fold increase over the 0.06% risk in the general population (Dolovich et al., 1998). Nonacs et al. (2005) recommended that clinicians should avoid 1st trimester use of benzodiazepines because major skeletal development occurs during this period of time.

Exposure to benzodiazepines in the 3rd trimester may be associated with withdrawal symptoms in infants after they are born. Symptoms of benzodiazepine withdrawal include mild sedation, hypotonia (i.e., low muscle tone), reluctance to suck, apnea (i.e., brief suspensions of breathing), cyanosis (i.e., bluish skin tone), and temperature dysregulation (March & Yonkers, 2001). Although many clinicians choose to discontinue benzodiazepine use for these reasons, Nonacs et al. (2005) recommended against this practice, noting that it puts women at risk for the worsening of anxiety symptoms in the post-partum period. Moreover, these withdrawal symptoms can be managed.

Hale (2008) classified the benzodiazepines listed in Table 9.1 as L3, or moderately safe, for use while breastfeeding. This classification means that risks to the nursing infant are likely to be minimal and nonthreatening but that clinicians and their patients should carefully weigh the risks and benefits of taking a benzodiazepine while breastfeeding. March and Yonkers (2001) indicated that benzodiazepines can be found in the breast milk of nursing mothers, but only in high doses will these medications have an effect on the infant.

The following sections summarize the research that has been conducted on specific benzodiazepines that are used to treat the anxiety disorders described in this volume. It must be noted that none of the research to date has examined the impact of medication exposure independently of the anxiety disorder for which it is being prescribed, and many of the studies involved women who were being treated for seizure disorders rather than anxiety. Thus, findings should be interpreted with these caveats in mind.

Alprazolam (Xanax)

Alprazolam is the most commonly prescribed medication for anxiety in women who are of reproductive age (Iqbal, Sobhan, & Ryals, 2002). Results from a 10-year prospective study of 542 women who took alprazolam during the 1st trimester of pregnancy found no clear pattern of congenital abnormalities or pregnancy loss (St. Clair & Schirmer, 1992). Another prospective study following 236 women who took alprazolam in the 1st trimester found identified congenital abnormalities in five infants (Schick-Boschetto & Zuber, 1992), but there was no evidence to conclude that alprazolam use caused these defects. Although the results from these large studies are encouraging, it should be noted that there are case studies that document major congenital abnormalities in infants exposed to alprazolam in utero (e.g., Barry & St. Clair, 1987).

Available data on the risk to nursing infants come only in the form of case studies. One case report suggested that infants who are weaned from breastfeeding mothers taking alprazolam exhibit withdrawal symptoms, including restlessness and irritability (Anderson & McGuire, 1989). Moreover, there is a case study of a nursing infant who exhibited mild drowsiness while his mother took alprazolam, though it later resolved even as the mother continued to use the medication (Ito, Blajchman, Stephenson, Eliopoulos, & Koren, 1993). Caution should be used when extrapolating from case reports, but given the paucity of data at present, they provide information of which clinicians should be aware.

Clonazepam (Klonopin)

There are case reports of congenital abnormalities, toxicity, and withdrawal symptoms in infants of women who took clonazepam during pregnancy (e.g., J. B. Fisher, Edgren, Mammel, & Coleman, 1985), but the majority of women in these reports were taking the medication as an anticonvulsant for epilepsy rather than as an anxiolytic for an anxiety disorder (Iqbal et al., 2002). Thus, it is not clear whether it was clonazepam or complications associated with maternal epilepsy that caused those problems. Moreover, many of these women were taking a combination of medications during pregnancy, making it difficult to attribute congenital abnormalities solely to the use of clonazepam. Iqbal et al. (2002) recommended that infants born to mothers who take clonazepam during pregnancy should be monitored for central nervous system depression and apnea.

There are even fewer case reports of clonazepam use in breastfeeding women. Birnbaum et al.'s (1999) case series of 11 new mothers taking between 0.25 and 2.0 mg of clonazepam found that 10 of the infants had no detectable traces of clonazepam or its metabolites in their serum, and none of the infants exhibited any side effects. In contrast, Hale (2008) noted that there are a few case studies of clonazepam-exposed infants who had breathing difficulties and hypotonia.

Diazepam (Valium)

Of all of the benzodiazepines, diazepam has been studied the most extensively in pregnant and postpartum women, although much of the research was published some time ago when diazepam was prescribed more frequently than it is today. Research has suggested that use of diazepam during the 1st trimester of pregnancy is associated with oral cleft (e.g., Saxen & Saxen, 1975). On the other hand, several reports of women who overdosed on diazepam at some point in their pregnancy indicated that rates of congenital abnormalities or nervous system dysfunction in their infants were no higher than would be expected by chance (e.g., Czeizel et al., 1984). Results from prospective studies raise the possibility that use of diazepam during pregnancy increases the risk of a benzodiazepine syndrome, which resembles fetal alcohol syndrome (Laegreid, Olegard, Wahlstrijm, & Comradi, 1987). Diazepam use during pregnancy has also been associated with low birth weight and small head circumference (Laegreid, Hagberg, & Lundberg, 1992). Infants of mothers who take diazepam during pregnancy exhibit withdrawal symptoms after they are born, including irritability, insomnia, crying, tremors, suckling difficulties, apnea, diarrhea, and vomiting. The onset of these symptoms occurs between a few days and a few weeks after birth, and they can last for several months (Iqbal et al., 2002). Although results from these studies suggest that diazepam is associated with an array of adverse neonatal outcomes, it should be acknowledged that many other studies have failed to find these associations (e.g., Rosenberg et al., 1983). Iqbal et al. (2002) concluded that the occasional use of diazepam is safe during pregnancy, but that it should be given at the lowest possible dose and should be avoided in the weeks before delivery in order to prevent neonatal withdrawal.

Spigset (1994) estimated that the infant dose of diazepam and its active metabolite is on average 0.78% to 9.1% that of the breastfeeding mother. Case studies have indicated that nursing infants of mothers who take diazepam in the postpartum period may exhibit lethargy, sedation, and weight loss (Patrick, Tilstone, & Reavey, 1972; Wesson et al., 1985). If postpartum women taking diazepam observe these symptoms in their infants, it is recommended that either the drug or breastfeeding be discontinued (Iqbal et al., 2002). Because diazepam is a longer acting benzodiazepine than alprazolam and lorazepam, it should not be the first benzodiazepine considered for lactating women (Hale, 2008).

Lorazepam (Ativan)

Lorazepam is recommended over diazepam for use during pregnancy because, in addition to the fact that it is shorter acting, it does not cross the placenta as easily (Cree, Meyer, & Hailey, 1973). Moreover, it metabolizes primarily to a pharmacologically inactive substance that does not accumulate (Iqbal et al., 2002). There is no evidence that use of lorazepam during pregnancy is associated with congenital abnormalities, although one study found that risk of atresia (i.e., a condition in which a bodily orifice or passage is abnormal, such as the failure of the ear canal to be fully formed) is increased in infants of mothers who took lorazepam (Godet, Damato, & Dalery, 1995). Research has suggested that oral administrations of lorazepam are not associated with neonatal toxicity, but these symptoms have been reported in premature infants or in infants of mothers who took lorazepam intravenously (Whitelaw, Cummings, & McFadyen, 1981). Case studies have documented neonatal withdrawal symptoms of respiratory depression, irritability, insomnia, and feeding difficulties (Erkkola, Kero, Kanto, & Aaltonen, 1983; McAuley, O'Neill, Moore, & Dundee, 1982; Sanchis, Rosique, & Catala, 1991).

Only a few studies have examined the effects of lorazepam on infants of lactating mothers. For example, one study found that infants of mothers who took lorazepam during pregnancy exhibited breathing problems, hypothermia, and feeding problems (Johnstone, 1981). In fact, infants in this study excreted lorazepam for up to 11 days following childbirth. However, Hale (2008) concluded that the amount of lorazepam secreted into breast milk is usually insignificant, and there have been no reports of adverse side effects in nursing infants.

Azapirones

Azapirones are anxiolytic medications that are associated with fewer adverse side effects than benzodiazepines and have no potential for physiologic addiction. Unlike benzodiazepines, they exert their action by activating serotonin receptors. However, they work more slowly than benzodiazepines, taking up to 4 weeks to fully exert their effects (Choy, 2007). As indicated in Table 9.1, one azapirone that is efficacious in treating generalized anxiety disorder is buspirone (BuSpar).

There is little research on the effects of buspirone use on the fetus and nursing infant. According to Hale (2008), there is evidence that it is secreted into animal breast milk, so it is likely that this would also be the case for human breast milk. He noted that buspirone has a relatively short half-life (i.e., 4.8 hr), which would decrease the probability that it would accumulate in an infant's plasma. Hale categorized buspirone as being L3, or moderately safe, to take while breastfeeding, largely because its concentration in breast milk is currently unknown. Thus, there are many features of buspirone that make it more attractive than a benzodiazepine for generally anxious women to take during pregnancy or while breastfeeding. However, these potential benefits must be weighed against the fact that its effects on the fetus and newborn have not been investigated systematically, and the drug's efficacy in pregnant and lactating women has not been documented even in case reports.

Serotonin Reuptake Inhibitors

Serotonin reuptake inhibitors are antidepressants that include two major categories of medications: (a) selective serotonin reuptake inhibitors

(SSRIs), and (b) serotonin-norepinephrine reuptake inhibitors (SNRIs). These medications delay the reuptake process, allowing greater time for serotonin (or in the case of the SNRIs, serotonin and norepinephrine) to exert action. Although serotonin reuptake inhibitors are classified as antidepressants, they are prescribed frequently in the pharmacological treatment of anxiety disorders and are currently regarded as the first-line medications for a number of anxiety and depressive disorders.

Most studies have failed to find an association between increases in the rate of risk of miscarriage and SSRI or SNRI use (e.g., Brunel, Vial, Roche, Bertolotti, & Evreux, 1994; McConnell, Linn, & Filkins, 1998; McElhatton et al., 1996). In the reports that did detect an increased risk (e.g., Kulin et al., 1998), the rates of miscarriage were in the range of that which would be expected of women in the general population. In fact, Sugiura-Ogasawara et al. (2002) raised the possibility that psychiatric symptoms such as depression, rather than antidepressant use per se, increase the risk of miscarriage.

A greater number of studies have examined the degree to which SSRI use is associated with organ malformation, the bulk of which have found that serotonin reuptake inhibitor use is not associated with congenital abnormalities above the baseline rate of 1% to 3% in the general population (see meta-analyses by A. Addis & Koren, 2000; Altshuler et al., 1996; and database studies by Malm, Klukka, & Neuvonen, 2005; Wen et al., 2006). However, some data suggest that paroxetine may be associated with an increased risk of cardiovascular malformations (Goldstein & Sundell, 1999; Nonacs et al., 2005). These data are described in greater length later in the chapter when we focus specifically on this medication.

Evidence exists that some infants born to mothers taking SSRIs during pregnancy exhibit neonatal toxicity and perinatal symptoms, which Nonacs et al. (2005) defined as "a spectrum of physical and behavioral symptoms observed in the acute neonatal period that are attributed to drug exposure at or near the time of delivery" (p. 30). For example, a large population-based study conducted in Vancouver, British Columbia, with 119,547 mothers and infants found that infants born to mothers who took SSRIs had shorter gestations, longer hospital stays, and lower birth weight than infants who were born to mothers who reported equally high levels of psychiatric symptoms but who did not take SSRIs (Oberlander, Warburton, Misri, Aghajanian, & Hertzman, 2006). Infants exposed to SSRIs in this study were more likely than infants of depressed mothers who did not take SSRIs to have respiratory distress, jaundice, and feeding difficulties. When they conducted analyses to account for the severity of mothers' depression, the researchers found that significant differences between the exposed and unexposed infants remained for an increased incidence of birth weight below the 10th percentile and respiratory distress. Although these results are noteworthy, it is likely that they are statistically significant largely because of the size of the database.

There is also a small possibility that infants of mothers who used SSRIs during pregnancy display withdrawal symptoms (Donnelly & Paton, 2007). Laine, Hekkinen, Ekblad, and Kero (2003) prospectively compared newborns of 20 mothers who took either fluoxetine or citalopram during pregnancy with newborns of 20 mothers who did not take medications during pregnancy. Relative to nonexposed infants, infants of mothers who took SSRIs exhibited more frequent tremor and restlessness and increased muscle tone. However, the symptoms declined after 1 to 4 days, and no group differences were detected at 2 weeks and again at 2 months. Laine et al. (2003) suggested that this symptom profile was more consistent with serotonergic overreactivity than withdrawal. However, some case studies have suggested that SSRI use during pregnancy is associated with withdrawal symptoms such as irritability and excessive crying (e.g., Costei, Kozer, Ho, Ito, & Koren, 2002). Nonacs et al. (2005) concluded that symptoms indicative of withdrawal or serotonergic overreactivity are short-lived and do not require medical attention.

Although it is important to be aware of studies documenting the risk of neonatal withdrawal symptoms and perinatal complications, Nonacs et al. (2005) warned that the implications of these findings should be kept in perspective. For example, Casper et al. (2003) found an association between SSRI use during pregnancy and lowered Apgar scores, but the difference between exposed and nonexposed babies was less than 1 point, and the mean Apgar score of the exposed babies was still in the healthy range. Similarly, Simon, Cunningham, and Davis (2002) found a difference in gestational age between newborns exposed to SSRIs during pregnancy (mean gestational age = 38.5 weeks) and newborns not exposed to SSRIs during pregnancy (mean gestational age = 39.4 weeks). Although statistically significant, many of these differences are small and posed only a small amount of risk to the health of the infant. To date, there have been no reports of fetal or infant death due to exposure, nor any long-term sequelae following 3rd-trimester exposure to SSRIs.

One specific infant outcome that has received recent attention is pulmonary hypertension of the newborn (PPHN)—a severe respiratory failure requiring intubation and mechanical ventilation. Chambers et al. (2006) matched 377 women whose infants had PPHN with 836 control infants. Relative to six control infants, 14 infants with PPHN had been exposed to an SSRI after the 20th week of gestation (adjusted odds ratio: 6.1). Neither the use of SSRIs before the 20th week nor the use of non-SSRI antidepressants at any time during pregnancy was associated with an increased risk of PPHN. Although this finding is concerning, it is important to remember that the rate of PPHN is low—one to two infants per 1,000 live births. SSRI use after the 20th week of gestation raised this rate to three to six infants per 1,000 live births. In addition to the low absolute level of risk associated with SSRI use after the 20th week of gestation, there are no other reports to date that have replicated this finding.

Collectively, results from the studies reviewed thus far suggest that there are slight risks to the fetuses and infants of childbearing women who take SSRIs. However, it is important to recognize that there are numerous studies that have not replicated the significant association between SSRI use during pregnancy and many of these variables (e.g., Zeskind & Stephens, 2004). Furthermore, important methodological variables could account for some of the significant results in this body of research. For example, levels of psychiatric symptoms and maternal mood are typically not controlled in these analyses, so it is unclear whether the SSRI or psychiatric symptoms themselves are associated with adverse birth outcomes (Nonacs et al., 2005; Yonkers et al., 2009). Moreover, most of the studies in this body of literature do not use blind raters to assess neonatal outcome, so it is possible that ratings are influenced by the a priori study hypotheses (Nonacs et al., 2005).

Most of the literature described to this point in the section focuses on problems with the newborn's physical health soon after delivery. Misri et al. (2006) raised the possibility that prenatal exposure to SSRIs during pregnancy has the potential to affect serotonin levels during neuronal development, which in turn could affect longer term emotional and behavioral functions related to serotonin (e.g., those associated with depression and anxiety). To investigate this possibility, these researchers prospectively compared emotional and behavioral expression and responsivity in children who were and were not exposed to SSRIs (and in some cases, additional treatment with clonazepam) in utero. At birth, a higher percentage of newborns exposed to SSRIs showed symptoms of poorer adaptation than did infants who were not exposed to SSRIs (Misri, Oberlander, et al., 2004; Oberlander et al., 2004). However, there were no differences between the exposed and unexposed groups at 4 years of age in symptoms of internalizing behaviors (i.e., emotional reactivity, depression, anxiety, irritability, withdrawal; Misri et al., 2006). Instead, children's internalizing symptoms were more strongly associated with current maternal anxiety. Taken together, results from this series of studies suggest that SSRI-exposed infants demonstrate some emotional and behavioral sequelae immediately following birth, but that later in development the mother's current psychiatric condition is much more important in its association with children's internalizing behavior. These results also suggest that getting treatment for an anxiety disorder at any time, not only during pregnancy or the immediate postpartum period, has the potential to benefit the child.

It should be acknowledged that these results with human subjects contrast with results from animal studies, which suggest that exposure to SSRIs at critical developmental periods in utero are associated with changes in brain circuitry and maladaptive behaviors, such as anxiety, depression, and aggression, that persist into adulthood. Specifically, animals exposed to SSRIs in utero have demonstrated abnormalities in sexual activity, locomotor activity, and sleep regulation. They also have exhibited reductions in tryptophan, the precursor to serotonin, and the activity of the serotonin transporter in specific areas of the brain (Borue, Chen, & Condron, 2007). Clearly, it is of utmost importance for researchers to identify precisely when these "critical" developmental periods occur throughout fetal and infant development, as well as for researchers to track prospectively the degree to which serotonin reuptake inhibitor use during pregnancy predicts children's maladaptive behaviors in adulthood. Although Borue et al.'s (2007) conclusions might cause alarm in some readers, it is important to acknowledge that animal subjects used in these studies are subjected to controlled environments in order to isolate the effects of the variables in question in the study (e.g., the effect of the SSRI on adult anatomy and behavior). These studies cannot account for variations in the quality of the environments in which humans are reared, which very well might protect (or exacerbate) any vulnerabilities posed by early alterations in serotonin levels.

As was seen in the section on benzodiazepines, there is far less literature on the effects of serotonin reuptake inhibitor use during lactation on the infant. Excretion of SSRIs into the breast milk is low, milk/plasma (M/P) drug concentrations are generally less than 1, and low infant plasma concentrations are usually reported (Eberhard-Gran, Eskild, & Opjordsmoen, 2006). M/P ratios reflect the ratio of drug concentration in the breast milk to drug concentration in the mother's plasma. A value less than 1 indicates that less of the drug is available in the breast milk than in the plasma, which is preferred so that the infant is exposed to the smallest amount of the psychotropic medication (Gentile, Rossi, & Bellantuono, 2007).

The likelihood of adverse infant outcomes associated with taking SSRIs while breastfeeding is low, but if they do occur, the effects are mainly colic, gastrointestinal problems, and sleep disturbance (Eberhard-Gran et al., 2006; Ragan, Stowe, & Newport, 2005). Gentile et al. (2007) found no association between M/P ratios and adverse infant outcomes in women who took SSRIs while breastfeeding. Hale (2008) categorized all of the SSRIs as being safer (i.e., Category L2) to take while breastfeeding, and he categorized the SNRI venlafaxine (Effexor) as moderately safe to take while breastfeeding.

The following sections summarize the research on specific serotonin reuptake inhibitors that are used to treat the anxiety disorders described in this volume.

Fluoxetine (Prozac)

The majority of the studies that have examined serotonin reuptake use in pregnant and postpartum women have focused on fluoxetine; there have been several prospective studies that have compared outcomes in the infants of women who took fluoxetine during pregnancy with the infants of women who did not take psychotropic medications during pregnancy (and in some cases, with the infants of women who took a different type of psychotropic medication; e.g., Brunel et al., 1994; Chambers, Johnson, Dick, Felix, & Jones, 1996; Goldstein, 1995; Goldstein, Corbin, & Sundell, 1997; McConnell et al., 1998; McElhatton et al., 1996; Nulman et al., 1997, 2002; Pastuszak et al., 1993). Results from early studies suggested that women medicated with fluoxetine during pregnancy had higher-than-average rates of miscarriage, but more recent studies have failed to replicate these findings (see Levine, Oandasan, Primeau, & Berenson, 2003, for a review). Chambers et al. (1996) found that women who took fluoxetine in the 3rd trimester had higher rates of premature labor and admission to special-care nurseries. However, those mothers also had higher rates of several characteristics that put women at risk of pregnancy complications, such as smoking, alcohol use, and low weight gain, raising the possibilities that factors other than use of fluoxetine could account for these findings (cf. Goldstein & Sundell, 1999).

No studies have found an association between fluoxetine and major organ malformations (Chambers et al., 1996; Goldstein, 1995; Nulman & Koren, 1996; Pastuszak et al., 1993), and most experts conclude that use of fluoxetine at any time during pregnancy is not teratogenic (Goldstein & Sundell, 1999). Other studies have examined the longer term consequences in children of mothers who took fluoxetine during pregnancy. For example, two prospective studies examining 55 infants whose mothers took fluoxetine during pregnancy through preschool found that there were no differences between exposed and nonexposed children in a number of cognitive (e.g., IQ), emotional (e.g., temperament), and behavioral (e.g., activity level) variables (Nulman et al., 1997; Nulman et al., 2002).

Most research that has examined the effects of exposure to fluoxetine during lactation has concluded that it is safe for breastfeeding infants. Infants' average daily intake of the fluoxetine is 5% to 9% of the maternal dose (Taddio, Ito, & Koren, 1996). In their review of studies examining a total of 190 infants who had been exposed to fluoxetine during lactation, Burt et al. (2001) concluded that there were no adverse effects. However, several case studies that have raised the possibility of an association between adverse effects in the infant and maternal use of fluoxetine have documented colic (Kristensen et al., 1999; Lester, Cucca, Andreozzi, Flanagan, & Oh, 1993), low weight gain (Chambers et al., 1999) and somnolence, lethargy, fever, and unresponsiveness (Hale, Shum, & Grossberg, 2001). Moreover, in another small study, infants who were being weaned from breastfeeding mothers who took fluoxetine demonstrated a clinical profile that was interpreted as withdrawal (i.e., crying, irritability, poor feeding; Kristensen et al., 1999). Despite the fact that most research has suggested that infants exposed to fluoxetine experienced no adverse effects, other serotonin reuptake inhibitors, such as sertraline, are often recommended over fluoxetine because these other serotonin reuptake inhibitors (a) have shorter half-lives, meaning that the risk of infant accumulation is reduced, and (b) have inert metabolites, in contrast to fluoxetine's active metabolite. Hale (2008) suggested that the risk of not breastfeeding far outweighs the risk of taking fluoxetine while breastfeeding and recommended that lactating women who take fluoxetine should continue to take the medication but monitor their infants for adverse side effects.

Sertraline (Zoloft)

Sertraline is the most frequently prescribed SSRI in pregnant women (Wichman et al., 2008). Results from studies to date provide no evidence to suggest that use of sertraline during pregnancy increases the risk of miscarriage, congenital abnormalities, premature birth, or low birth weight (e.g., Kulin et al., 1998; McConnell et al., 1998). Studies also suggest that there are no adverse effects in newborns exposed to sertraline through breast milk. Ragan et al. (2005) reviewed 18 studies (with 180 exposed infants) that examined the effects of sertraline on exposed infants and found that one infant was agitated, another infant had a number of problems such as low muscle tone and hearing problems, and seven infants had an unspecified adverse reaction, which was more likely explained by in utero exposure than by exposure through breast milk. Moreover, Brandes, Soares, and Cohen (2004) found that the serum levels of sertraline or its metabolite, N-desmethylsertraline, were either undetectable or too low to be qualified in nursing infants of mothers taking this medication.

Paroxetine (Paxil)

Paroxetine is the serotonin reuptake inhibitor that, outside of fluoxetine, has received the most attention in the research literature. Case studies have indicated that use of paroxetine during pregnancy is associated with withdrawal symptoms in the newborn (i.e., respiratory distress, jitteriness, irritability; Dahl, Olhager, & Ahlner, 1997; Nordeng, Lindemann, Perminov, & Reikvam, 2001). Costei et al. (2002) reported that infants of women who took paroxetine in the 3rd trimester of pregnancy were more likely to have neonatal complications (e.g., respiratory distress) than infants of mothers who took paroxetine only during the 1st or 2nd trimesters. Moreover, infants born to mothers who took paroxetine in the 3rd trimester as well as while breastfeeding showed adverse effects, such as decreased alertness and constipation, relative to infants in a control group.

In 2005, GlaxoSmithKline published on its website the results of a claims database study ($N = 815$) that suggested that infants exposed to

paroxetine in the 1st trimester may have a higher risk of congenital malformations, particular cardiovascular defects (2%, which was later adjusted to 1.5%;
Cole, Ephross, Cosmatos, & Walker, 2007). As a result, the FDA issued a warning that use of paroxetine during pregnancy is associated with congenital abnormalities and changed it from a Category C to a Category D medication, which
led to a dramatic reduction in the frequency with which it has been prescribed
to pregnant women (Wichman et al., 2008). A great deal of subsequent research
has been conducted to verify this claim, and interestingly, these studies
have yielded mixed results. Bar-Oz et al. (2007) conducted a meta-analysis of
case-control and cohort studies examining malformations in infants whose
mothers took paroxetine during the 1st trimester. The overall increase in risk of
cardiac deficits was 7.4%, whereas the overall risk of other major malformations
was not elevated. Although these results seem consistent with the FDA warn-
ings, they should be interpreted in light of the fact that Bar-Oz et al. found a
similar rate of increased risk of cardiac deficits in infants of women who took
other SSRIs during the 1st trimester of pregnancy. The authors made the
interesting speculation that women who take SSRIs are more depressed and
anxious than women who do not take these medications, and therefore are
more likely to bring their infants for early testing. Thus, the higher rates of
cardiac deficits may be explained, at least in part, by a detection bias, as it is
possible that a percentage of infants of mothers who did not take paroxetine
during pregnancy have cardiac deficits but that they have not been identified
because their mothers are less likely to seek testing for these problems.

Subsequently, many of the same authors who contributed to the Bar-Oz
(2007) meta-analysis analyzed unpublished data collected around the world
on a total sample of 1,174 infants (Einarson et al., 2008). In contrast to the
results from the meta-analysis, they found that the rates of cardiac deficits in
infants who were and were not exposed to paroxetine in the 1st trimester
were 0.7%, which falls within the incidence of cardiac deficits in the general
population. An additional 2,061 cases obtained from database studies revealed
an incidence of cardiac defects of 1.5% in paroxetine-exposed infants. Einarson
et al. (2008) concluded that the incidence in more than 3,000 infants was
well within the range of the population incidence of approximately 1%.

Paroxetine has the potential to be safer than fluoxetine for use in lactating women because it has a shorter half-life and a slightly higher molecular
weight, which accounts for its decreased diffusion in breast milk (Hendrick,
Stowe, Altshuler, Hostetter, & Fukuchi, 2000). Brandes et al. (2004) reviewed
five studies that examined the effects of paroxetine in the infants of breastfeeding women and found that the serum levels of paroxetine were either
undetectable or too low to be quantified. Ragan et al. (2005) identified
13 studies (with 105 infants) that examined the effects of paroxetine in the
infants of breastfeeding women and found that only one infant was documented

as being agitated and unsettled, and another had an unspecified adverse reaction that might have been more related to exposure to paroxetine in utero than through breast milk.

Citalopram (Celexa)

Very few studies have examined the effects of use of citalopram during pregnancy and the postpartum period and its effects on the infant. Ericson, Kallen, and Wilholm (1999) conducted a prospective study of the effects of 1st-trimester exposure to SSRIs in 969 infants (375 of whom were exposed specifically to citalopram) and found no elevation in the rate of major congenital abnormalities. Laine et al. (2003)'s analysis of withdrawal symptoms in infants whose mother took either fluoxetine or citalopram during pregnancy found that exposed infants had a four-fold increase in withdrawal symptoms compared with unexposed infants. However, Condon (2003) later pointed out that these symptoms were limited to infants who had been exposed to fluoxetine.

In a study of seven lactating women taking citalopram, their infants' average daily intake of the drug was approximately 3.7% of the maternal dose (Rampono et al., 2000). Ragan et al. (2005) identified 10 studies (with a total of 69 infants) that examined the effects of citalopram on breastfeeding women's infants and found only a single instance of the following issues: colic, decreased feeding, irritability/restlessness, and uneasy sleep (i.e., K. Schmidt, Olesen, & Jensen, 2000). Although this small bit of research suggests that citalopram is safe to use while breastfeeding, Eberhard-Gran et al. (2006) cautioned against the use of high doses of citalopram while breastfeeding on the basis of the K. Schmidt, Olesen, & Jensen (2000) case study.

Escitalopram (Lexapro)

Of all of the SSRIs, escitalopram has received the least attention in the literature. No prospective or retrospective studies have examined the effects of exposure to escitalopram during pregnancy on the infant, and most large studies examining the SSRIs as a group include few, if any, women who are taking escitalopram. However, escitalopram is an active metabolite of citalopram, so the research on citalopram is likely to be relevant in understanding potential risks posed by use of the medication during pregnancy and lactation.

In a study of eight lactating women (Rampono et al., 2006), the average weight of the dose of the drug in the infant was 5.3% of the mother's dose. Traces of escitalopram and its metabolite were undetectable in the infants, and no adverse side effects in the infant were reported. Castberg and Spigset (2006) described the case of a woman who began taking escitalopram immediately after giving birth, and there were no adverse effects in the infant. Thus, escitalopram seems safe for use during pregnancy and while breastfeeding and is preferred over citalopram because its metabolite is inert.

Fluvoxamine (Luvox)

Subgroup analyses from a major study designed to examine congenital abnormalities associated with a variety of SSRIs indicated that there was no increased risk in the infants whose mothers were taking fluvoxamine while pregnant (Malm et al., 2005). Thus, at this time there is no evidence to conclude that use of fluvoxamine is associated with adverse side effects or complications in the newborn, although more research is needed to verify this observation. Case studies have indicated that the infant dose of fluvoxamine and its metabolites range from 0.5% to 1.58% of the maternal dose (Hagg, Granberg, & Carleborg, 2000; S. Wright, Dawling, & Ashford, 1991). No case studies have identified any adverse effects in the infants of lactating women (e.g., Arnold, Suckow, & Lichtenstein, 2000; Piontek, Wisner, Perel, & Peindl, 2001).

Venlafaxine (Effexor)

A large study of 150 pregnant women who took venlafaxine during pregnancy indicated that there was no elevation in the rate of major congenital abnormalities in the newborns of these women relative to comparison samples of women who took various SSRIs during pregnancy and women who did not take medications during pregnancy (Einarson et al., 2001). Results from case studies investigating adverse effects in newborns exposed to venlafaxine in utero have been mixed. For example, Moses-Kolko et al. (2005) referenced a case study of a newborn who had been exposed to venlafaxine in utero and exhibited symptoms of jitteriness, increased muscle tone, feeding disturbances, and irritability. On the other hand, Hendrick, Altshuler, Wertheimer, and Dunn (2001) indicated that there were no abnormalities in a newborn of a woman who took venlafaxine during pregnancy, although a low dose of its metabolite was detected in the infant.

In a study of three lactating women (Ilett et al., 2002), the average weight of the dose of venlafaxine in the infants' serum was 3.2% of the maternal dose. None of the infants had any adverse side effects. Hendrick et al. (2001) also described the case of a woman who began taking venlafaxine on the day of her delivery, and there were no adverse effects in her nursing infant. Despite the fact that these case reports provide preliminary evidence that venlafaxine is safe for lactating women, Hale (2008) regarded venlafaxine's risk to nursing infants as one category higher than the SSRIs because of recent unpublished evidence documenting adverse effects that include respiratory distress, cyanosis, apnea, seizures, and temperature instability.

Tricyclic Antidepressants

Tricyclic antidepressants (TCAs; imipramine [Tofranil], clomipramine [Anafranil]) are medications that inhibit reuptake of serotonin, norepinephrine, and dopamine and that have been prescribed for several decades in the treatment of emotional disturbances such as depression and many anxiety disorders. Despite the longevity of these medications, there is surprisingly little research on the effects of their use during pregnancy and lactation. At present, TCAs are prescribed less than the serotonin reuptake inhibitors because their use is often associated with many side effects, such as dry mouth, blurry vision, constipation, urinary retention, cognitive impairments, and increased body temperature. In fact, some of these side effects are also experienced during pregnancy, so it has been recommended that TCAs should not be the first medication of choice for pregnant women (March & Yonkers, 2001). Nevertheless, we briefly discuss research that has examined the safety of TCA use during pregnancy and while breastfeeding, as these medications are still prescribed on occasion for co-occurring anxiety and depression, panic disorder, and obsessive–compulsive disorder (OCD).

The meta-analyses described earlier indicating that there was no significant association between use of SSRIs during pregnancy and congenital malformations found similar results for the use of TCAs during pregnancy (A. Addis & Koren, 2000; Altshuler et al., 1996). In a large-scale study comparing outcome in infants exposed to SSRIs, TCAs, or no medications in utero, Simon et al. (2002) found that infants exposed to TCAs and control infants who were not exposed to medications had similar Apgar scores. Research by Nulman and colleagues (Nulman et al., 1997; Nulman et al., 2002) indicated that TCA use during pregnancy is not associated with disturbances in children's mood, behavior, temperament, distractibility, or activity level. However, research has documented that infants born to mothers taking TCAs during pregnancy exhibited symptoms associated with withdrawal, such as jitteriness, irritability, and infrequent seizures (e.g., Webster, 1973). Moreover, animal studies have documented a range of behavioral abnormalities over the first 30 days of life in offspring born to mothers who were taking TCAs, but similar studies have not been conducted with humans (L. S. Cohen & Rosenbaum, 1998). Most studies have found no adverse effects of maternal TCA use in nursing infants (Llewellyn & Stowe, 1998). The FDA regards the pregnancy risk of imipramine as Category D and the pregnancy risk of clomipramine as Category C, and Hale (2008) classified both of these drugs as L2, or safer, to take while breastfeeding.

Monoamine Oxidase Inhibitors

Monoamine oxidase inhibitors (MAOIs) are antidepressants that work by inhibiting the activity of the enzyme monoamine oxidase, which in turn prevents the breakdown of neurotransmitters such as serotonin and norepinephrine. Research shows that one MAOI, phenelzine (Nardil), has been particularly efficacious in the treatment of social anxiety disorder (Blanco et al., 2003), although very little research has been done on the effects of MAOI use in pregnant and lactating women. Nonacs et al. (2005) identified one study that used a small sample size and found that MAOI use was associated with organ malformation and noted that MAOIs may induce a hypertensive crisis if certain medications are used to prevent delivery. Thus, they recommended that MAOIs should be avoided during pregnancy. Moreover, no research has examined effects of phenelzine use on nursing infants, so Hale (2008) did not assign it a lactation risk category code. Thus, phenelzine should be used to treat social anxiety disorder in lactating women with extreme caution, and other medications that are efficacious in treating social anxiety disorder should be considered before phenelzine.

EFFICACY

There is a paucity of research on the efficacy of pharmacotherapy in the treatment of perinatal anxiety disorders (Dennis & Stewart, 2004), as most empirical inquiry on this topic centers on the degree to which use of psychotropic medications affects the development of the fetus and nursing baby, rather than the degree to which these medications are efficacious in pregnant and lactating women. In fact, most efficacy studies of medications for anxiety disorders in general might not apply to women with prenatal anxiety disorders, as pregnant women are generally excluded from clinical trials designed to evaluate these medications (Birndorf & Sacks, 2008). No studies have specifically examined the efficacy of psychotropic medication in the treatment of depression or anxiety in pregnant and postpartum women (Yonkers et al., 2009).

There are, however, a number of case reports that provide very preliminary evidence for the efficacy of some psychotropic medications in the treatment of perinatal anxiety disorders. For example, these studies indicate that imipramine may be effective in treating prenatal (Ware & DeVane, 1990) and postpartum (Metz, Sichel, & Goff, 1988) panic disorder. In addition, SSRIs have been used in the treatment of perinatal OCD (see Altemus, 2001; and Ross & McLean, 2006, for a review). Clearly, larger scale research is needed to evaluate the efficacy of various psychotropic medications for the treatment of perinatal anxiety disorders.

PRACTICAL IMPLICATIONS

Research on the safety of psychotropic medications and their effects on the fetus or infant in pregnant and lactating women is incomplete. Broadly speaking, SSRIs have the most empirical evidence supporting their safety. Despite this research base, childbearing women and medical professionals alike are understandably reluctant to medicate for perinatal emotional disturbances because it is known that these medications do indeed pass through the placenta, trace amounts are found in breast milk, and some of the studies have found an association between psychotropic medication use and adverse effects in the infant. Most of the perinatal complications documented in empirical research seem to be short-lived and able to be managed (Moses-Kolko et al., 2005; Nonacs et al., 2005). However, there are no long-term studies of fetuses exposed to psychotropic medications in utero or infants exposed to psychotropic medications through breast milk.

There are no expert consensus guidelines for the recommendation of treatment for perinatal anxiety. However, there are guidelines for the treatment of depression during pregnancy and the postpartum period, which is often treated with many of the same medications as perinatal anxiety. The expert guidelines recommend psychotherapy for pregnant and breastfeeding women with mild to moderate symptoms and pharmacotherapy for pregnant and breastfeeding women with severe symptoms, such as a history of suicidal behavior, psychosis, recurrent episodes, or comorbidity (Yonkers et al., 2009). Until expert guidelines for the treatment of perinatal anxiety are drafted, it is reasonable to consult the depression guidelines in the decision-making process.

Several scholar–clinicians have made important observations and suggestions regarding pharmacotherapy for pregnant and postpartum women. Many clinicians consider the severity of women's symptoms, comorbid psychiatric symptoms, and the extent of their psychiatric history, reasoning that women who present with severe symptoms, comorbidity, or an extensive psychiatric history are likely to benefit from medication, whereas women with less severe symptoms or no psychiatric history may be referred for psychotherapy (cf. Yonkers et al., 2009). In addition, clinicians intending to prescribe medications to pregnant and lactating women should consider their patients' responses to previous treatment. Interventions that successfully reduced symptoms in the past would be logical choices for intervention during pregnancy and the postpartum period (Birndorf & Sacks, 2008). If a woman took a particular type of medication during pregnancy, then that same medication should be used in the postpartum period because the infant has already been exposed to it (Ragan et al., 2005).

If a clinician proceeds with pharmacotherapy, he or she should be mindful of several observations from the research literature. For example,

Nonacs and Cohen (1998) pointed out that physicians who treat postpartum mood disturbance with pharmacotherapy often do so less intensely than they do nonpostpartum mood disturbance and cautioned that this approach has the potential to be ineffective. Clinicians should use the lowest dose possible to achieve a therapeutic effect, but it is important that the dose is significant enough that it will have a tangible effect on the woman's clinical presentation. In addition, Nonacs et al. (2005) indicated that some clinicians discontinue psychotropic medications in the weeks leading up to delivery in order to minimize the risk of physical and behavioral symptoms of toxicity or withdrawal in the newborn, but there is little evidence that this practice indeed reduces risk to the newborn, and it has the potential to instead exacerbate symptoms in the mother. Ragan et al. (2005) indicated that much of the concern about exposure of the infant to psychotropic medications through breastfeeding is overstated, noting that infants have metabolic enzymes that are comparable with those in adults, and that a child would have to breastfeed for more than 2 years to get the same exposure to antidepressants that occurs during only 1 month of pregnancy. On the other hand, others have cautioned that infants less than 2 months old may be susceptible to the effects of psychotropic medication passed through breast milk, as their hepatic and renal functions are still developing as is their blood-brain barrier, which might increase the passage of drugs into their central nervous system (Eberhard-Gran et al., 2006).

In all cases, clinicians should keep in mind the following suggestions as they medicate pregnant and lactating women: (a) document all exposures to medications and other substances that have the potential to affect fetal development; (b) choose the medication that has the greatest amount of research documenting its efficacy and adverse effects in these populations (Nonacs et al., 2005); and (c) if at all possible, choose monotherapy over polytherapy (Birndorf & Sacks, 2008). If a woman taking benzodiazepines learns that she is pregnant and wishes to discontinue medication, she should gradually discontinue the medication, as the abrupt discontinuation of anxiolytics can put women at risk of rebound symptoms. Instead, it is suggested that medications be tapered over a period of time greater than 2 weeks, accompanied by adjunctive psychotherapy (L. S. Cohen & Rosenbaum, 1998; Nonacs et al., 2005). Moreover, lactating women who use psychotropic medications should be aware that concentrations of the drug in their breast milk vary according to the concentration of the drug in the plasma, which is determined in part by the amount of time that has passed since ingestion. It is recommended that they feed their infant immediately before they take the drug, when their plasma concentration is presumably at its lowest (Eberhard-Gran et al., 2006).

As clinicians and consumers, we are left with these conflicting recommendations that are both based on scientific observation but that lead to very different decisions. The variety of recommendations in the research literature underscore the need for clinicians who work with pregnant and lactating women to be familiar with biological processes associated with pregnancy and lactation and the use of psychotropic medication as well as the ever-changing literature that investigates the effects on the newborn and nursing infant. Ultimately, the decision to medicate should be made in collaboration with the woman after she weighs the advantages of disadvantages of psychotropic medications and other treatment options for her perinatal anxiety disorder (Nonacs et al., 2005). On the basis of their personal values and the weight given to the risks and benefits, many mothers elect avenues other than medication, such as psychotherapy. These choices, barring overt and immediate risk to the woman or her child, should be supported.

10

PSYCHOTHERAPY FOR PERINATAL ANXIETY

Many pregnant and postpartum women with psychiatric symptoms opt for psychotherapy instead of psychotropic medications, as they want to avoid exposing their baby to medication in utero or through breast milk. More than 20 years ago, Barnett and Parker (1985) demonstrated that psychotherapy targeting social support, anxiety management, self-esteem and self-confidence, and healthy parent–infant interactions was more effective than no treatment in reducing state and trait anxiety in postpartum women. Since that time, many different approaches to psychotherapy have been evaluated for perinatal depression, but researchers are only now turning their attention back to examining the efficacy of psychotherapy for perinatal anxiety.

In this chapter, I describe some psychotherapeutic approaches for treating anxiety disorders that empirical research has found to be efficacious. It is generally assumed that these therapeutic approaches would be effective in treating pregnant and postpartum women (Ross & McLean, 2006), but empirical research is needed to test this notion. When relevant research or scholarly discussion is available, I present the manner in which these approaches have been implemented with pregnant and postpartum women and data that speak to their efficacy. I focus on the manner in which the interventions described in this chapter could proceed with the cases presented in Chapters 2 through 6.

COGNITIVE BEHAVIORAL THERAPY

Cognitive behavioral therapy (CBT) is a short-term, time-limited approach to psychotherapy that uses an active problem-solving framework to help patients develop concrete strategies to manage stressors that they encounter in their lives. There are two main targets in CBT: cognitions and behaviors. Maladaptive cognitions that exacerbate anxiety are targeted through *cognitive restructuring,* a process in which the clinician works with the patient to develop skills to identify, evaluate, and if necessary, modify problematic thoughts, images, and beliefs that are associated with life interference and/or distress. For example, many people with anxiety disorders predict that the "worst-case scenario" will happen to them. Through the process of cognitive restructuring, these individuals develop tools to evaluate the likelihood that these predictions will occur, how bad it would be if the worst case scenario were realized, and the most likely outcome. Moreover, many anxious individuals underestimate their ability to cope with adversity (A. T. Beck & Emery, 1985), and the cognitive restructuring process helps them to realistically evaluate their ability to do so.

Maladaptive behaviors are targeted through a number of strategies. Because a core feature of anxiety is avoidance behavior, many CBT protocols for anxiety disorders incorporate *exposure,* in which patients systematically confront a feared stimulus in order to habituate to the discomfort, learn that the stimulus is not as dangerous as expected, and implement strategies for managing distress. People with social anxiety disorder, for instance, often experience anxiety when interacting with others whom they assume will judge them negatively. Exposure with socially anxious patients often requires them to intentionally place themselves in these situations and remain there until their anxiety dissipates—a process called *in vivo exposure.* People with panic disorder usually fear the experience of internal bodily symptoms that resemble a panic attack, such as racing heart, sweating, or dizziness. *Interoceptive exposure* with panic patients requires them to gain experience tolerating these internal sensations by intentionally provoking them. In contrast, people with post-traumatic stress disorder (PTSD) often go to great lengths to avoid thinking about a previous trauma. These patients benefit from *imaginal exposure,* in which they systematically imagine vivid details of the trauma in order to habituate to the distress associated with memories and reminders of the trauma. Other behavioral components that are often incorporated into CBT include assertiveness training, goal setting, problem solving, muscle relaxation, and controlled breathing (J. H. Wright, Basco, & Thase, 2006).

The following sections describe CBT approaches for treating each of the anxiety disorders described in this volume, with an eye toward illustrating the manner in which they could be applied to the treatment of pregnant and post-partum women. This section ends with a description of preliminary research conducted to establish the efficacy of CBT in reducing anxiety in pregnant and postpartum women.

CBT for Generalized Anxiety Disorder

CBT for the treatment of generalized anxiety disorder (GAD) is multifaceted (Robichaud & Dugas, 2009). In many instances, it incorporates awareness and self-monitoring, which helps generally anxious patients identify triggers of anxiety and the manner in which they respond to those triggers (Borkovec, 2006). Cognitive restructuring helps patients to make accurate appraisals of situations as they encounter them, refrain from forming expectations for the future, and evaluate faulty beliefs about the degree to which worry is helpful. Imaginal exposure helps patients face vivid images of feared catastrophes, and in vivo exposure can be used to purposefully place patients in situations associated with uncertainty or ambiguity (Dugas & Robichaud, 2007). In addition, some CBT protocols for GAD incorporate relaxation techniques to help patients achieve a state of calmness in the present moment, amid the triggers of anxiety (Borkovec, 2006), and problem-solving skills in order to address their problems and lack of confidence in their problem-solving ability (Dugas & Robichaud, 2007). Moreover, imagery rehearsal can be used to help these patients practice applying the coping skills in managing their anxiety. Empirical research has shown that this CBT for GAD is more efficacious than a waiting-list control condition (Dugas et al., 2003; Ladouceur et al., 2000) and nondirective therapy, and that it is at least as effective as pure cognitive therapy and pure behavior therapy approaches (Borkovec & Costello, 1993; Borkovec, Newman, Pincus, & Lytle, 2002).

Recall the case of Carla from Chapter 2. Carla experienced an increase in worry during her fourth pregnancy and participated in psychotherapy during late pregnancy and throughout the 1st year postpartum.

> Carla's therapist implemented many of these cognitive behavioral strategies when she resumed treatment at 8 weeks postpartum. During her first post-partum session, she was instructed to monitor the triggers of her anxiety. However, when she returned for her next session, she admitted that she did not complete this homework assignment because she was too consumed with caring for her newborn and attending to her other children. Thus, her therapist modified the homework to work more effectively with the reality of her life circumstances. Together in session, they identified the most common triggers for her anxiety and created a checklist, so that

before going to bed Carla could quickly check off the triggers that she had experienced that day. They used that information to identify concrete strategies for coping with triggers she encountered most frequently in her life. In addition, her therapist conducted muscle relaxation with her in session so that she could learn to center herself and acquire the skills to invoke relaxation when she encountered triggers. She discovered that she could apply principles of relaxation while she was nursing her baby, and she began to look forward to turning on soft music and spending quiet time while breastfeeding. Carla also learned several strategies for cognitive restructuring, so that when she had negative thoughts associated with a trigger, she could take a step back and ask herself questions such as: What is the worst thing that will happen? What is the most realistic thing that will happen? What is the likelihood that the worst thing will happen? If it did happen, how bad would it be? What would I do to handle it? After Carla acquired these skills, she engaged in imaginal exposure exercises with her therapist, such that she imagined how she would handle perceived catastrophes, such as her husband losing his job, her baby being sick, and her older children getting into trouble. By the end of treatment, Carla reported a substantial decrease in her anxiety symptoms and improvement in her ability to handle stressors.

CBT holds great promise for work with pregnant and postpartum women, as it offers tangible strategies for identifying and modifying worries; provides practice in dealing with life's problems through exposure; and offers behavioral skills to manage stressors, such as relaxation and problem-solving. However, it has not yet been evaluated in samples of pregnant or postpartum women. In my clinical work with anxious postpartum women, I find that many of my patients have difficulty finding the time to do standard CBT homework assignments, such as self-monitoring, because of the demands of new motherhood. Thus, clinicians should be creative in working collaboratively with patients to develop homework assignments that can be implemented effectively on the spot or that take only a small amount of time at one point in the day, such as Carla's checklist of triggers.

CBT for Obsessive–Compulsive Disorder

A standard cognitive behavioral treatment for obsessive–compulsive disorder (OCD) is exposure and response prevention (ERP), which involves in vivo and imaginal exposure to distressing stimuli and the acquisition of response prevention strategies. Patients participate in exposure exercises in session under the clinician's direction, and they complete self-guided exposures as homework in between sessions (Abramowitz, Braddock, & Moore, 2009). Exposure weakens the link between obsessive thinking and distress because it (a) provides evidence that the feared outcomes will not occur and (b) demonstrates to the person that distress eventually decreases without performing a compulsive ritual or avoiding reminders of the intrusive thought (Abramowitz, Schwartz, Moore, & Luenzmann, 2003). Some researchers have combined ERP and cognitive restructuring, particularly for the treatment of OCD characterized by obsessive thoughts that are not accompanied by behavioral rituals (Freeston et al., 1997). Cognitive restructuring with obsessive–compulsive patients focuses on the misinterpretation of obsessive thoughts as being highly significant and the rigid need to control the thoughts (Abramowitz, Braddock, et al., 2009). Results from randomized controlled trials indicate that ERP is more efficacious in treating OCD than waiting-list (Van Balkom et al., 1998) and pill placebo (Foa et al., 2005) conditions.

Abramowitz and his colleagues have posited that theoretically, the cognitive behavioral treatment of perinatal OCD should not proceed any differently from OCD expressed at other times in a person's life (Abramowitz, Schwartz, Moore, & Luenzmann, 2003). In fact, Abramowitz, Moore, Carmin, Wiegartz, and Purdon (2001) described the successful treatment of four new fathers who had developed postpartum OCD using a CBT protocol that incorporated education about the nature of intrusive thoughts and their relation to emotional distress, exposure exercises, and response prevention. It is important for clinicians to know that although ERP is very effective in the treatment of OCD, it requires a great deal of time and commitment on the part of the patient. Intensive ERP protocols typically include 15 treatment sessions over the course of 3 weeks (Franklin, Abramowitz, Kozak, Levitt, & Foa, 2000). Less intensive interventions have been evaluated and found to be efficacious, but even then these interventions rely on twice-weekly 2-hr sessions (Abramowitz, Foa, & Franklin, 2003), which is substantially more time than the typical 50-min weekly therapy session that is often used to treat other psychological disorders. The amount of time spent in session is strongly associated with short- and long-term reductions in symptoms (Abramowitz, Braddock, et al., 2009). Thus, women who exhibit moderate to severe symptoms of OCD and who choose to participate in ERP will likely need to solicit the assistance of close others to provide child care as they participate in this treatment protocol.

Recall the case of Diane from Chapter 3, whose avoidance of her baby because of intrusive thoughts and images of harming him caused such life interference that her family encouraged her to seek inpatient care, followed by weekly outpatient psychotherapy.

> In her outpatient sessions, Diane's therapist reinforced the gains she had made during her inpatient stay by leading her through imaginal exposures of caring for her baby, such as feeding him, bathing him, and rocking him to sleep. In addition, he accompanied her to her home, where she actually engaged in these activities. She resisted the urge to count to five before

she picked up the baby, as well as the impulse to avoid him when she was experiencing acute anxiety. Diane also developed cognitive strategies to address her belief that having these thoughts made her a bad person and that there was a high likelihood that she would actually act on them. She was given information about the prevalence of intrusive thoughts in new parents to normalize her experience. Each time she interacted with her baby without harming him (which occurred in every instance), Diane recorded it on a piece of paper so that she could see evidence accumulating that she was not going to act on her frightening thoughts. She worked with her therapist to construct the adaptive self-statement, "Having these thoughts in no way guarantees that I am going to harm my baby, and the fact that I am feeling anxious means that I am not actually going to act upon them." After 2 months of outpatient treatment, her obsessive–compulsive symptoms decreased substantially, and she began providing care for her baby without the supervision of others.

CBT for Panic Disorder

The American Psychiatric Association (1998) regards CBT as a first-line treatment for panic disorder. A typical CBT protocol for panic disorder includes five components (McCabe & Gifford, 2009). *Psychoeducation* is typically conducted in the early sessions to orient patients to the CBT model and help them understand the manner in which certain cognitions and behaviors maintain and exacerbate panic symptoms. *Cognitive restructuring* targets the misinterpretation of bodily sensations and exaggerated consequences of having a panic attack. *Interoceptive exposure* exercises induce feared physical sensations and allow patients to habituate to them. *In vivo exposure* is used particularly when patients exhibit agoraphobic avoidance and involves exposure to situations that are avoided for fear of having a panic attack. Finally, some CBT protocols for panic disorder involve *muscle relaxation* or *controlled breathing* strategies, although some evidence suggests that these strategies can actually interfere with treatment because they are used by patients as safety cues during exposures, which prevents them from learning to tolerate their anxiety (N. B. Schmidt et al., 2000). Results from a recent meta-analysis suggest that CBT for panic disorder is more efficacious than waiting-list and placebo control conditions in reducing anxiety and depression and improving quality of life; that it is equally as efficacious as psychotropic medication in reducing symptoms posttreatment; and on some measures, that it is more efficacious than psychotropic medication in reducing symptoms at longer term follow-up assessments (Mitte, 2005).

Most of the CBT protocols described in this book are appropriate for pregnant and postpartum women, provided that the therapist modifies between-session homework assignments to account for the demands associated with the transition to parenthood. The same cannot be said for aspects of the CBT protocol for panic disorder as would be conducted with pregnant women. As stated in Chapter 4, a case study has documented placental abruption associated with a severe panic attack (L. S. Cohen, Rosenbaum, & Heller, 1989). Although this finding needs to be replicated in a study with a multiple research participants before one can conclude that having a panic attack leads to such severe consequences, clinicians should proceed with caution when they design exposure exercises that have a strong likelihood of simulating panic attacks. In fact, I recommend that clinicians who prefer to implement interoceptive exposure exercises with pregnant women do so in close collaboration with the woman's physician.

One case report describes the application of CBT to a childbearing woman with panic disorder (Robinson, Walker, & Anderson, 1992). A 26-year-old woman presented for treatment 4 months before the delivery of her first child. After a 3-week monitoring period, she participated in a 6-week trial of CBT. The full course of CBT was administered while she was still pregnant, and it included psychoeducation, self-monitoring, cognitive restructuring, and in vivo exposure. Her panic attacks declined from 1.5 per week during the baseline period to 0.33 per week during the treatment period, 0.33 per week during the first 9 weeks of follow-up, and 0.06 times per week during the following 16 weeks. The protocol did not have any obvious adverse effects on her health or the health of her child. However, she did not participate in any interoceptive exposure exercises.

Recall Becca from Chapter 4, who experienced a dramatic increase in the frequency of panic attacks after weaning her baby from breastfeeding at 6 months postpartum.

> Becca attended weekly CBT sessions for 4 months and learned an array of strategies to manage her panic attacks, including cognitive restructuring, muscle relaxation, and controlled breathing. Through a self-monitoring exercise, she learned that she was most likely to experience panic attacks when her baby was doing something that she did not think she could handle (e.g., when he was unable to be soothed). Her therapist helped her to acquire strategies to evaluate the notion that she cannot handle her baby, such as having her estimate the percentage of first-time mothers who have had difficulty soothing their babies and having her remember times when she successfully handled instances in which her baby did something unexpected. In addition, she engaged in interoceptive exposure exercises, such as running in place to elevate her heart rate and spinning in a chair to provoke dizziness. Her husband attended two sessions so that he could gain familiarity with the strategies and have the ability to coach Becca in between sessions as she did her homework assignments. At the end of 4 months, the frequency of her panic attacks dropped to two to three minor episodes per week. Although by this time Becca's functioning

was close to normal, she was still unsettled by the course of events over the previous few months. She continued to see her clinician on a biweekly basis, who continued to use a cognitive behavioral approach to address guilt, shame, and low self-esteem.

CBT for Social Anxiety Disorder

Like cognitive behavioral interventions for panic disorder and OCD, CBT for social anxiety disorder incorporates exposure and cognitive restructuring (L. Magee, Erwin, & Heimberg, 2009). Exposure exercises with socially anxious patients are typically done in vivo through actual or simulated situations in sessions and self-guided practice in between sessions. Cognitive restructuring usually focuses on patients' tendencies to assume that they know what others are thinking about them and to predict negative outcomes for the future. Some CBT approaches for social anxiety disorder also incorporate social skills training and relaxation. Meta-analyses have found that CBT is more effective in reducing social anxiety than waiting-list control conditions and that exposure with cognitive restructuring, in particular, is more effective in reducing social anxiety than placebo control conditions (e.g., Fedoroff & Taylor, 2001). Although one of the most widely studied CBT interventions is conducted in a group format (Heimberg & Becker, 2002), it is also efficacious when delivered in individual formats (Stangier, Heidenreich, Peitz, Lauterbach, & Clark, 2003). However, these CBT protocols have yet to be evaluated in samples of pregnant and postpartum women.

Recall the case of Lily from Chapter 5. Lily avoided interaction with friends and colleagues for fear that she would have nothing interesting to contribute to conversation.

> As stated in Chapter 5, Lily chose not to seek treatment for social anxiety disorder, but she used a self-help book that helped her to acquire cognitive behavioral strategies to manage social anxiety. She learned to identify instances in which she assumes that others are thinking negatively of her (i.e., mind reading) and developed an awareness that she takes these assumptions as fact, when she has little evidence to support them. She began to get perspective on these thoughts by identifying the likelihood that others have formed negative opinions of her, and if they have, whether their opinions are indicative of everyone else's opinions. Lily also constructed a schedule of exposure exercises, beginning with situations that caused moderate distress and working toward situations that were very difficult for her. The first exposure exercise that she undertook was to contact a coworker with whom she was close to arrange a lunch date. Contrary to her prediction, this coworker expressed delight that Lily had gotten in touch with her, and when they met for lunch, Lily was pleasantly surprised that this woman asked many questions about the baby.

Other exposures completed by Lily included meeting her law school friends at their monthly gathering, surprising a large group of coworkers by showing up at a happy hour, and bringing the baby into the office. In all of these instances, Lily took care to remain in each situation until her anxiety subsided, and she used her cognitive restructuring tools to evaluate and modify any negative thoughts that had no evidence to support them.

CBT for Specific Phobia

The gold standard treatment for specific phobia is exposure therapy, in which patients are systematically confronted in vivo with the feared stimulus (L. Magee et al., 2009; Van Ameringen, Mancini, & Patterson, 2009; Wolitzky-Taylor, Horowitz, Powers, & Telch, 2008). Exposure therapy has the potential to be a bit more difficult with a woman with a specific phobia of childbirth than with people who have other specific phobias, as it occurs on only a single occasion; thus, exposure to actual childbirth cannot take place on multiple trials across the course of several sessions, nor can it be practiced in between sessions as a homework assignment. Clinicians who conduct exposure therapy with women who report clinically significant fears of childbirth must be creative in designing exposures. For example, they could conduct vivid imaginal exposures of the sequence of events that occur throughout the various stages of labor and delivery. They also could conduct in vivo exposures by having phobic women talk with other mothers about their birth experiences and view graphic movies of childbirth. The aim of these creative exposures is to create circumstances that are as relevant as possible to childbirth so that the anxiety reduction achieved during exposures will generalize to the actual experience of childbirth.

In addition to exposure therapy, it can be helpful to implement a cognitive behavioral approach to pain management. The majority of CBT protocols for pain management are targeted toward chronic pain, rather than acute pain associated with an event such as labor. Nevertheless, some strategies that are typically included in these protocols, such as controlled breathing, relaxation, and guided imagery, are taught to women in birthing classes as they prepare for labor and delivery. As stated in the Introduction, results from one of my studies suggest that women's confidence in their ability to use these techniques during labor partially accounts for the amount of pain that they report when they are in the midst of labor (Larsen, O'Hara, Brewer, & Wenzel, 2001). Thus, pregnant women with a specific phobia of childbirth could work with their therapist to hone these strategies and ensure that they can be accessed in times of stress and pain. Moreover, cognitive restructuring would likely be a useful strategy for clinicians to use with phobic pregnant women to identify, evaluate, and modify catastrophic thoughts (e.g., "I will die," "Labor will go on forever").

Recall the case of Samantha from Chapter 6, whose specific phobia of childbirth was interfering with consistent attendance at her prenatal visits.

> Samantha began working with a cognitive behavioral therapist with she was 7 months pregnant. The early sessions were 2 hr long, rather than the typical 50 min, and occurred twice a week to facilitate intensive exposure to the events that occur during childbirth. They watched home videos of some of Samantha's relatives who recorded the births of their children and documentaries of childbirth produced by The Learning Channel. At the beginning of each exposure, her therapist obtained a Subjective Unit of Discomfort rating, and he continued to obtain ratings throughout the exposure to monitor the degree to which Samantha's anxiety decreased. Furthermore, her therapist coached her in using controlled breathing as she viewed these depictions of birth. He also worked with Samantha to develop tools so that she could catch herself when she began to make catastrophic predictions about horrible things happening during labor and delivery. She became armed with statistics showing that the majority of deliveries occur with no complications as well as knowledge of typical complications that do occur and the ease with which they can be handled by medical staff. After 6 weeks of twice-weekly exposures, although she continued to report higher than average anxiety and fear about childbirth, Samantha's avoidance behavior decreased substantially, and she attended all of the weekly prenatal appointments that were scheduled for the last month of her pregnancy.

CBT for Posttraumatic Stress Disorder

There are a variety of CBT interventions for PTSD, most of which involve the two main components of exposure and cognitive restructuring (Riggs & Foa, 2009). Exposure can proceed in a number of ways, including writing about the trauma, using imaginal exposure to relive the trauma, and practicing in vivo exposure to environmental cues that trigger distress or memories of the trauma. Cognitive restructuring focuses on maladaptive thoughts and beliefs about the trauma, themselves, or the world. Some CBT protocols also include psychoeducation, relaxation, and breathing strategies. Empirical research that compared different CBT interventions has generally found no difference between those that primarily use exposure strategies and those that primarily use cognitive strategies (e.g., Marks, Lovell, Noshirvani, Livanou, & Thrasher, 1998). However, Riggs and Foa (2009) suggested that the combination of in vivo and imaginal exposure is essential in the treatment of PTSD and that treatments that combine exposure and cognitive restructuring are just as efficacious as those that use exposure alone.

Twohig and O'Donohue (2007) described the successful application of exposure therapy to treat PTSD in a woman who was in her 3rd trimester of pregnancy, with no adverse effects on the health of the patient or the baby. The trauma of focus in this treatment was not a difficult childbirth experience, but this case report demonstrated that exposure therapy was safe and effective in a pregnant women. Moreover, Ayers, McKenzie-McHarg, and Eagle (2007) described the successful application of in vivo exposure, imaginal exposure, and cognitive restructuring exercises in two cases of women who had been diagnosed with childbirth-related PTSD.

Recall the case of Kellie from Chapter 6. She experienced a number of stressors surrounding the birth of her third child, most notably an instance in which medical staff exclaimed that the baby was not breathing but would not give her more information about her newborn's health.

> As stated in Chapter 6, Kellie was not treated with CBT for PTSD because there were no qualified therapists in the surrounding area. Had she worked with a therapist who used this approach, she would have engaged in several exposure exercises. To help Kellie overcome her fear and avoidance, the therapist would have accompanied her back to the hospital where she gave birth. She would have led Kellie through a number of imaginal exposure exercises to relive the birth experience. Through cognitive restructuring, she and her therapist would have identified the central beliefs that maintain and exacerbate her symptoms, such as "I am ineffective" and "I don't deserve to be treated well." Together, these exercises would have reduced her anxious arousal and the self-deprecating thoughts that prevented her from being assertive in a number of areas of her life, such as with insensitive medical staff, her extended family, her children, or her estranged husband.

Efficacy

There is preliminary evidence that CBT has the potential to be efficacious in reducing various manifestations of anxiety in pregnant and postpartum women. To date, four studies have examined the degree to which anxiety symptoms in childbearing women decrease after participating in a trial of CBT. Because each of the CBT interventions in these studies was unique, I describe the design, components of the CBT intervention, and outcome in each of these studies.

In one study (Milgrom, Negri, Gemmill, McNeil, Martin, 2005), 192 depressed postpartum women were randomly assigned to one of four conditions: (a) CBT group, (b) group counseling, (c) individual counseling, or (d) routine primary care. Women in all three active therapy conditions participated in nine weekly 90-min sessions and an additional three sessions with their partners. The CBT intervention focused on relaxation, engagement in pleasant activities, and time management. The group and individual counseling interventions focused on supportive listening, history taking, problem clarification, goal formation, and problem solving. Women in the primary care condition received routine case management by a maternal and child health nurse, who referred them for additional services in the community when appropriate. Results indicated that women's Beck Anxiety Inventory (BAI; A. T. Beck & Steer, 1990) scores declined significantly and to a similar degree in all three psychotherapy groups. Thus, CBT was efficacious in reducing physical and emotional symptoms of anxiety in depressed postpartum women, although it did not outperform supportive psychotherapy conditions.

Austin et al. (2008) recruited 191 at-risk women who were at the end of their 1st trimester of pregnancy and randomly assigned them to the CBT intervention or a control condition. Women assigned to the CBT condition participated in six weekly 2-hr CBT group sessions that focused on behavioral strategies for managing stress, anxiety, and depression associated with pregnancy and the early postpartum period. Women assigned to the control condition received an information booklet that described risk factors and triggers for postpartum mood disturbance, strategies to manage postpartum distress, and resources that they could access. Results indicated that 28% of those in the CBT group met diagnostic criteria for an anxiety disorder during pregnancy, a value that dropped to 18% at approximately 2 months postpartum and 16% at approximately 4 months postpartum. However, this decline was not statistically significant, nor was it different from the decline in anxiety disorder diagnoses in the control group. The mean State-Trait Anxiety Inventory (Spielberger, Gorsuch, & Lushene, 1970) score declined slightly in the women who participated in the CBT group, but it remained stable in the women who were assigned to the control condition.

Griffiths and Barker-Collo (2008) recruited a small sample (N = 45) of pregnant and postpartum women who were regarded as having antenatal adjustment problems to participate in eight twice weekly 2-hr group CBT sessions. Unlike the other studies reviewed in this section, there was no control group. The CBT intervention consisted of psychoeducation, relaxation, stress management, communication training, decision making, problem solving, and relapse prevention. Scores on the BAI dropped significantly from pre- to posttreatment. Specifically, 35% of the sample fell in the moderate or severe range on this measure at the pretreatment assessment, compared with only 17.5% at the posttreatment assessment. Although these results suggest that this type of CBT group is efficacious in reducing physical and emotional symptoms of anxiety, it is limited by the absence of a control condition. Thus, the degree to which CBT was efficacious in reducing anxiety above and beyond the passage of time or a nonspecific attention control condition cannot be determined.

Finally, Misri, Reebye, Corral, and Milis (2004) examined the degree to which the combination of paroxetine and CBT would be more efficacious in reducing symptoms of emotional disturbance than paroxetine alone. They recruited a small sample ($N = 35$) of women diagnosed with moderate to severe major depression and a comorbid anxiety disorder and randomly assigned them to one of these two conditions. Women who received CBT in addition to paroxetine received weekly hour-long sessions for 12 weeks. The CBT intervention was tailored from manuals on depression, anxiety, and eating disorders and focused on education about the interrelation among thoughts, feelings, and behaviors, providing strategies to target each of these areas. Women in both conditions exhibited similar reductions in anxiety symptoms, as measured by the Hamilton Rating Scale for Anxiety (Hamilton, 1959) and the Yale-Brown Obsessive Compulsive Scale (Goodman, Price, Rasmussen, Mazure, Fleischman, et al., 1989; Goodman, Price, Rasmussen, Mazure, Delgado, et al., 1989).

Collectively, results from these studies suggest that women who participate in a trial of CBT during late pregnancy or during the postpartum period can expect to experience reductions in anxiety symptoms. However, at present there is no evidence to suggest that CBT is more efficacious than other interventions. One factor that might explain the absence of significant differences between groups in the Milgrom et al. (2005) and the Austin et al. (2008) studies is that the control conditions likely incorporated principles of CBT, rendering the two conditions more equivalent than the researchers had intended. Specifically, Milgrom et al.'s counseling intervention incorporated a focus on goal formation and problem solving, which are common strategies used in CBT. The control condition in Austin et al.'s study was an information booklet that described many mood management strategies that were consistent with the cognitive behavioral skills that are targeted in psychotherapy. One could conceptualize the information booklet condition as cognitive behavioral bibliotherapy, which, as is described in Chapter 11, is efficacious in reducing symptoms of emotional distress.

Additional caveats must be considered when interpreting the results of these studies. None of these studies was designed with the sole purpose of evaluating the efficacy of CBT for a particular anxiety disorder in childbearing women. Thus, the interventions did not proceed according to the protocols described earlier in this section. Moreover, most participants in these studies had primary diagnoses of depression, and the purpose of these studies was to examine the degree to which a range of symptoms, only one being anxiety, were reduced by CBT in depressed women. I strongly encourage researchers to conduct efficacy studies with samples of pregnant and postpartum women who have primary diagnoses of anxiety disorders and examine changes in anxiety disorder diagnoses and symptoms as primary dependent variables. I also recommend that researchers evaluate the efficacy of the specific protocols described earlier in this section, as these have the most empirical support for their efficacy in samples of patients with anxiety disorders.

INTERPERSONAL PSYCHOTHERAPY

Interpersonal psychotherapy (IPT) is a brief, time-limited psychotherapy that focuses on problems in interpersonal relationships and their association with mood disturbance (Weissman, Markowitz, & Klerman, 2000). The clinician and patient work actively and collaboratively to identify problematic patterns in current relationships; express affect associated with those patterns; and change maladaptive expectations, communication styles, or other relationship behaviors. Therapeutic work often falls into one of four interpersonal problem areas: (a) grief, (b) role disputes, (c) role transitions, or (d) interpersonal deficits.

Although the majority of empirical research on the efficacy of IPT has focused on patients with depressive disorders, there is preliminary evidence that it is efficacious in the treatment of some anxiety disorders, particularly panic disorder (Lipsitz et al., 2006), social anxiety disorder (Borge et al., 2008; Lipsitz, Markowitz, Cherry, & Fyer, 1999), and PTSD (Bleiberg & Markowitz, 2005; Krupnick et al., 2008; Robertson, Rushton, Batrim, Moore, & Morris, 2007). IPT is an appealing therapeutic approach for use with childbearing women, as they are going through a significant role transition that is often accompanied by role disputes (Weissman et al., 2000). In addition, childbirth can stir up grief about close others who have passed away and who will be unable to play a role in the child's life. Randomized controlled trials indicate that IPT is efficacious in reducing depression during pregnancy (Spinelli & Endicott, 2003) and the postpartum period (O'Hara, Stuart, Gorman, & Wenzel, 2000). In one study (Grote, Bledsoe, Swartz, & Frank, 2004), a brief eight-session adaptation of IPT was associated with a significant reduction in BAI scores posttreatment and at a 6-month follow-up assessment in depressed, low-income patients. In the following sections, I discuss the manner in which IPT might be useful in treating anxiety in childbearing women with panic disorder, social anxiety disorder, and PTSD.

IPT for Panic Disorder

According to Lipsitz et al. (2006), IPT has the potential to be useful in treating panic disorder because many people experience interpersonal conflict, transition, or loss in the time immediately preceding the onset of panic. The birth of a child would certainly fall into the domain of interpersonal transition. In the case of Becca, described in Chapter 4, it appears that problems in her relationship with her husband appeared only after her panic attacks began to cause significant life interference. In other words, interpersonal distress seemed to be a consequence of her anxiety disorder, rather than a cause. I would recommend CBT as the first-line psychotherapeutic approach in these cases, as it has the most empirical evidence that supports its efficacy. However, IPT could be considered an alternative when childbearing women (a) are nonresponsive to CBT, (b) have difficulty implementing the structured CBT homework assignments, (c) have medical issues that contraindicate participation in exposure exercises, (d) develop panic attacks only after it is clear that they are having difficulty transitioning to the role of mother, (e) develop panic attacks only after significant conflict or tension with a close other has escalated, or (f) express a preference for this modality.

IPT for Social Anxiety Disorder

Weissman et al. (2000) noted that IPT is a logical choice to treat social anxiety disorder because a deficit in interpersonal functioning is the core feature of the clinical presentation of most socially anxious patients. Many socially anxious individuals present for treatment when their anxiety intensifies in the midst of a role transition. Some IPT protocols for social anxiety disorder include additional problem areas, such as role insecurity (e.g., lack of assertiveness, conflict avoidance; Lipsitz et al., 1999) and interpersonal sensitivity (e.g., over-interpreting perceived negative communications; Weissman et al., 2000).

IPT would be a logical choice for the case of Lily, described in Chapter 5, as she demonstrated insecurity in her role as a working mother employed at a powerful law firm. Nevertheless, it is important to recognize that although research has demonstrated that IPT is associated with significant reductions in socially anxious symptoms posttreatment (Lipsitz et al., 1999), data have suggested that it does not outperform other modalities of treatment and yields a lower percentage of treatment responders than CBT (Borge et al., 2008; Lipsitz et al., 2008). Thus, I recommend CBT as the first-line psychotherapeutic approach for social anxiety disorder but would consider IPT as an alternative when childbearing women (a) are nonresponsive to CBT, (b) have difficulty implementing the structured CBT homework assignments, or (c) express a preference for this modality.

IPT for Posttraumatic Stress Disorder

Bleiberg and Markowitz (2005) adapted IPT for PTSD, with the rationale that (a) many patients find exposure-based therapies aversive, which can deter them from seeking treatment; (b) IPT is a treatment that focuses on life events, and PTSD is a disorder that stems from life events; and (c) people with PTSD often exhibit interpersonal difficulties, such as problems trusting others and establishing boundaries. In their sample of 13 patients, symptoms in all three clusters (i.e., reexperiencing, avoidance and numbing, increased arousal) decreased significantly 14 weeks following baseline. In the only study comparing IPT with a control condition, Krupnick et al. (2008) found that IPT was more efficacious than a waiting-list control condition in reducing posttraumatic stress and depressive symptoms and in improving scores on scales of interpersonal sensitivity, need for social approval, lack of sociability, and interpersonal ambivalence in low-income women who had experienced a sexual assault. The rate of patients no longer receiving a diagnosis of PTSD posttreatment was similar to rates obtained in studies examining the efficacy of CBT. However, Robertson et al. (2007) found that an 8-week group adaptation for patients with PTSD was associated with a reduction in avoidance but not reexperiencing or arousal symptoms, although it appeared to facilitate improvement in psychosocial functioning and general psychological distress.

Kellie, whose case was described in Chapter 6, might have benefitted from IPT because she had significant interpersonal problems with her children, estranged husband, and extended family members. Krupnick et al. (2008) noted that IPT was especially useful in helping women to identify feelings and behaviors that contribute to interpersonal problems, recognize the tendency to isolate socially, and avoid revictimization by becoming involved with others who are abusive. All of these themes are relevant to Kellie's clinical presentation. Although data from at least two of the three empirical studies are encouraging, it should be acknowledged that there is a more extensive body of literature with studies using much larger sample sizes that support the efficacy of CBT for PTSD. Thus, I recommend CBT as the first-line psychotherapeutic approach for PTSD but would consider IPT as an alternative when childbearing women (a) are nonresponsive to CBT; (b) have difficulty implementing the structured CBT homework assignments; (c) express a preference for this modality; or (d) describe interpersonal impairment as their primary problem, rather than symptoms of reexperiencing, avoidance and numbing, or increased arousal.

DEBRIEFING AND SUPPORTIVE COUNSELING

Substantial attention has been given to the efficacy of debriefing and supportive counseling, particularly in women who have had difficult childbirths (e.g., those who required emergency cesarean sections). *Debriefing* is an opportunity for people who have gone through a traumatic experience to describe their experience in detail and express their feelings about it in the days following the traumatic experience. However, most research on samples of people who have gone through various traumas has shown that debriefing is not helpful in preventing later emotional disturbances, and that, at times, it is associated with a later increase in psychiatric symptoms (Wessely & Deahl, 2003).

The research on debriefing and supportive counseling specifically with women who have undergone traumatic birth experiences is also mixed. Components of debriefing in these studies include (a) supportive listening, (b) encouraging emotional expression, (c) answering questions, (d) encouraging women to utilize their social support system, (e) reinforcing adaptive coping strategies, and (f) identifying solutions for emotional distress (Gamble & Creedy, 2004; Gamble et al., 2005). Results from some studies suggest that women receiving debriefing and supportive counseling following a traumatic childbirth report fewer posttraumatic stress symptoms, less depression, and less self-blame in the postpartum period than women receiving standard postpartum care (Gamble et al., 2005; Lavender & Walkinshaw, 1998; Ryding, Wijma, & Wijma, 1998a). However, results from other studies suggest that debriefing and supportive counseling are not associated with a reduction in posttraumatic stress or depressive symptoms (Priest, Henderson, Evans, & Hagan, 2003; Ryding, Wirén, Johansson, Ceder, & Dahlström, 2004), and one study reported that it is associated with nonsignificant elevations in psychiatric symptoms (Small, Lumley, Donohue, Potter, & Waldenström, 2000). Interestingly, in these latter studies, a substantial majority of the women perceived these interventions to be helpful.

Gamble et al. (2005) speculated that debriefing is most effective when two factors are in place. First, they suggested that it should be offered only to women who perceived that their health or their baby's health was in danger and experienced fear, horror, or helplessness (i.e., Criterion A for a diagnosis of PTSD). These are the women at greatest risk of developing psychiatric symptoms in the postpartum period, and they might benefit from an intervention that will help them to gain an accurate perspective on the events that they experienced. Second, they suggested that more than one debriefing session should be offered, as women might not have fully processed the traumatic experience in the first few days following childbirth, the time at which many debriefing interventions take place (Gamble & Creedy, 2004).

At present, the empirical literature does not support the use of a systematic debriefing or supportive counseling intervention for women who had difficult childbirths. It is possible that focusing to such a large degree on the course of events associated with the difficult childbirth would actually retraumatize the woman (cf. Wessely & Deahl, 2003), or that women who undergo a traumatic childbirth are experiencing numbing symptoms to the degree that they cannot benefit from debriefing in the days following childbirth. If women desire to discuss their childbirth experiences postdelivery, it is recommended that the health care professional with whom they are talking (a) be one who was involved with the delivery, and (b) provide an opportunity to discuss the positive aspects of the delivery as well as the negative aspects. According to Boyce and Condon (2000), focusing solely on the negative aspects of delivery pathologizes the experience and could lay the groundwork for distorting their recollections of the experience in the future, which could interfere with normal adaptation during the postpartum period.

OTHER THERAPEUTIC CONSIDERATIONS

Some scholar–clinicians in the field have advanced other considerations in conducting psychotherapy with anxious pregnant and postpartum women. Although these recommendations are not incorporated into a formal school of psychotherapy, they may nevertheless be helpful for clinicians to keep in mind when working with this population.

Education

The provision of education allows childbearing women to have access to factual information about the risks and procedures associated with pregnancy, labor, delivery, and beyond. It also allows women to ask questions that are relevant to their personal situation and gather information to dispel unrealistic worries. Many scholar–clinicians strongly urge health care professionals to give as much information to women as possible so that women can form accurate expectations for their progression through gestation and the course of events that they will experience during childbirth. For example, Glazer (1980) suggested that nurses and midwives should educate pregnant women about normal fetal growth and development. In addition, she suggested that health care providers should discuss the fetus's continued growth at each prenatal visit, informing women of height measurements, fetal heart rate, and weight gain. Because her research demonstrated that anxiety and concern about fetal well-being increase significantly in the 3rd trimester, she encouraged health care professionals to take extra time to address the concerns and associated anxiety during this time period. Moreover, women who report traumatic childbirth experiences have indicated that their expectations were violated and that they had much less control over the experience than they thought they would (Allen, 1998). When they were not informed of what was happening, they assumed that something was going wrong. Thus, education about the course of labor and delivery, the complications that might arise, and the typical procedures invoked to address complications should be reviewed carefully with women during their 3rd trimester (Olde, van der Hart, Kleber, & van Son, 2006).

It is equally important for mental health professionals who work with anxious childbearing women to provide psychoeducation about their symptoms and the course of psychotherapeutic intervention in ways that are understandable. Clinicians should communicate a conceptualization of patients' clinical presentation that incorporates genetic, biological, and psychological vulnerabilities, as well as the life stress that they are experiencing. Emphasis on the importance of receiving treatment for a perinatal anxiety disorder should be balanced with normalization of the difficulties that often accompany the transition to parenthood. Before proceeding with treatment, clinicians should describe what therapy will involve, the activities in which they will engage in session, and a flexible estimation of the time it will take to see some improvement in symptoms. Women should be encouraged to ask questions about the treatment to determine whether it is a good match for them. Psychoeducation is one part of the CBT and IPT protocols described earlier in this chapter.

Self-Care Strategies

It is crucial that childbearing women engage in adequate self-care across the transition to parenthood in order to give themselves the best chance to manage the physical and emotional stress associated with childbirth. Common self-care targets include the reduction of caffeine, implementation of healthy sleep hygiene strategies, provision of time for relaxation, and healthy eating (Ross & McLean, 2006). Of course, many of these things are easier said than done when a new mother is nursing her infant every 2 hr. Clinicians should brainstorm ways to implement as regular a schedule as possible and identify solutions to potential obstacles. When necessary, partners can be brought into treatment so that they can be educated about the importance of self-care and commit to supporting the new mother in any way that they can.

PRACTICAL IMPLICATIONS

Aside from the study described by Barnett and Parker (1985) over 20 years ago, no empirical research has been conducted specifically to evaluate the efficacy of psychotherapy in reducing anxiety in a sample of anxious pregnant or postpartum women. The few studies that have examined the efficacy of CBT or IPT for depressed childbearing women have indicated that these therapeutic approaches significantly reduce anxiety from pre- to posttreatment, though not to a greater degree than a comparison intervention. What is needed are studies that (a) recruit samples of pregnant or postpartum women who are diagnosed with *Diagnostic and Statistical Manual of Mental Disorders* (4th ed., text revision;

American Psychiatric Association, 2000) anxiety disorders; (b) implement the well-established protocols described in this chapter; (c) include a comparison intervention that does not overlap with the psychotherapeutic approach under investigation; and (d) administer standard measures of anxiety symptoms, the scores of which will serve as the primary dependent variables to be analyzed.

I recommend that clinicians adopt evidence-based treatments for perinatal anxiety disorders. Psychotherapeutic approaches such as CBT and IPT are active and collaborative, which would work well for childbearing women who hope to obtain immediate relief from their symptoms. At present, the greatest body of empirical research supports the use of CBT with anxiety disorder patients, and for the most part, there is nothing to suggest that CBT would be contraindicated in pregnant and postpartum women. The one exception might be the implementation of interoceptive exposure with pregnant women who suffer from panic disorder, as this exercise involves the intentional provocation of physical symptoms that resemble panic and that in rare cases might cause a pregnancy complication. However, there are circumstances in which IPT might be considered as an alternative treatment, such as instances in which a woman is nonresponsive to CBT or when the conceptualization of clinical presentation clearly indicates that interpersonal dysfunction precipitated the onset of anxiety. One advantage of IPT is that it has been used successfully with many samples of depressed childbearing women, so we know it is well received by women as they transition to parenthood.

In contrast, the literature on debriefing after a difficult childbirth is mixed at best, and there is evidence with samples of people who have been exposed to different traumas that it has the potential to be harmful. It is logical that some women who have gone through a difficult childbirth will want to talk with a health care professional about their experience soon thereafter. In these cases, a health care professional who was involved in the delivery should meet with them, taking care to attend to their concerns with respect and sensitivity as well as to focus on the positive aspects of the delivery so that women leave with as balanced a perspective as is possible.

Perhaps the most important point clinicians must keep in mind when conducting psychotherapy with pregnant and postpartum women is that they are vulnerable, overwhelmed, and unsure of themselves. They are often desperate for validation that they are good mothers and wives, and in many instances their symptoms are so foreign that they do not recognize themselves (Kleiman, 2009). Regardless of the theoretical framework a clinician adopts as he or she proceeds with psychotherapy, attention to the therapeutic relationship is imperative in order to create a safe, validating environment for the childbearing woman to work through her struggles with anxiety.

11

SELF-HELP RESOURCES
FOR PERINATAL ANXIETY

Although many childbearing women wish to seek professional help for their distress, they often face barriers as they attempt to follow through with doing so. In my practice, two major obstacles that postpartum women face in attending regular psychotherapy sessions are lack of available time and lack of child care. This clinical observation is supported by the fact that some intervention studies examining psychosocial treatments for postpartum emotional distress suffer from significant attrition (e.g., 52%; Austin et al., 2008). Thus, it is sensible that women who experience perinatal anxiety would benefit from self-help resources that provide education and specific strategies to manage distress without requiring travel to a health care professional's office. Much of the existing self-help materials fall under the label of *bibliotherapy*, defined as written materials, computer or Internet programs, and or audio- or videotaped materials for addressing specific problems that a person might experience or for meeting therapeutic needs (Marrs, 1995).

Professionals who recommend bibliotherapy to any patient, including childbearing women, must be aware of the advantages and disadvantages of this approach to treatment and clearly articulate these to their patient. According to Rosen (1987), advantages of these self-help materials are that they (a) can reach a large number of people, (b) are cost-effective, (c) allow people to address problems and issues on their own without the reliance on a trained professional, and (d) provide education that can in turn prevent the exacerbation of mental illness. However, there are also drawbacks to many self-help materials. Use of self-help resources requires focused attention and consistent practice, and there is a chance that users might not implement the intervention strategies effectively. The vast majority of self-help resources have not been evaluated empirically, which means there are few data that can speak to their efficacy. Moreover, many authors of self-help resources exaggerate claims of their effectiveness, promising that people will be "cured" if they follow the self-help program (Rosen, 1987).

How, then, does a professional know which books to recommend, and how does a consumer know which books to select? Recently, Redding, Herbert, Forman, and Gaudiano (2008) rated the top 50 best-selling self-help books for depression, anxiety, and posttraumatic stress on Amazon.com on the basis of their overall usefulness as well as the degree to which the books (a) were grounded in psychological science, (b) offered reasonable expectations to the reader, (c) provided specific (vs. vague or general) guidance, and (d) offered suggestions that had the potential to be harmful. The characteristics of the books that they regarded as being of the highest quality included the following: (a) the self-help resource has a cognitive behavioral orientation or is otherwise grounded in psychological theory and research; (b) the primary author is a recognized mental health professional; (c) the primary author holds a doctoral degree; (d) one or more specific problems are targeted, rather than general distress or multiple problems; (e) the self-help resource does not include claims that are too good to be true; and (f) guidelines for monitoring progress and seeking professional help are provided. The full list of books is included in their article. Although no books on managing perinatal distress were included in this sample, Redding et al.'s guidelines have the potential to provide helpful guidance for professionals and consumers who are recommending or purchasing self-help resources.

SELF-HELP RESOURCES FOR ANXIETY DISORDERS

Some scholars have evaluated the efficacy of self-help resources specifically for anxiety disorders. Although the self-help resources evaluated in these studies are not geared toward perinatal anxiety disorders, results from these studies identify the factors that increase the likelihood that self-help programs for perinatal anxiety disorders will be effective. Results from qualitative and quantitative reviews suggest that self-help treatments for anxiety are more effective than waiting-list control and placebo control conditions, although they are less effective than treatments delivered face-to-face by a mental health professional (Hirai & Clum, 2006; Newman, Erickson, Przeworski, & Dzus,

2003). These reviews indicate that people who participate in self-help programs for the treatment of anxiety disorders are more likely to be successful if they (a) find the treatment credible, (b) are motivated, (c) are accountable to someone for this progress (e.g., a spouse or partner), (d) spend a longer amount of time with the self-help materials, and (e) have at least minimal contact with a mental health professional to provide support and guidance (Newman, Erickson, Przeworski, & Dzus, 2003; van Boeijen et al., 2005). Self-help programs seem to be most effective in the treatment of specific phobias (Newman, Erickson, et al., 2003), panic disorder (Carlbring, Westling, & Andersson, 2000; Hirai & Clum, 2006), and social anxiety disorder (Abramowitz, Moore, Braddock, & Harrington, 2008), although in some cases more than half of the participants still score in the dysfunctional range on the measure of relevant anxiety symptoms when they are evaluated posttreatment. In contrast, few studies have examined the effectiveness of self-help programs in the treatment of generalized anxiety disorder (GAD), posttraumatic stress disorder (PTSD), and obsessive–compulsive disorder (OCD).

One implication of this body of literature is that if childbearing women with anxiety disorders hope to acquire strategies to manage their anxiety, then it is preferable for them to meet face-to-face with a mental health professional. However, following a self-help program is preferable to doing nothing. For those who opt to use a self-help program, having minimal contact with a mental health professional to provide support and guidance will increase the probability of success. Nevertheless, childbearing women who do not have access to a mental health professional to provide support and guidance can still attain significant symptom reduction through a self-help program by staying motivated and spending as much quality time as possible on the self-help exercises.

MAXIMIZING THE EFFECTIVENESS OF SELF-HELP RESOURCES

In addition to determining the most appropriate self-help resources to consult, consumers often have questions about the most appropriate ways to use the materials. In this section, I provide suggestions for maximizing the effectiveness of self-help materials.

- *Set aside time on a regular basis to read and use the self-help material.* This suggestion will undoubtedly be challenging for women who are adjusting to parenting a newborn child. However, the importance of persistent exposure to the self-help material cannot be understated. The challenges of new motherhood will already create circumstances that are not optimal for the retention of unfamiliar material because of sleep deprivation, high stress, and a newborn whose needs must be addressed as soon as the mother is aware of them. Spending time with the self-help material on a daily basis will help new mothers retain important concepts, see a thread that relates the material they read at previous sittings with material they are reading that day, and have the opportunity to implement mood management strategies in their lives sooner rather than later. Childbearing women who use self-help resources are encouraged to talk with their partners or other family members to identify an opportunity each day in which they can read the material without having to supervise their newborn or other children.

- *Determine whether the material needs to be read sequentially or as relevant.* When a person is tired, stressed, and struggling with symptoms of anxiety and depression, it is tempting to "cut corners" and jump to the most relevant chapters of self-help books. However, this strategy may or may not be the most effective way to use the self-help resource. If a book is meant to be read sequentially, a person who jumps to the most interesting or relevant chapter will risk not being able to fully understand or appreciate it because it assumes that the reader knows the definitions of concepts introduced earlier in the book. At the beginning of many self-help books, there is a guide for the reader that will specify whether it is intended to be read sequentially or whether chapters can be read out of order. Childbearing women are strongly encouraged to follow the approach suggested by the author to maximize the effectiveness of the self-help resource.

- *Read actively.* New material is almost always retained to a greater degree when it is read actively rather than passively. Active reading means that the individual engages in behaviors such as underlining, highlighting, taking notes, and/or writing personally relevant comments in the margins. Not only will this approach help a new mother stay actively engaged with the material, it will also help her identify the points that are most relevant to the symptoms that she is experiencing and allow her to remember these points the next time she experiences distress.

- *Complete the suggested exercises.* All too often, people who use self-help resources will skip suggested exercises because they attach a negative judgment to them—they view the exercise as silly, they predict that the exercise will not be helpful, or they dismiss the exercise as requiring too much time and effort. Childbearing women who use self-help materials are strongly encouraged to keep an open mind, suspend their preconceived expectations, and complete the suggested exercises. Studies that have evaluated the efficacy of self-help resources base their conclusions on the assumption that readers complete the entire program. The goal is to maximize the number of mood management strategies that are available to new mothers so that they can evaluate the strategies that are most effective on the basis of their experiences with implementing them.

- *Use accompanying audio- or videotaped materials.* The rationale for this suggestion is similar to the rationale for the suggestion to complete the exercises included in the written self-help materials—that it is important for childbearing women to be exposed to and practice the full array of strategies for managing anxiety and depression before drawing a conclusion about the strategies that work best for them. In fact, there is a strong possibility that new mothers will respond particularly well to audio- and/or videotaped materials because they often provide sensory soothing and an opportunity to learn strategies to manage distress through experiential means, rather than through reading and retaining written information. Many new mothers find that listening to and/or watching audio- or videotaped materials provides a pleasurable break from the stress of caring for a newborn.

- *Discuss the reading and exercises with a trusted individual.* One way to promote retention and understanding of new material is to present what one has learned to another individual and engage in discussion about it. Thus, childbearing women are encouraged to talk about the self-help material with a trusted individual, such as their partner, a close friend, a close family member, or another new mother. Such discussion has the potential to illustrate specific ways in which the new mother can use the self-help strategies in her daily life and may even uncover new, related strategies or potential obstacles for which she might be vigilant in implementing the strategies on her own. In addition, sharing what she has learned from the self-help material with a trusted individual has the potential create a partnership in which the other individual can check in with her from time to time and help ensure that she stays on track.

- *Do not hesitate to contact a professional.* One danger of using a self-help resource is that a person may not seek appropriate professional help when her clinical presentation clearly indicates that she should do so. High-quality self-help resources usually include guidance on when it is relevant to contact a professional for help. Women who have many of the characteristics of those who are recommended to seek professional help are strongly encouraged to do so, as their symptoms may require a multimodal approach to treatment (e.g., psychotherapy and psychotropic medications) or a greater intensity of treatment (e.g., twice-weekly sessions with a mental health professional). For example, women who are suicidal or who are exhibiting symptoms consistent with a postpartum psychotic episode should always contact a mental health professional as soon as possible, rather than try to resolve their symptoms through a self-help resource. There are other reasons for childbearing women who use self-help materials to consult with professionals. Contacting a professional would be appropriate in instances in which women diligently use self-help materials and practice suggested strategies, but their symptoms do not improve or worsen after several weeks. In addition, it is appropriate to contact a professional when much of the material is not understandable or seems too difficult to implement. There are several self-help resources that are, in fact, meant to be read in conjunction with seeing a professional (Redding et al., 2008).

- *Read online reviews of the self-help material.* Admittedly, there are advantages and disadvantages of reading online reviews. For example, one disadvantage is that the reviews are not truly representative of the experiences of the full sample of people who have used the self-help material—those who post reviews tend to be either quite satisfied with the material or quite unsatisfied. Thus, it is important for readers of online reviews to keep this in mind as they evaluate the reviews. Nevertheless, online reviews can be helpful because people often explain the specific manner in which the self-help material benefitted them. Not only does this instill hope in a person who has just purchased or otherwise accessed the self-help resource, but it also provides useful tips for maximizing the effectiveness of the material. Moreover, people who submit online reviews often reference other self-help material that was helpful for them, which provides additional resources for new mothers to consult.

- *Do not expect immediate relief.* Finally, it is important for new mothers to have accurate expectations for what the self-help material can and cannot provide, as well as the time frame in which they can expect to see some change. Many new mothers are in such distress that they want immediate relief (Kleiman, 2009). Most other treatment modalities take some time for effects to be noticed; for example, people who take selective serotonin reuptake inhibitors (see Chapter 9, this volume) often do not notice changes until the medications have taken some time to build up in their system (i.e.,

2–8 weeks). It usually takes even longer for people to notice the effects of psychotherapeutic approaches, such as cognitive behavioral therapy (CBT). There is no reason to expect that self-help approaches would take less time for their effects to be noticed, and in fact, it might take longer for them to be noticed because they are not accompanied by some of the nonspecific ingredients of change associated with seeing a professional in person, such as a sound therapeutic relationship (Horvath & Symonds, 1991). Nevertheless, research has shown that self-help approaches are indeed effective in reducing symptoms of anxiety and depression, so it will be important for childbearing women to formulate the expectation that symptom relief is expected but probably will only be attained after several weeks of consistent reading and practicing of the mood-management skills.

SELF-HELP RESOURCES FOR PERINATAL ANXIETY DISORDERS

In this section, I describe a number of self-help resources that professionals can recommend to women who experience perinatal anxiety. I do not provide a comprehensive review of each book, but I highlight some of the aspects of each book that would be particularly relevant to pregnant and postpartum women who are experiencing troubling anxiety symptoms. This list is not exhaustive, as self-help resources are continually published and revised. Nevertheless, these resources should provide a starting point for women who suffer with perinatal anxiety to consult. In general, I recommend that when consumers purchase resources on emotional disturbances associated with the transition to parenthood, they should take the time to ensure that the resource covers anxiety, specifically, in addition to depression.

Becoming a Calm Mom: How to Manage Stress and Enjoy the First Year of Motherhood (Deborah Roth Ledley; American Psychological Association, 2009)

Ledley is an expert clinician and researcher who specializes in anxiety disorders and who brought her strong training in CBT to the management of postpartum anxiety. In the early chapters, she describes six cognitive behaviorally based strategies for managing postpartum anxiety: (a) restructuring unhelpful thoughts, (b) changing behavioral responses to meet goals, (c) communicating assertively, (d) making sound decisions, (e) using breathing and relaxation, and (f) attending to relationships. In subsequent chapters, she applies these six anxiety management strategies to parenting; self-care; the decision to go back to work; and partner, family, and friend relationships.

Although the book is geared toward postpartum mothers, pregnant women may wish to read this book in order to hone their skills to manage postpartum distress. Ledley has developed a website (http://www.thecalmmom.com/) as a companion to the book, which includes tips for new mothers that pertain to caring for their newborns, taking care of themselves, and maintaining a healthy relationship with their partners. It also contains information about "hot topics" relevant to postpartum anxiety.

Beyond the Blues: A Guide to Understanding and Treating Prenatal and Postpartum Depression (Shoshana S. Bennett and Pec Indman; Moodswings Press, 2006)

Bennett, a clinical psychologist, founded Postpartum Assistance for mothers and is a former president of Postpartum Support International. Following the birth of her first child, she struggled with postpartum OCD. Indman is a marriage and family therapy counselor whose practice specializes in perinatal depression and anxiety. They differentiate among depression and the various manifestation of perinatal anxiety, including OCD, panic disorder, and PTSD, providing descriptions, identifying risk factors, and describing cases of these various perinatal emotional disturbances and their treatment. In addition, the authors provide tips for self-care. They answer frequently asked questions about the course of perinatal psychiatric illness, breastfeeding and infant attachment, medication use while breastfeeding, and ways to communicate their struggles to close others. They include chapters for partners as well as a chapter written specifically for various health care professionals who might be working with postpartum women. Moreover, they provide an extensive list of books, articles, organizations, and websites to consult for more information. Advantages of this book are that the authors recognize anxiety as well as depression, cover emotional disturbances in both pregnancy and the postpartum period, and present their information in a very brief, easy-to-read format. Its disadvantage is that the book might not contain enough information for women to truly understand the nature of their perinatal emotional disturbance, which will necessitate that they consult other sources. Thus, this book might be most useful as an introduction to postpartum emotional disturbance that can help women identify the specific type of follow-up information that would be most helpful for them to seek.

Overcoming Postpartum Depression and Anxiety (Linda Sebastian; Addicus Books, 1998)

Sebastian is a psychiatric nurse who specializes in working with postpartum women with emotional disturbances. She devotes an entire chapter to anxiety disorders in this book and includes many chapters that pertain to both anxiety and depression, including a discussion of various types of mental health professionals who provide psychotherapy with postpartum women, medications, and the course of recovery. There is also a chapter geared specifically toward fathers and families. The advantages and disadvantages of this book are similar to those associated with the Bennett and Indman (2006) book—it provides basic information in easy-to-understand language, but women who want more specific information might need to consult additional sources.

Pregnancy Blues: What Every Woman Needs to Know About Depression During Pregnancy (Shaila Mulkarni Misri; Bantam Dell, 2005)

Misri is a psychiatrist and clinical professor of psychiatry and obstetrics and gynecology at the University of British Columbia. She is also the founder and director of Reproductive Mental Health Program at two hospitals in Vancouver, British Columbia, Canada. Some of her scholarly work was cited in Chapters 2 and 10. Misri includes an easy-to-understand discussion of the neurochemical changes associated with pregnancy that have an impact on emotional disturbances as well as a chapter that summarizes the research on the effects of maternal stress and anxiety on the baby. She includes a chapter on emotional disturbances other than depression, including anxiety disorders, and a discussion on the use of psychotropic medications during pregnancy and lactation. Moreover, she includes chapters outlining options for treatment that weigh the advantages and disadvantages of various treatment modalities. The main focus of this book is on providing information to childbearing women who are struggling with emotional disturbances, rather than on providing strategies for managing perinatal psychiatric symptoms. Nevertheless, this book stands out because it includes a discussion of cultural factors and other background variables (e.g., marital violence, history of infertility) that exacerbate the risk of perinatal emotional distress. Women who are seeking information that is based on scientific research will appreciate this resource.

The Pregnancy and Postpartum Anxiety Workbook: Practical Skills to Help You Overcome Anxiety, Worry, Panic Attacks, Obsessions, and Compulsions (Pamela S. Wiegartz and Kevin L. Gyoerkoe; New Harbinger, 2009)

Wiegartz and Gyoerkoe are experts in anxiety disorders and CBT; thus, it is no surprise that this book includes an array of cognitive and behavioral strategies to manage anxiety symptoms that occur during pregnancy and the postpartum period. Specifically, it describes the application of relaxation, cognitive restructuring, exposure, and problem-solving strategies. Moreover, it applies these strategies to the management of symptoms associated with GAD, OCD, panic disorder, and PTSD. The book includes additional chapters on relapse prevention and comorbid depression. There is a chapter dedicated to fathers who are transitioning to parenthood and supporting their partners as they are struggling with postpartum anxiety. The book provides space for readers to record their symptoms and track their progress with the anxiety management strategies described. Of all of the resources described in this section, this book is most directly related to clinically significant expressions of perinatal anxiety disorders.

This Isn't What I Expected: Overcoming Postpartum Depression (Karen R. Kleiman and Valerie D. Raskin; Bantam Books, 1994).

Kleiman is a psychotherapist and the founder of the Postpartum Stress Center in the Philadelphia suburbs, and Raskin (who now goes by Davis-Raskin) is a psychiatrist who specializes in women's mental health. This book is regarded as a classic self-help resource for postpartum depression, but what makes it relevant here is that the authors refer to postpartum depression as encompassing both depression and anxiety, particularly panic attacks and obsessive–compulsive symptoms. Information in this book provides a great deal of validation and support for women who are going through postpartum depression and anxiety as well as specific cognitive, behavioral, and relational strategies for managing these symptoms. The authors highlight warning signs for clinically significant symptoms of depression and anxiety that warrant attention from a professional, discuss the advantages and disadvantages of various treatments for postpartum depression and anxiety, and include a chapter meant to be read by the spouses or partners of women with postpartum depression and anxiety. This book is especially suited to postpartum women who are experiencing symptoms of both anxiety and depression and who are trying to learn more about the postpartum emotional experience and determine how best to manage their symptoms.

Understanding Your Moods When You're Expecting: Emotions, Mental Health, and Happiness—Before, During, and After Pregnancy (Lucy J. Puryear; Houghton Mifflin, 2007)

Puryear is a practicing psychiatrist who specializes in perinatal emotional disturbances and who served as an expert witness for the defense in the trial of Andrea Yates (see Chapter 3, this volume). This book provides advice on coping with fears of childbirth and obsessive–compulsive symptoms in the postpartum period. Puryear describes the range of emotions that women experience during each trimester of pregnancy, labor and delivery, and the postpartum period, ending each chapter with tips for adapting to the demands associated with that stage of the transition to parenthood. This book contains less information about anxiety than the other books described in this section, but its advantage is that it targets the entire transition to parenthood.

PRACTICAL IMPLICATIONS

There are literally hundreds of self-help resources available for anxiety disorders, which makes it daunting for childbearing women who are already overwhelmed and exhausted to choose the one that they believe will be the best match for them. Although the research on self-help resources for anxiety disorders indicates that at least some contact with a mental health professional is helpful to obtain support and guidance while using self-help materials, there are plenty of ways to attain benefits without the help of a mental health professional. There are several self-help books that were written for childbearing women who are struggling with anxiety and depression. Moreover, there is a much larger market of self-help books for anxiety disorders that are not necessarily geared toward the transition to parenthood. Many of these latter books are based on the cognitive behavioral model, which has been referenced in other places in this volume and has been most often demonstrated to be efficacious in the treatment of anxiety disorders. These resources might be useful in cases in which the nature of the anxiety that the childbearing woman is experiencing is unrelated to fears associated with the transition to parenthood.

I strongly believe that childbearing women who experience anxiety or depression should receive treatment in order to develop strategies for managing their distress and to minimize the impact these symptoms have on their and their child's well-being. Nevertheless, I have come across women in my clinical practice who would very much like to attend regular psychotherapy sessions, but when they commit to a course of psychotherapy, they feel even more overwhelmed and pressured than they did before they sought treatment. The use of self-help resources has the potential to be one way for them to obtain the help they need in a manner that fits with the demands of new motherhood. Because research has shown that self-help resources for anxiety disorders are most effective when people can check in with a mental health professional for support and guidance, I strongly recommend that clinicians adapt their practices to allow for this modality of treatment in conjunction with a decreased frequency of visits, relative to their practices with nonperinatal patients.

CONCLUSION:
WHERE DO WE GO FROM HERE?

Research on the nature and prevalence of perinatal anxiety disorders has expanded tremendously over the past 10 to 15 years. The majority of studies show that rates of generalized anxiety disorder and obsessive–compulsive disorder are elevated in pregnant and postpartum women. Findings are mixed with regard to perinatal panic disorder, but it appears that some pregnant and postpartum women experience an exacerbation of panic symptoms during the transition to parenthood and that the postpartum period is a time when the probability of a new onset of panic disorder is greater than that which would be expected on the basis of chance alone. Although the prevalence of social anxiety disorder is lower in the postpartum period than what is typically observed in large epidemiological samples, some new cases of social anxiety disorder appear to develop during the transition to parenthood. Moreover, a large percentage of women report some fear of labor and delivery as well as negative experiences during childbirth, and some of these women go on to develop posttraumatic stress symptoms during the postpartum period. It is my hope that this volume has helped clinicians to understand these different expressions of perinatal anxiety disorders and recognize that even subsyndromal manifestations can cause childbearing women great distress (cf. Abramowitz, Schwartz, Moore, & Luenzmann, 2003).

AVENUES FOR FUTURE RESEARCH

Although we now have a solid understanding of the clinical presentations of pregnant and postpartum women with these anxiety disorders, very little systematic research has been conducted to identify the specific sociodemographic, biological, psychological, and environmental factors that predispose women to experience an onset or exacerbation of anxiety during the transition to parenthood. The research described in Chapter 1 on the consequences of maternal anxiety during pregnancy has made significant advances in understanding the pathways through which anxiety exerts adverse effects on the child. It will be important to translate those research designs to samples of women with the anxiety disorders described in this volume in order to understand the manner in which particular anxiety expressions are associated with particular types of maternal and child maladjustment. I view this as the primary agenda as research in this field progresses.

In addition, there are several other aspects of perinatal anxiety disorders that are associated with more questions than there are answers. In this section, I identify some of these areas of inquiry and propose additional areas for future research.

Role of Biological and Psychological Variables

In the biopsychosocial model of perinatal anxiety described in Chapter 7, I proposed that sensitivity to changes in particular hormone levels has the potential to make women vulnerable to anxiety during the transition to parenthood. Although this hypothesis is in line with contemporary thinking on this topic (e.g., Altemus, 2001), confirmation with empirical research is needed. Unfortunately, what often happens in this literature is that a biological variable that is found to be significant in one study is not replicated in another. The key will be to obtain multiple measurements of biological variables at critical periods of fetal and infant development. In addition, my biopsychosocial model of perinatal anxiety includes many psychological vulnerability factors that characterize people in general with anxiety disorders but that, for the most part, have not been confirmed empirically to characterize pregnant and postpartum women with anxiety disorders. Not only should research demonstrate that these variables are elevated in pregnant and postpartum women with anxiety disorders compared with pregnant and postpartum women without anxiety disorders, but ideally it should also show that these variables are present before the anxiety disorder has its onset or exacerbation during the transition to parenthood.

Perinatal Anxiety Disorders in Fathers

Some scholars referenced in this volume have identified elevated rates of anxiety in postpartum fathers (e.g., Abramowitz, Schwartz, & Moore, 2003; Ballard, Davis, Handy, & Mohan, 1993). I encourage researchers in this field to conduct a large epidemiological study of the prevalence of anxiety symptoms and disorders in both mothers and fathers throughout the entire transition to parenthood (e.g., from the end of the 1st trimester through the 1st year postpartum). Such a study would not only provide more definitive rates on the prevalence of these emotional disturbances during pregnancy and the postpartum period but would also allow us to begin to tease apart the role of various factors (e.g., biological, psychological) in the manifestation of perinatal anxiety, as fathers do not endure the tremendous hormonal changes that mothers do during the transition to parenthood.

Culture and Ethnicity

There has been virtually no research on the prevalence and phenomenology of perinatal anxiety in different ethnic and cultural groups, which is a major omission in this literature to date. Not only is it important for large epidemiological research to identify the prevalence of perinatal anxiety disorders as a function of race and ethnicity, it is also important for other research to identify the manner in which variables that are related to a new mother's culture (e.g., the presence of extended family in the home, participation in religious services) affect the manifestation of various types of anxiety disorders.

Women at Risk

It has been proposed that women with fertility problems or who have had a pregnancy loss are at particular risk of developing perinatal anxiety disorders (e.g., Geller, Kerns, & Klier, 2004; Ross & McLean, 2006). These are but two of a number of variables that have the potential to make women vulnerable to the development of anxiety disorders during the transition to parenthood. As was seen in Chapter 6, variables that are likely to put women at risk particularly for perinatal posttraumatic stress disorder are previous sexual trauma and interpersonal violence. It will be important for future research to identify groups of women who are at high risk of developing perinatal anxiety disorders.

Pharmacotherapy for Anxiety Disorders During Pregnancy and Lactation

Most of the research on the effects of pharmacotherapy on the fetus, newborn, and developing child has been conducted using retrospective case study designs or chart reviews, and in those studies that are prospective, the participants in the sample are depressed but not necessarily anxious. Furthermore, a large prospective study of children exposed to medication while breastfeeding is sorely needed, as most of our knowledge in this area comes from case studies. I encourage scholars to conduct a large prospective study that identifies the effects in children of mothers taking various types of psychotropic medication for anxiety disorders during pregnancy and lactation. The key feature of such a study would be to include a comparison group of children whose mothers experienced a similar degree of anxiety and/or depression but who were not exposed to medication (L. S. Cohen & Rosenbaum, 1998; Gentile & Bellantuono, 2009).

Efficacy of Evidence-Based Psychotherapeutic Approaches

There are clearly evidence-based treatments for anxiety disorders that are available, particularly those that fall under cognitive behavioral and interpersonal approaches. What is less clear is the degree to which these treatments are relevant to and efficacious for pregnant and postpartum women with anxiety disorders. Although most scholars have suggested that there is no reason to believe that these protocols would be ineffective or harmful in treating women during this transition to parenthood (e.g., Abramowitz, Schwartz, Moore, & Luenzmann, 2003; Ross & McLean, 2006), this remains an empirical question. I strongly encourage scholars to evaluate the efficacy of evidence-based psychotherapy protocols in samples of pregnant and postpartum women. When adaptations must be made to accommodate the physical changes through which these women are going (e.g., with interoceptive exposure for panic disorder) or the time constraints they are under (e.g., with cognitive behavioral therapy homework assignments), a clear rationale must be provided, and data must illustrate the specific manner in which the adaptation enhances treatment outcome.

CONCLUDING THOUGHTS

As I was preparing this volume, I was struck by just how much the body of literature on perinatal anxiety and depression is focused on the *negative*—suffering and distress; adverse effects on pregnancy, labor, delivery, and postpartum maladjustment; problems in the marital or partner relationship; disrupted mother–infant attachment; and problems in the child's emotional and cognitive development. These sequelae are very real and warrant serious attention. However, it is equally important to acknowledge the meaning that can come from the experience of perinatal anxiety and depression. Women who successfully deal with such emotional distress have the potential to build hope and resiliency that will prepare them for significant life transitions or stressors that they may encounter in the future. Moreover, by developing adaptive coping skills for managing their emotional disturbance, they will be able to model a balanced approach to handling life stressors for their children. Although no new mother would choose to endure this kind of suffering, it is hoped that women with perinatal anxiety disorders will gain some wisdom that will help to center them as they face the challenges associated with subsequent stages of their child's development.

Moreover, it is important to keep in mind that some degree of anxiety is functional, as long as it is in moderation (Affonso, Liu-Chiang, & Mayberry, 1999). It keeps new mothers alert for danger or threat so that they can ensure the survival of their offspring. Although clinicians should be vigilant for signs that perinatal anxiety is causing life interference and distress in their patients, they should be equally as mindful to not overpathologize it. There is an abundance of factors that contribute to the risk of poor birth outcomes and problematic infant and child development, and focusing solely on maternal anxiety has the potential to induce shame and self-blame (Oates, 2002). Pregnant and postpartum women are in a vulnerable time in their lives, and their anxiety must be identified and addressed with sensitivity, balance, care, and concern. Anxiety during the transition to parenthood is normal and to be expected, and anxiety that is at a level that warrants a diagnosis or otherwise causes excessive distress is treatable. The most important issues are that new mothers engage in healthy behaviors during pregnancy and the postpartum period, accept the support from close others, and seek treatment when necessary.

REFERENCES

Abramowitz, J. S., Braddock, A. E., & Moore, E. L. (2009). Psychological treatment of obsessive-compulsive disorder. In M. M. Antony & M. B. Stein (Eds.), *Oxford handbook of anxiety and related disorders* (pp. 391–404). New York, NY: Oxford University Press.

Abramowitz, J. S., Foa, E. B., & Franklin, M. E. (2003). Exposure and ritual prevention for obsessive-compulsive disorder: Effects of intensive versus twice-weekly sessions. *Journal of Consulting and Clinical Psychology, 71*, 394–398. doi:10.1037/0022-006X. 71.2.394

Abramowitz, J. S., Khandker, M., Nelson, C. A., Deacon, B. J., & Rygwall, R. (2006). The role of cognitive factors in obsessive-compulsive symptoms: A prospective study. *Behaviour Research and Therapy, 44*, 1361–1374. doi:10.1016/j.brat. 2005.09.011

Abramowitz, J. S., Moore, E. L., Braddock, A. E., & Harrington, D. L. (2008). Self-help cognitive behavioral therapy for social phobia: A controlled trial. *Journal of Behavior Therapy and Experimental Psychiatry, 40*, 98–105. doi:10.1016/j.jbtep. 2008.04.004

Abramowitz, J., Moore, K., Carmin, C., Wiegartz, P. S., & Purdon, C. (2001). Acute onset of obsessive-compulsive disorder in males following childbirth. *Psychosomatics, 42*, 429–431. doi:10.1176/appi.psy.42.5.429

Abramowitz, J. S., Nelson, C. A., Rygwall, R., & Khandker, M. (2007). The cognitive mediation of obsessive compulsive symptoms: A longitudinal study. *Journal of Anxiety Disorders, 21*, 91–104. doi:10.1016/j.janxdis.2006.05.003

Abramowitz, J. S., Schwartz, S. A., & Moore, M. K. (2003). Obsessional thoughts in postpartum females and their partners: Content, severity, and relationship with depression. *Journal of Clinical Psychology in Medical Settings, 10*, 157–164. doi:10.1023/A:1025454627242

Abramowitz, J. S., Schwartz, S. A., Moore, K. M., & Luenzmann, K. R. (2003). Obsessive-compulsive symptoms in pregnancy and the puerperium: A review of the literature. *Journal of Anxiety Disorders, 17*, 461–478. doi:10.1016/S0887-6185 (02)00206-2

Addis, A., & Koren, G. (2000). Safety of fluoxetine during the first trimester of pregnancy: A meta-analytic review of epidemiological studies. *Psychological Medicine, 30*, 89–94. doi:10.1017/S0033291799001270

Addis, M. E., & Martell, C. R. (2004). *Overcoming depression one step at a time: The new behavioral activation approach to getting your life back*. Oakland, CA: New Harbinger.

Adewuya, A. O., Ola, B. A., Aloba, O. O., & Mapayi, B. M. (2006). Anxiety disorders among Nigerian women in late pregnancy: A controlled study. *Archives of Women's Mental Health, 9*, 325–328. doi:10.1007/s00737-006-0157-5

Affonso, D. D., Liu-Chiang, C.-Y., & Mayberry, L. J. (1999). Worry: Conceptual dimensions and relevance to childbearing women. *Health Care for Women International, 20,* 227–236. doi:10.1080/073993399245728

Albert, U., Maina, G., & Bogetto, F. (2000). Obsessive compulsive disorder (OCD) and triggering life events. *European Journal of Psychiatry, 14,* 180–188.

Alehagen, S., Wijma, K., & Wijma, B. (2001). Fear during labor. *Acta Obstetricia et Gynecologica Scandinavica, 80,* 315–320.

Allen, S. (1998). A qualitative analysis of the process, mediating variables, and impact of traumatic childbirth. *Journal of Reproductive and Infant Psychology, 16,* 107–131. doi:10.1080/02646839808404563

Altemus, M. (2001). Obsessive compulsive disorder during pregnancy and postpartum. In K. Yonkers & B. Little (Eds.), *Management of psychiatric disorders in pregnancy* (pp. 149–163). New York, NY: Oxford University Press.

Altemus, M., & Brogan, K. (2004). Pregnancy and postpartum. *CNS Spectrums, 9,* 10–11.

Altemus, M., Deuster, P., Galliven, E., Carter, S., & Gold, P. W. (1995). Suppression of hypothalamic-pituitary-adrenal axis response to stress in lactating women. *The Journal of Clinical Endocrinology and Metabolism, 80,* 2954–2959. doi:10.1210/jc.80.10.2954

Altshuler, L. L., Cohen, L. S., Szuba, M. P., Burt, V. K., Gitlin, M., & Mintz, J. (1996). Pharmacologic management of psychiatric illness in pregnancy: Dilemmas and guidelines. *The American Journal of Psychiatry, 153,* 592–606.

Altshuler, L. L., & Hendrick, V. (1996). Pregnancy and psychotropic medication: Changes in blood levels. *Journal of Clinical Psychopharmacology, 16,* 78–80. doi:10.1097/00004714-199602000-00015

American Psychiatric Association. (1987). *Diagnostic and statistical manual of mental disorders* (3rd ed., rev.). Washington, DC: Author.

American Psychiatric Association. (1998). Practice guideline for the treatment of patients with panic disorder. Work group on panic disorder. *The American Journal of Psychiatry, 155*(Suppl. 5), 1–34.

American Psychiatric Association. (2000). *Diagnostic and statistical manual of mental disorders* (4th ed., text revision). Washington, DC: Author.

Anderson, P. O., & McGuire, G. G. (1989). Neonatal alprazolam withdrawal: Possible effects of breastfeeding [Letter to the editor]. *DICP: the Annals of Pharmacotherapy, 23,* 614.

Antony, M. M. (2002a). Measures for obsessive compulsive disorder. In M. M. Antony, S. M. Orsillo, & L. Roemer (Eds.), *Practitioner's guide to empirically based measures of anxiety* (pp. 219–243). New York, NY: Kluwer Academic/Plenum.

Antony, M. M. (2002b). Measures for panic disorder and agoraphobia. In M. M. Antony, S. M. Orsillo, & L. Roemer (Eds.), *Practitioner's guide to empirically based measures of anxiety* (pp. 95–132). New York, NY: Kluwer Academic/Plenum.

Antony, M. M., & Barlow, D. H. (2002). Specific phobias. In D. H. Barlow (Ed.), *Anxiety and its disorders: The nature and treatment of anxiety and panic* (2nd ed.; pp. 380–417). New York, NY: Guilford Press.

Antony, M. M., Orsillo, S. M., & Roemer, L. (Eds.). (2002). *Practitioner's guide to empirically based measures of anxiety*. New York, NY: Kluwer Academic/Plenum. doi:10.1007/b108176

Areskog, B., Kjessler, B., & Uddenberg, N. (1982). Identification of women with significant fear of childbirth during late pregnancy. *Gynecologic and Obstetric Investigation, 13*, 98–107. doi:10.1159/000299490

Areskog, B., Uddenberg, N., & Kjessler, B. (1981). Fear of childbirth in late pregnancy. *Gynecologic and Obstetric Investigation, 12*, 262–266. doi:10.1159/000299611

Areskog, B., Uddenberg, N., & Kjessler, B. (1983a). Background factors in pregnant women with and without fear of childbirth. *Journal of Psychosomatic Obstetrics and Gynaecology, 2*, 102–108. doi:10.3109/01674828309081267

Areskog, B., Uddenberg, N., & Kjessler, B. (1983b). Experience of delivery in women with and without antenatal fear of childbirth. *Gynecologic and Obstetric Investigation, 16*, 1–12. doi:10.1159/000299205

Arizmendi, T. G., & Affonso, D. D. (1987). Stressful events related to pregnancy and postpartum. *Journal of Psychosomatic Research, 31*, 743–756. doi:10.1016/0022-3999(87)90023-7

Arnold, L. M., Suckow, R. F., & Lichtenstein, P. K. (2000). Fluvoxamine concentrations in breast milk and in maternal and infant sera [Letter to the editor]. *Journal of Clinical Psychopharmacology, 20*, 491–493. doi:10.1097/00004714-200008000-00018

Austin, M.-P., Frilingos, M., Lumley, J., Hadzi-Pavlovic, D., Roncolato, W., Acland, S., . . . Parker, G. (2008). Brief antenatal cognitive behavior therapy group intervention for the prevention of postnatal depression and anxiety: A randomised controlled trial. *Journal of Affective Disorders, 105*, 35–44. doi:10.1016/j.jad.2007.04.001

Austin, M.-P., Tully, L., & Parker, G. (2007). Examining the relationship between antenatal anxiety and postnatal depression. *Journal of Affective Disorders, 101*, 169–174. doi:10.1016/j.jad.2006.11.015

Ayers, S., McKenzie-McHarg, K., & Eagle, A. (2007). Cognitive behaviour therapy for postnatal post-traumatic stress disorder: Case studies. *Journal of Psychosomatic Obstetrics and Gynaecology, 28*, 177–184. doi:10.1080/01674820601142957

Ayers, S., & Pickering, A. D. (2001). Do women get posttraumatic stress disorder as a result of childbirth? A prospective study of incidence. *Birth, 28*, 111–118. doi:10.1046/j.1523-536X.2001.00111.x

Bailham, D., & Joseph, S. (2003). Post-traumatic stress following childbirth: A review of the emerging literature and directions, for research and practice. *Psychology Health and Medicine, 8*, 159–168. doi:10.1080/1354850031000087537

Ballard, C. G., Davis, R., Handy, S., & Mohan, R. N. C. (1993). Postpartum anxiety in mothers and fathers. *European Journal of Psychiatry, 7*, 117–121.

Ballard, C. G., Stanley, A. K., & Brockington, I. F. (1995). Post-traumatic stress disorder (PTSD) after childbirth. *The British Journal of Psychiatry, 166*, 525–528. doi:10.1192/bjp.166.4.525

Bandelow, B. (1999). *Panic and Agoraphobia Scale (PAS)*. Seattle, WA: Hogrefe & Huber.

Bandelow, B., Sojka, F., Broocks, A., Hajak, G., Bleich, S., & Rüther, E. (2006). Panic disorder during pregnancy and the postpartum period. *European Psychiatry, 21*, 495–500. doi:10.1016/j.eurpsy.2005.11.005

Bar-Oz, B., Einarson, T., Einarson, A., Boskovic, R., O'Brien, L., Malm, H., . . . Koren, G. (2007). Paroxetine and congenital malformations: Meta-analysis and consideration of potential confounding factor. *Clinical Therapeutics, 29*, 918–926. doi:10.1016/j.clinthera.2007.05.003

Barlow, D. H. (2000). Unraveling the mysteries of anxiety and its disorders from the perspective of emotion theory. *American Psychologist, 55*, 1247–1263. doi:10.1037/0003-066X.55.11.1247

Barlow, D. H. (2002). *Anxiety and its disorders: The nature and treatment of anxiety and panic* (2nd ed.). New York, NY: Guilford Press.

Barlow, D. H., Vermilyea, J., Blanchard, E. B., Vermilyea, B. B., Di Nardo, P. A., & Cerny, J. A. (1985). The phenomenon of panic. *Journal of Abnormal Psychology, 94*, 320–328. doi:10.1037/0021-843X.94.3.320

Barnett, B., & Parker, G. (1985). Professional and non-professional intervention for highly anxious primiparous mothers. *The British Journal of Psychiatry, 146*, 287–293. doi:10.1192/bjp.146.3.287

Barnett, B., & Parker, G. (1986). Possible determinants, correlates, and consequences of high levels of anxiety in primiparous mothers. *Psychological Medicine, 16*, 177–185. doi:10.1017/S0033291700002610

Barnett, B., Schaafmsa, M. F., Guzman, A.-M., & Parker, G. B. (1991). Maternal anxiety: A 5-year review of an intervention study. *Journal of Child Psychology and Psychiatry, and Allied Disciplines, 32*, 423–438. doi:10.1111/j.1469-7610.1991.tb00321.x

Barr, J. A., & Beck, C. T. (2008). Infanticide secrets: Qualitative study on postpartum depression. *Canadian Family Physician, 54*, 1716–1717.e1–e5.

Barry, W. S., & St. Clair, S. M. (1987). Exposure to benzodiazepines in utero. *Lancet, 329*, 1436–1437. doi:10.1016/S0140-6736(87)90629-5

Beck, A. T., & Emery, G. (1985). *Anxiety disorders and phobias: A cognitive perspective*. New York, NY: Basic Books.

Beck, A. T. (1970). *Depression: Causes and treatment*. Philadelphia: University of Pennsylvania Press.

Beck, A. T., & Steer, R. A. (1990). *Beck Anxiety Inventory manual*. San Antonio, TX: The Psychological Corporation.

Beck, C. T. (1996). A concept analysis of panic. *Archives of Psychiatric Nursing, 10,* 265–275. doi:10.1016/S0883-9417(96)80035-5

Beck, C. T. (1998). Postpartum onset of panic disorder. *Image—the Journal of Nursing Scholarship, 30,* 131–135. doi:10.1111/j.1547-5069.1998.tb01267.x

Beck, C. T. (2001). Predictors of postpartum depression: An update. *Nursing Research, 50,* 275–285. doi:10.1097/00006199-200109000-00004

Beck, C. T. (2004). Post-traumatic stress disorder due to childbirth: The aftermath. *Nursing Research, 53,* 216–224. doi:10.1097/00006199-200407000-00004

Beck, C. T., & Driscoll, J. W. (2006). *Postpartum mood and anxiety disorders: A clinician's guide.* Boston, MA: Jones and Bartlett.

Beebe, K. R., Lee, K. A., Carrieri-Kohlman, V., & Humpherys, J. (2007). The effects of childbirth self-efficacy and anxiety during pregnancy and prehospitalization labor. *Journal of Obstetric, Gynecologic, and Neonatal Nursing, 36,* 410–418.

Beech, B. A., & Robinson, J. (1985). Nightmares following childbirth [Letter to the editor]. *The British Journal of Psychiatry, 147,* 586.

Bennett, H. A., Einarson, A., Taddio, A., Koren, G., & Einarson, T. R. (2004). Prevalence of depression during pregnancy: Systematic review. *Obstetrics and Gynecology, 103,* 698–709.

Bennett, S. S., & Indman, P. (2006). *Beyond the blues: A guide to understanding and treating prenatal and postpartum depression* (2nd ed.). San Jose, CA: Moodswings Press.

Besiroglu, L., Uguz, F., Saglam, M., Agargun, M. Y., & Cilli, A. S. (2007). Factors associated with major depressive disorder occurring after the onset of obsessive compulsive disorder. *Journal of Affective Disorders, 102,* 73–79. doi:10.1016/j.jad.2006.12.007

Birnbaum, C. S., Cohen, L. S., Bailey, J. W., Grush, L. R., Robertson, L. M., & Stowe, Z. M. (1999). Serum concentrations of antidepressants and benzodiazepines in nursing infants: A case series. *Pediatrics, 104,* e11. doi:10.1542/peds.104.1.e11

Birndorf, C. A., & Sacks, A. C. (2008). To medicate or not: The dilemma of pregnancy and psychiatric illness. In S. D. Stone & A. E. Menken (Eds.), *Perinatal and postpartum mood disorders: Perspectives and treatment guide for the health care practitioner* (pp. 237–265). New York, NY: Springer.

Birtchnell, J., Evans, C., & Kennard, J. (1988). The total score of the Crown-Crisp Experiental Index: A useful and valid measure of psychoneurotic pathology. *The British Journal of Medical Psychology, 61,* 255–266.

Blake, D. D., Weathers, F. W., Nagy, L. M., Kaloupek, D. G., Gusman, F. D., Charney, D., & Keane, T. M. (1995). The development of a clinician-administered PTSD scale. *Journal of Traumatic Stress, 8,* 75–90. doi:10.1002/jts.2490080106

Blanchard, E. B., Buckley, T. C., Hickling, E. J., & Taylor, A. E. (1998). Posttraumatic stress disorder and comorbid major depression: Is the correlation an illusion? *Journal of Anxiety Disorders, 12,* 21–37. doi:10.1016/S0887-6185(97)00047-9

Blanchard, E. B., Jones-Alexander, J., Buckley, T. C., & Forneris, C. A. (1996). Psychometric properties of the PTSD Checklist (PCL). *Behaviour Research and Therapy, 34,* 669–673. doi:10.1016/0005-7967(96)00033-2

Blanco, C., Schenier, F. R., Schmidt, A., Blanco-Jerez, C. R., Marshall, R. D., Sánchez-Lacay, A., & Liebowitz, M. R. (2003). Pharmacological treatment of social anxiety disorder: A meta-analysis. *Depression and Anxiety, 18,* 29–40. doi:10.1002/da.10096

Bleiberg, K. L., & Markowitz, J. C. (2005). A pilot study of interpersonal psychotherapy for posttraumatic stress disorder. *The American Journal of Psychiatry, 162,* 181–183. doi:10.1176/appi.ajp.162.1.181

Bobes, J., González, M. P., Bascarán, M. T., Arango, C., Sáiz, P. A., & Bousoño, M. (2001). Quality of life and disability in patients with obsessive-compulsive disorder. *European Psychiatry, 16,* 239–245. doi:10.1016/S0924-9338(01)00571-5

Borge, F.-M., Hoffart, A., Sexton, H., Clark, D. M., Markowitz, J. C., & McManus, F. (2008). Residential cognitive therapy versus residential interpersonal therapy for social phobia: A randomized clinical trial. *Journal of Anxiety Disorders, 22,* 991–1010. doi:10.1016/j.janxdis.2007.10.002

Borkovec, T. D. (2006). Applied relaxation and cognitive therapy for pathological worry and generalized anxiety disorder. In G. C. L. Davey & A. Wells (Eds.), *Worry and psychological disorders: Theory, assessment, and treatment* (pp. 273–287). Chichester, England: Wiley. doi:10.1002/9780470713143.ch16

Borkovec, T. D., & Costello, E. (1993). Efficacy of applied relaxation and cognitive behavioral therapy in the treatment of generalized anxiety disorder. *Journal of Consulting and Clinical Psychology, 61,* 611–619. doi:10.1037/0022-006X.61.4.611

Borkovec, T. D., & Lyonfields, J. D. (1993). Worry: Thought suppression of emotional processing. In H. W. Krohne (Ed.), *Attention and avoidance* (pp. 101–118). Seattle, WA: Hogrefe & Huber.

Borkovec, T. D., Newman, M. G., Pincus, A. L., & Lytle, R. (2002). A component analysis of cognitive behavioral therapy for generalized anxiety and the role of interpersonal problems. *Journal of Consulting and Clinical Psychology, 70,* 288–298. doi:10.1037/0022-006X.70.2.288

Borkovec, T. D., Robinson, E., Pruzinsky, T., & DePree, T. A. (1983). Preliminary exploration of worry: Some characteristics and processes. *Behaviour Research and Therapy, 21,* 9–16. doi:10.1016/0005-7967(83)90121-3

Borue, X., Chen, J., & Condron, B. G. (2007). Developmental effects of SSRIs: Lessons learned from animal studies. *International Journal of Developmental Neuroscience, 25,* 341–347. doi:10.1016/j.ijdevneu.2007.06.003

Boyce, P., & Condon, J. (2000). Traumatic childbirth and the role of debriefing. In B. Raphael & J. P. Wilson (Eds.), *Psychological debriefing: Theory, practice, and evidence* (pp. 272–280). New York, NY: Cambridge University Press. doi:10.1017/CBO9780511570148.020

Brace, M., & McCauley, E. (1997). Oestrogens and psychological well-being. *Annals of Medicine, 29,* 283–290. doi:10.3109/07853899708999349

Brandes, M., Soares, C. N., & Cohen, L. S. (2004). Postpartum onset obsessive compulsive disorder: Diagnosis and management. *Archives of Women's Mental Health, 7,* 99–110. doi:10.1007/s00737-003-0035-3

Brandt, K. R., & MacKenzie, T. B. (1987). Obsessive-compulsive disorder exacerbated during pregnancy: A case report. *International Journal of Psychiatry in Medicine, 17,* 361–366.

Breitkopf, C. R., Primeau, L. A., Levine, R. E., Olson, G. L., Wu, Z. H., & Berenson, A. B. (2006). Anxiety symptoms during pregnancy and postpartum. *Journal of Psychosomatic Obstetrics and Gynaecology, 27,* 157–162. doi:10.1080/01674820500523521

Brouwers, E. P. M., van Baar, A. L., & Pop, V. J. M. (2001a). Does the Edinburgh Postnatal Depression Scale measure anxiety? *Journal of Psychosomatic Research, 51,* 659–663. doi:10.1016/S0022-3999(01)00245-8

Brouwers, E. P. M., van Baar, A. L., & Pop, V. J. M. (2001b). Maternal anxiety during pregnancy and subsequent infant development. *Infant Behavior and Development, 24,* 95–106. doi:10.1016/S0163-6383(01)00062-5

Brown, T. A., Campbell, L. A., Lehman, C. L., Grisham, J. R., & Mancill, R. B. (2001). Current and lifetime comorbidity of the *DSM–IV* anxiety and mood disorders in a large clinical sample. *Journal of Abnormal Psychology, 110,* 585–599. doi:10.1037/0021-843X.110.4.585

Brozovich, F., & Heimberg, R. G. (2008). An analysis of post-event processing social anxiety disorder. *Clinical Psychology Review, 28,* 891–903. doi:10.1016/j.cpr.2008.01.002

Bruce, S. E., Vasile, R. G., Goisman, R. M., Salzman, C., Spencer, M., Machan, J. T., & Keller, M. B. (2003). Are benzodiazepines still the medication of choice for patients with panic disorder with or without agoraphobia? *The American Journal of Psychiatry, 160,* 1432–1438. doi:10.1176/appi.ajp.160.8.1432

Brunel, P., Vial, T., Roche, I., Bertolotti, E., & Evreux, J. (1994). Follow-up of 151 pregnant women exposed to antidepressant treatment (MAOI excluded) during organogenesis. *Therapie, 49,* 117–122.

Burns, G. L., Keortge, S. G., Formea, G. M., & Sternberger, L. G. (1996). Revision of the Padua Inventory of Obsessive Compulsive Disorder Symptoms: Distinctions between worry, obsessions, and compulsions. *Behaviour Research and Therapy, 34,* 163–173. doi:10.1016/0005-7967(95)00035-6

Burt, V. K., Suri, R., Altshuler, L., Stowe, Z., Hendrick, V. C., & Muntean, E. (2001). The use of psychotropic medication during breastfeeding. *The American Journal of Psychiatry, 158,* 1001–1009. doi:10.1176/appi.ajp.158.7.1001

Buttolph, M. L., & Holland, A. D. (1990). Obsessive-compulsive disorders in pregnancy and childbirth. In M. Jenike, L. Baer, & W. Minichiello (Eds.), *Obsessive-compulsive disorders, theory and management* (1st ed., pp. 89–97). Chicago: Yearbook Medical Publishers.

Bybee, P. (1989). Postpartum anxiety disorder [Letter to the editor]. *The Journal of Clinical Psychiatry, 50,* 268.

Callahan, J. L., Borja, S. E., & Hynan, M. T. (2006). Modification of the Perinatal PTSD Questionnaire to enhance clinical utility. *Journal of Perinatology, 26*, 533–539. doi:10.1038/sj.jp.7211562

Callahan, J. L., & Hynan, M. T. (2002). Identifying mothers at risk for postnatal emotional distress: Further evidence for the validity of the Perinatal Posttraumatic Stress Disorder Questionnaire. *Journal of Perinatology, 22*, 448–454. doi:10.1038/sj.jp.7210783

Canals, J., Esparó, G., & Fernández-Ballart, J. D. (2002). How anxiety levels during pregnancy are linked to personality and sociodemographic factors. *Personality and Individual Differences, 33*, 253–259. doi:10.1016/S0191-8869(01)00149-0

Carlbring, P., Westling, B. E., & Andersson, G. (2000). A review of self-help books for panic disorder. *Scandinavian Journal of Behaviour Therapy, 29*, 5–13. doi:10.1080/028457100439827

Carrera, M., Herrán, A., Ayuso-Mateos, J. L., Sierra-Bidde, D., Ramírez, M. L., Ayestarán, A., . . . Vázquez-Barquero, J. L. (2006). Quality of life in early phases of panic disorder: Predictive factors. *Journal of Affective Disorders, 94*, 127–134. doi:10.1016/j.jad.2006.03.006

Casper, R. C., Fleisher, B. E., Lee-Ancajas, J. C., Gilles, A., Gaylor, E., DeBattista, A., & Hoyme, H. E. (2003). Follow-up of children of depressed mothers exposed or not exposed to antidepressant drugs during pregnancy. *The Journal of Pediatrics, 142*, 402–408. doi:10.1067/mpd.2003.139

Castberg, I., & Spigset, O. (2006). Excretion of escitalopram in breast milk. *Journal of Clinical Psychopharmacology, 26*, 536–538. doi:10.1097/01.jcp.0000231607.45402.b4

Cattell, R. B., & Scheier, I. H. (1963). *Handbook for the IPAT Anxiety Scale Questionnaire (Self-Analysis Form)*. Champaign, IL: Institute for Personality & Ability Testing.

Chambers, C. D., Anderson, P. O., Thomas, R. G., Dick, L. M., Felix, R. J., Johnson, K. A., & Jones, K. L. (1999). Weight gain in infants breastfed by mothers who take fluoxetine. *Pediatrics, 104*, e61. doi:10.1542/peds.104.5.e61

Chambers, C. D., Hernandez-Diaz, S., Van Marter, L. J., Werler, M. M., Louik, C., & Jones, K. L., & Mitchell, A. A. (2006). Selective serotonin-reuptake inhibitors and risk of persistent pulmonary hypertension of the newborn. *The New England Journal of Medicine, 354*, 579–587. doi:10.1056/NEJMoa052744

Chambers, C. D., Johnson, K., Dick, L., Felix, R. J., & Jones, K. L. (1996). Birth outcomes in pregnant women taking fluoxetine. *The New England Journal of Medicine, 335*, 1010–1015. doi:10.1056/NEJM199610033351402

Chang, H. L., Chang, T. C., Lin, T. Y., & Kuo, S. S. (2002). Psychiatric morbidity and pregnancy outcome in a disaster area of Taiwan 921 earthquake. *Psychiatry and Clinical Neurosciences, 56*, 139–144. doi:10.1046/j.1440-1819.2002.00948.x

Chelmow, D., & Halfin, V. P. (1997). Pregnancy complicated by obsessive-compulsive disorder. *The Journal of Maternal-Fetal Medicine, 6*, 31–34.

Choi, Y., Bishai, D., & Minkovitz, C. S. (2009). Multiple births are a risk factor for postpartum maternal depressive symptoms. *Pediatrics, 123,* 1147–1154. doi:10.1542/peds.2008-1619

Choy, Y. (2007). Managing side effects of anxiolytics. *Primary Psychiatry, 14,* 68–76.

Choy, Y., Fyer, A. J., & Goodwin, R. D. (2007). Specific phobia and comorbid depression: A close look at the National Comorbidity Survey data. *Comprehensive Psychiatry, 48,* 132–136. doi:10.1016/j.comppsych.2006.10.010

Clark, D. A., & Claybourn, M. (1997). Process characteristics of worry and obsessive intrusive thoughts. *Behaviour Research and Therapy, 35,* 1139–1141. doi:10.1016/S0005-7967(97)10007-9

Clark, D. M., Salkovskis, P. M., Öst, L.-G., Breitholtz, E., Koehler, K. A., Westling, B. E., . . . Gelder, M. (1997). Misinterpretation of body sensations in panic disorder. *Journal of Consulting and Clinical Psychology, 65,* 203–213. doi:10.1037/0022-006X.65.2.203

Clark, D. M., & Wells, A. (1995). A cognitive model of social phobia. In R. G. Heimberg, M. R. Liebowitz, D. A. Hope, & F. R. Schneier (Eds.), *Social phobia: Diagnosis, assessment, and treatment* (pp. 69–93). New York, NY: Guilford Press.

Cohen, L. S., & Rosenbaum, J. F. (1998). Psychotropic drug use during pregnancy: Weighing the risks. *The Journal of Clinical Psychiatry, 59*(Suppl. 2), 18–28.

Cohen, L. S., Rosenbaum, J. F., & Heller, V. L. (1989). Panic attack-associated placental abruption: A case report. *The Journal of Clinical Psychiatry, 50,* 266–267.

Cohen, L. S., Sichel, D. A., Dimmock, J. A., & Rosenbaum, J. F. (1994a). Impact of pregnancy on panic disorder: A case series. *The Journal of Clinical Psychiatry, 55,* 284–288.

Cohen, L. S., Sichel, D. A., Dimmock, J. A., & Rosenbaum, J. F. (1994b). Postpartum course in women with preexisting panic disorder. *The Journal of Clinical Psychiatry, 55,* 289–292.

Cohen, L. S., Sichel, D. A., Faraone, S. V., Robertson, L. M., Dimmock, J. A., & Rosenbaum, J. F. (1996). Course of panic disorder during pregnancy and the puerperium: A preliminary study. *Biological Psychiatry, 39,* 950–954. doi:10.1016/0006-3223(95)00300-2

Cohen, M. M., Ansara, S., Shei, B., Stuckless, N., & Stewart, D. E. (2004). Posttraumatic stress disorder after pregnancy, labor, and delivery. *Journal of Women's Health, 13,* 315–324. doi:10.1089/154099904323016473

Cole, J. A., Ephross, S. A., Cosmatos, I. S., & Walker, A. M. (2007). Paroxetine in the first trimester and the prevalence of congenital malformations. *Pharmacoepidemiology and Drug Safety, 16,* 1075–1085. doi:10.1002/pds.1463

Coleman, V. H., Carter, M. M., Morgan, M. A., & Schulkin, J. (2008). Obstetrician-gynecologists' screening patterns for anxiety during pregnancy. *Depression and Anxiety, 25,* 114–123. doi:10.1002/da.20278

Condon, J. (2003). Serotonergic symptoms in neonates exposed to SSRIs during pregnancy [Letter to the editor]. *The Australian and New Zealand Journal of Psychiatry, 37,* 777–778. doi:10.1111/j.1440-1614.2003.01282.x

Connor, K. M., & Davidson, J. R. T. (1998). Generalized anxiety disorder: Neurobiological and pharmacotherapeutic perspectives. *Biological Psychiatry, 44*, 1286–1294. doi:10.1016/S0006-3223(98)00285-6

Cooper, P. J., & Murray, L. (1995). Course and recurrence of postnatal depression: Evidence for the specificity of the diagnostic concepts. *The British Journal of Psychiatry, 166*, 191–195. doi:10.1192/bjp.166.2.191

Costei, A. M., Kozer, E., Ho, T., Ito, S., & Koren, G. (2002). Perinatal outcome following third trimester exposure to paroxetine. *Archives of Pediatrics & Adolescent Medicine, 156*, 1129–1132.

Côté-Arsenault, D. (2003). The influence of perinatal loss on anxiety in multigravidas. *Journal of Obstetric, Gynecologic, and Neonatal Nursing, 32*, 623–629. doi:10.1177/0884217503257140

Cowley, D. S., & Roy-Byrne, P. P. (1989). Panic disorder and pregnancy. *Journal of Psychosomatic Obstetrics and Gynaecology, 10*, 193–210. doi:10.3109/01674828909016694

Cox, J. L., Holden, J. M., & Sagovsky, R. (1987). Detection of postnatal depression: Development of the 10-item Edinburgh Postnatal Depression Scale. *The British Journal of Psychiatry, 150*, 782–786. doi:10.1192/bjp.150.6.782

Cox, D. N., & Reading, A. E. (1989). Fluctuations in state anxiety over the course of pregnancy and the relationship to outcome. *Journal of Psychosomatic Obstetrics and Gynaecology, 10*, 71–78. doi:10.3109/01674828909016679

Crandon, A. J. (1979a). Maternal anxiety and neonatal well-being. *Journal of Psychosomatic Research, 23*, 113–115. doi:10.1016/0022-3999(79)90015-1

Crandon, A. J. (1979b). Maternal anxiety and obstetric complications. *Journal of Psychosomatic Research, 23*, 109–111. doi:10.1016/0022-3999(79)90014-X

Cree, J. E., Meyer, J., & Hailey, D. M. (1973). Diazepam in labour: Its metabolism and effect on the clinical condition and thermogenesis of the newborn. *British Medical Journal, 4*, 251–255. doi:10.1136/bmj.4.5887.251

Creedy, D. K., Shochet, I. M., & Horsfall, J. (2000). Childbirth and the development of acute trauma symptoms: Incidence and contributing factors. *Birth, 27*, 104–111. doi:10.1046/j.1523-536x.2000.00104.x

Crompton, J. (1996a). Post-traumatic stress disorder and childbirth. *British Journal of Midwifery, 4*, 290–294.

Crompton, J. (1996b). Post-traumatic stress disorder and childbirth: 2. *British Journal of Midwifery. 4*, 354–373.

Curran, S., Nelson, T. E., & Rodgers, R. J. (1995). Resolution of panic disorder during pregnancy. *Irish Journal of Psychological Medicine, 12*, 107–108.

Czarnocka, J., & Slade, P. (2000). Prevalence and predictors of post-traumatic stress symptoms following childbirth. *The British Journal of Clinical Psychology, 39*, 35–51. doi:10.1348/014466500163095

Czeizel, A., Szentesi, I., Szekeres, I., Glauber, A., Bucski, P., & Molnár, C. (1984). Pregnancy outcome and health condition of offspring of self-poisoned pregnant women. *Acta Paediatrica Academiae Scientiarum Hungaricae, 25*, 209–236.

Dahl, M. L., Olhager, A. J., & Ahlner, J. (1997). Paroxetine withdrawal syndrome in a neonate. *The British Journal of Psychiatry, 171*, 391–392. doi:10.1192/bjp.171.4.391c

Davis, E. P., Snidman, N., Wadhwa, P. D., Glynn, L. M., Dunkel-Schetter, C., & Sandman, C. A. (2004). Prenatal maternal anxiety and depression predict negative behavioral reactivity in infancy. *Infancy, 6*, 319–331. doi:10.1207/s15327078in0603_1

Dayan, J., Creveuil, C., Herlicoviez, M., Herbel, C., Baranger, E., Savoye, C., & Thouin, A. (2002). Role of anxiety and depression in the onset of spontaneous preterm labour. *American Journal of Epidemiology, 155*, 293–301. doi:10.1093/aje/155.4.293

DeMier, R. L., Hynan, M. T., Harris, H. B., & Manniello, R. L. (1996). Perinatal stressors as predictors of symptoms of posttraumatic stress in mothers of infants at high risk. *Journal of Perinatology, 16*, 276–280.

Dennis, C.-L. E., & Stewart, D. E. (2004). Treatment of postpartum depression, part I: A critical review of biological interventions. *The Journal of Clinical Psychiatry, 65*, 1242–1251. doi:10.4088/JCP.v65n0914

Dent, M. F., & Bremner, J. D. (2009). Pharmacotherapy for posttraumatic stress disorder and other trauma-related disorders. In M. M. Antony & M. B. Stein (Eds.), *Oxford handbook of anxiety and related disorders* (pp. 405–416). New York, NY: Oxford University Press.

Denys, D., Tenney, N., van Megen, H. J., de Geus, F., & Westenberg, H. G. (2004). Axis I and II comorbidity in a large sample of patients with obsessive-compulsive disorder. *Journal of Affective Disorders, 80*, 155–162. doi:10.1016/S0165-0327(03)00056-9

Diaz, S. F., Grush, L. R., Sichel, D. A., & Cohen, L. S. (1997). Obsessive-compulsive disorder in pregnancy and the puerperium. In M. T. Pato & G. Steketee (Eds.), *OCD across the life cycle* (pp. 97–112). Washington, DC: American Psychiatric Association Press.

Ditkoff, E. C., Crary, W. G., Cristo, M., & Lobo, R. A. (1991). Estrogen improves psychological function in asymptomatic postmenopausal women. *Obstetrics and Gynecology, 78*, 991–995.

Dolovich, L. R., Addis, A., Vaillancourt, J. M., Power, J. D., Koren, G., & Einarson, T. R. (1998). Benzodiazepine use in pregnancy and major malformations or oral cleft: Meta-analysis of cohort and case-control studies. *British Medical Journal, 317*, 839–843.

Donnelly, A., & Paton, C. (2007). Safety of selective serotonin reuptake inhibitors in pregnancy. *Psychiatric Bulletin, 31*, 183–186. doi:10.1192/pb.bp.106.012898

Dugas, M. J., Freeston, M. J., & Ladouceur, R. (1997). Intolerance of uncertainty and problem orientation in worry. *Cognitive Therapy and Research, 21*, 593–606. doi:10.1023/A:1021890322153

Dugas, M. J., Gagnon, F., Ladouceur, R., & Freeston, M. H. (1998). Generalized anxiety disorder: A preliminary test of a conceptual model. *Behaviour Research and Therapy, 36*, 215–226. doi:10.1016/S0005-7967(97)00070-3

Dugas, M. J., Ladouceur, R., Léger, E., Freeston, M., Langlois, F., Provencher, M. D., & Boisvert, J.-M. (2003). Group cognitive behavioral therapy for generalized anxiety disorder: Treatment outcome and long-term follow-up. *Journal of Consulting and Clinical Psychology, 71*, 821–825. doi:10.1037/0022-006X.71.4.821

Dugas, M. J., & Robichaud, M. (2007). *The cognitive behavioral treatment of generalized anxiety disorder: From science to practice*. New York, NY: Routledge.

Eberhard-Gran, M., Eskild, A., & Opjordsmoen, S. (2006). Use of psychotropic medications in treating mood disorders during lactation: Practical recommendation. *CNS Drugs, 20*, 187–198. doi:10.2165/00023210-200620030-00002

Edlund, M. J., & Swann, A. C. (1987). The economic and social costs of panic disorder. *Hospital & Community Psychiatry, 38*, 1277–1279.

Eggleston, A. M., Calhoun, P. S., Svikis, D. S., Tuten, M., Chisolm, M. S., & Jones, H. E. (2009). Suicidality, aggression, and other treatment considerations among pregnant, substance-dependent women with posttraumatic stress disorder. *Comprehensive Psychiatry, 50*, 415–423. doi:10.1016/j.comppsych.2008.11.004

Einarson, A., Fatoye, B., Sarkar, M., Lavinge, S. V., Brochu, J., Chambers, C., . . . Koren, G. (2001). Pregnancy outcome following gestational exposure to venlafaxine: A multicenter prospective controlled study. *The American Journal of Psychiatry, 158*, 1728–1730. doi:10.1176/appi.ajp.158.10.1728

Einarson, A., Pistelli, A., DeSantis, M., Malm, H., Paulus, W. D., Panchaud, A., . . . Koren, G. (2008). Evaluation of the risk of congenital cardiovascular defects associated with the use of paroxetine during pregnancy. *The American Journal of Psychiatry, 165*, 749–752. doi:10.1176/appi.ajp.2007.07060879

Elhai, J. D., Grubaugh, A. L., Kashdan, T. B., & Frueh, B. C. (2008). Empirical examination of a proposed refinement to DSM-V posttraumatic stress disorder symptom criteria using the National Comorbidity Survey Replication data. *The Journal of Clinical Psychiatry, 69*, 597–602. doi:10.4088/JCP.v69n0411

Emmelkamp, P. M. G., & Gerlsma, C. (1994). Marital functioning and the anxiety disorders. *Behavior Therapy, 25*, 407–429. doi:10.1016/S0005-7894(05)80155-8

Engelhard, I. M., van den Hout, M. A., & Arntz, A. (2001). Posttraumatic stress disorder after pregnancy loss. *General Hospital Psychiatry, 23*, 62–66. doi:10.1016/S0163-8343(01)00124-4

Engelhard, I. M., van Rij, M., Boullart, I., Ekhart, T. H. A., Spaanderman, M. E. A., van den Hout, M. A., & Peeters, L. L. H. (2002). Posttraumatic stress disorder after pre-eclampsia: An exploratory study. *General Hospital Psychiatry, 24*, 260–264. doi:10.1016/S0163-8343(02)00189-5

Erkkola, R., Kero, P., Kanto, J., & Aaltonen, L. (1983). Severe abuse of psychotropic drugs during pregnancy with good perinatal outcome. *Annals of Clinical Research, 15*, 88–91.

Ericson, A., Kallen, B., & Wilholm, B. (1999). Delivery outcome after the use of antidepressants in early pregnancy. *European Journal of Clinical Pharmacology, 55*, 503–508. doi:10.1007/s002280050664

Evans, S., Ferrando, S., Findler, M., Stowell, C., Smart, C., & Haglin, D. (2008). Mindfulness-based cognitive therapy for generalized anxiety disorder. *Journal of Anxiety Disorders, 22,* 716–721. doi:10.1016/j.janxdis.2007.07.005

Fairbrother, N., & Abramowitz, J. S. (2007). New parenthood as a risk factor for the development of obsessional problems. *Behaviour Research and Therapy, 45,* 2155–2163. doi:10.1016/j.brat.2006.09.019

Fairbrother, N., & Woody, S. R. (2007). Fear of childbirth and obstetrical events as predictors of postnatal symptoms of depression and post-traumatic stress disorder. *Journal of Psychosomatic Obstetrics and Gynaecology, 28,* 239–242. doi:10.1080/01674820701495065

Fedoroff, I. C., & Taylor, S. (2001). Psychological and pharmacological treatments for social anxiety disorder: A meta-analysis. *Journal of Clinical Psychopharmacology, 21,* 311–324. doi:10.1097/00004714-200106000-00011

Fehm, L., Beesdo, K., Jacobi, F., & Fiedler, A. (2008). Social anxiety disorder above and below the diagnostic threshold: Prevalence, comorbidity, and impairment in the general population. *Social Psychiatry and Psychiatric Epidemiology, 43,* 257–265. doi:10.1007/s00127-007-0299-4

Field, T., Diego, M., & Hernandez-Reif, M. (2006). Prenatal depression effects on the fetus and newborn: A review. *Infant Behavior and Development, 29,* 445–455. doi:10.1016/j.infbeh.2006.03.003

Field, T., Diego, M., Hernandez-Reif, M., Schanberg, S., Kuhn, C., Yando, R., & Bendell, D. (2003). Pregnancy anxiety and comorbid depression and anger: Effects on the fetus and neonate. *Depression and Anxiety, 17,* 140–151. doi:10.1002/da.10071

Field, T., Hernandez-Reif, M., Diego, M., Figueiredo, B., Schanberg, S., & Kuhn, C. (2006). Prenatal cortisol, prematurity, and low birthweight. *Infant Behavior and Development, 29,* 268–275. doi:10.1016/j.infbeh.2005.12.010

First, M. B., Spitzer, R. L., Gibbon, M., & Williams, J. B. W. (1997). *Structured Clinical Interview for DSM-IV Axis I Disorders, Research Version, Non-Patient Edition (SCID-I/NP).* New York, NY: New York State Psychiatric Institute, Biometrics Research.

Fisher, J. B., Edgren, B. E., Mammel, C., & Coleman, J. M. (1985). Neonatal apnea associated with maternal clonazepam therapy: A case report. *Obstetrics and Gynecology, 66,* 345–355.

Fisher, P. L., & Wells, A. (2009). Psychological models of worry and generalized anxiety disorder. In M. M. Antony & M. B. Stein (Eds.), *Oxford handbook of anxiety and related disorders* (pp. 225–237). New York, NY: Oxford University Press.

Foa, E. B., Huppert, J. D., Leiberg, S., Langner, R., Kichic, R., Hajcak, G., & Salkovskis, P. M. (2002). The Obsessive-Compulsive Inventory: Development and validation of a short version. *Psychological Assessment, 14,* 485–496. doi:10.1037/1040-3590.14.4.485

Foa, E. B., Liebowitz, M. R., Kozak, M. J., Davies, S., Campeas, R., Franklin, M. E., . . . Tu, X. (2005). Randomized, placebo-controlled trial of exposure and ritual prevention, clomipramine, and their combination in the treatment of obsessive-compulsive disorder. *The American Journal of Psychiatry, 162,* 151–161. doi:10.1176/appi.ajp.162.1.151

Fones, C. (1996). Posttraumatic stress disorder occurring after painful childbirth. *Journal of Nervous and Mental Disease, 184,* 195–196. doi:10.1097/00005053-199603000-00012

Ford, E., Ayers, S., & Bradley, R. (2010). Exploration of a cognitive model to predict post-traumatic stress symptoms following childbirth. *Journal of Anxiety Disorders, 24,* 353–359.

Franklin, C. L., & Zimmerman, M. (2001). Posttraumatic stress disorder and major depressive disorder: Investigating the role of overlapping symptoms in diagnostic comorbidity. *Journal of Nervous and Mental Disease, 189,* 548–551. doi:10.1097/00005053-200108000-00008

Franklin, M. E., Abramowitz, J. S., Kozak, M. K., Levitt, J. T., & Foa, E. B. (2000). Effectiveness of exposure and ritual prevention for obsessive-compulsive disorder: Randomized compared with nonrandomized samples. *Journal of Consulting and Clinical Psychology, 68,* 594–602. doi:10.1037/0022-006X.68.4.594

Freeston, M. H., Dugas, M. J., & Ladouceur, R. (1996). Thoughts, images, worry, and anxiety. *Cognitive Therapy and Research, 20,* 265–273. doi:10.1007/BF02229237

Freeston, M. H., Ladouceur, R., Gagnon, F., Thibodeau, N., Rhéaume, J., Letarte, H., & Bujold, A. (1997). Cognitive behavioral treatment of obsessive thoughts: A controlled study. *Journal of Consulting and Clinical Psychology, 65,* 405–413. doi:10.1037/0022-006X.65.3.405

Freeston, M. H., Rhéaume, J., Letarte, H., Dugas, M. H., & Ladouceur, R. (1994). Why do people worry? *Personality and Individual Differences, 17,* 791–802. doi:10.1016/0191-8869(94)90048-5

Fresco, D. M., Mennin, D. M., Heimberg, R. G., & Turk, C. L. (2003). Using the Penn State Worry Questionnaire to identify individuals with generalized anxiety disorder: A receiver operating characteristic analysis. *Journal of Behavior Therapy and Experimental Psychiatry, 34,* 283–291. doi:10.1016/j.jbtep.2003.09.001

Gamble, J., & Creedy, D. (2004). Content and processes of postpartum counseling after a distressing birth experience: A review. *Birth, 31,* 213–218. doi:10.1111/j.0730-7659.2004.00307.x

Gamble, J., Creedy, D., Moyle, W., Webster, J., McAllister, M., & Dickson, P. (2005). Effectiveness of a counseling intervention after a traumatic childbirth: A randomized controlled trial. *Birth, 32,* 11–19. doi:10.1111/j.0730-7659.2005.00340.x

Geissbuehler, V., & Eberhard, J. (2002). Fear of childbirth during pregnancy: A study of more than 8000 pregnant women. *Journal of Psychosomatic Obstetrics and Gynaecology, 23,* 229–235. doi:10.3109/01674820209074677

Geller, P. A., Kerns, D., & Klier, C. M. (2004). Anxiety following miscarriage and the subsequent pregnancy: A review of the literature and future directions. *Journal of Psychosomatic Research, 56,* 35–45. doi:10.1016/S0022-3999(03)00042-4

Gentile, S., & Bellantuono, C. (2009). Selective serotonin reuptake inhibitor exposure during early pregnancy and risk of fetal major malformations: Focus on paroxetine. *The Journal of Clinical Psychiatry, 70,* 414–422. doi:10.4088/JCP.08r04468

Gentile, S., Rossi, A., & Bellantuono, C. (2007). SSRIs during breastfeeding: Spotlight on milk-to-plasma ratio. *Archives of Women's Mental Health, 10,* 39–51. doi:10.1007/s00737-007-0173-0

George, D. T., Ladenheim, J. A., & Nutt, D. J. (1987). Effect of pregnancy on panic attacks. *The American Journal of Psychiatry, 144,* 1078–1079.

Gitau, R., Fisk, N. M., Cameron, A., Teixeira, J., & Glover, V. (2001). Fetal HPA stress responses to invasive procedures are independent of maternal responses. *The Journal of Clinical Endocrinology and Metabolism, 86,* 104–109. doi:10.1210/jc.86.1.104

Gladstone, G. L., Parker, G. B., Mitchell, P. B., Malhi, G. S., Wilhelm, K. A., & Austin, M.-P. (2005). A brief measure of worry severity (BMWS): Personality and clinical correlates of severe worriers. *Journal of Anxiety Disorders, 19,* 877–892. doi:10.1016/j.janxdis.2004.11.003

Glazer, G. (1980). Anxiety levels and concerns among pregnant women. *Research in Nursing & Health, 3,* 107–113. doi:10.1002/nur.4770030305

Glover, V., Bergman, K., & O'Connor, T. G. (2008). The effects of maternal stress, anxiety, and depression during pregnancy on the neurodevelopment of the child. In S. D. Stone & A. E. Menkin (Eds.), *Perinatal and postpartum mood disorders: Perspectives and treatment for the health care practitioner* (pp. 3–15). New York, NY: Springer.

Glover, V., & Kammerer, M. (2004). The biology and pathophysiology of peripartum psychiatric disorders. *Primary Psychiatry, 11,* 37–41.

Glynn, L. M., Dunkel-Schetter, C., Hobel, C. J., & Sandman, C. A. (2008). Pattern of perceived stress and anxiety in pregnancy predicts preterm birth. *Health Psychology, 27,* 43–51. doi:10.1037/0278-6133.27.1.43

Glynn, L. M., Wadhwa, P. D., Dunkel-Schetter, C., Chicz-Demet, A., & Sandman, C. A. (2001). When stress happens matters: Effects of earthquake timing on stress responsivity during pregnancy. *American Journal of Obstetrics and Gynecology, 184,* 637–642. doi:10.1067/mob.2001.111066

Godet, P. F., Damato, T., & Dalery, J. (1995). Benzodiazepines in pregnancy: Analysis of 187 exposed infants drawn from a population-based birth defects registry. *Reproductive Toxicology, 9,* 585. doi:10.1016/0890-6238(96)81380-3

Goldbeck-Wood, S. (1996). Post-traumatic stress disorder may follow childbirth. *British Medical Journal, 313,* 774.

Goldberg, D. P., & Hillier, V. F. (1979). A scaled version of the General Health Questionnaire. *Psychological Medicine, 9,* 139–145. doi:10.1017/S0033291700021644

Golding, J., Pembrey, M., Jones, R., & the ALSPAC Study Team. (2001). ALSPAC—The Avon Longitudinal Study of Parents and Children I. Study methodology. *Paediatric and Perinatal Epidemiology, 15*, 74–87. doi:10.1046/j.1365-3016.2001.00325.x

Goldstein, D. J. (1995). Effects of third trimester fluoxetine exposure on the newborn. *Journal of Clinical Psychopharmacology, 15*, 417–420. doi:10.1097/00004714-199512000-00005

Goldstein, D. J., Corbin, L., & Sundell, K. (1997). Effects of first trimester fluoxetine exposure on the newborn. *American Journal of Obstetrics and Gynecology, 89*, 713–718. doi:10.1016/S0029-7844(97)00070-7

Goldstein, D. J., & Sundell, K. (1999). A review of the safety of selective serotonin reuptake inhibitors. *Human Psychopharmacology, 14*, 319–324. doi:10.1002/(SICI)1099-1077(199907)14:5<319::AID-HUP99>3.0.CO;2-D

Goodman, W. K., Price, L. H., Rasmussen, S. A., Mazure, C., Delgado, P., Heninger, G. R., & Charney, D. S. (1989). The Yale-Brown Obsessive-Compulsive Scale II: Validity. *Archives of General Psychiatry, 46*, 1012–1016.

Goodman, W. K., Price, L. H., Rasmussen, S. A., Mazure, C., Fleischman, R. L., Hill, C. L., . . . Charney, D. S. (1989). The Yale-Brown Obsessive-Compulsive Scale I: Development, use, and reliability. *Archives of General Psychiatry, 46*, 1006–1011.

Grant, B. F., Hasis, D. S., Stinson, F. S., Dawson, D. A., Ruan, W. J., Goldstein, R. B., . . . Huang, B. (2005). Prevalence, correlates, co-morbidity, and comparative disability of DSM-IV generalized anxiety disorder in the USA: Results from the National Epidemiologic Survey on Alcohol and Related Conditions. *Psychological Medicine, 35*, 1747–1759. doi:10.1017/S0033291705006069

Green, B. L., Lindy, J. D., Grace, M. C., & Leonard, A. C. (1992). Chronic posttraumatic stress disorder and diagnostic comorbidity in a disaster sample. *Journal of Nervous and Mental Disease, 180*, 760–766. doi:10.1097/00005053-199212000-00004

Green, J. M., Kafetsios, K., Statham, H. E., & Snowdon, C. M. (2003). Factor structure, validity, and reliability of the Cambridge Worry Scale in a pregnant population. *Journal of Health Psychology, 8*, 753–764. doi:10.1177/13591053030086008

Griffiths, P., & Barker-Collo, S. (2008). Study of a group treatment program for postnatal adjustment difficulties. *Archives of Women's Mental Health, 11*, 33–41. doi:10.1007/s00737-008-0220-5

Groome, L. J., Swiber, M. J., Bentz, L. S., Holland, S. B., & Atterbury, J. L. (1995). Maternal anxiety during pregnancy: Effect on fetal behavior at 38 to 40 weeks of gestation. *Developmental and Behavioral Pediatrics, 16*, 391–396.

Grote, N. K., Bledsoe, S. E., Swartz, H. A., & Frank, E. (2004). Feasibility of providing culturally relevant, brief interpersonal psychotherapy for antenatal depression in an obstetrics clinic: A pilot study. *Research on Social Work Practice, 14*, 397–407. doi:10.1177/1049731504265835

Guler, O., Sahin, F. K., Emul, M., Ozbulut, O., Gecici, O., Uguz, F., . . . Askin, R. (2008). The prevalence of panic disorder in pregnant women during the third

trimester of pregnancy. *Comprehensive Psychiatry, 49*, 154–158. doi:10.1016/
j.comppsych.2007.08.008

Gunter, N. C. (1986). Maternal perceptions of infant behavior as a function of
trait anxiety. *Early Child Development and Care, 23*, 185–196. doi:10.1080/
0300443860230208

Gunthert, K. C., Conner, T. S., Armelli, S., Tennen, H., Covault, J., & Kranzler, H. R.
(2007). Serotonin transporter gene polymorphism (5-HTTLPR) and anxiety
reactivity in daily life: A daily process approach to gene-environment interaction.
Psychological Medicine, 69, 762–768. doi:10.1097/PSY.0b013e318157ad42

Hagg, S., Granberg, K., & Carleborg, L. (2000). Excretion of fluvoxamine into
breast milk. *British Journal of Clinical Pharmacology, 49*, 286–288. doi:10.1046/
j.1365-2125.2000.00142-3.x

Halbreich, U. (1997). Hormonal interventions with psychopharmacological potential:
An overview. *Psychopharmacology Bulletin, 33*, 281–286.

Hale, T. W. (2008). *Medications and mother's milk* (13th ed.). Amarillo, TX: Hale.

Hale, T. W., Shum, S., & Grossberg, M. (2001). Fluoxetine toxicity in a breastfed infant.
Clinical Pediatrics, 40, 681–684. doi:10.1177/000992280104001207

Hamilton, M. (1959). The assessment of anxiety states by rating. *The British Journal
of Medical Psychology, 32*, 50–55.

Harris-Britt, A., Martin, S. L., Li, Y., Casanueva, C., & Kupper, L. L. (2004). Post-
traumatic stress disorder and associated functional impairments during pregnancy:
Some consequences of violence against women. *Journal of Clinical Psychology in
Medical Settings, 11*, 253–264. doi:10.1023/B:JOCS.0000045345.72671.5e

Haugen, E. N. (2003). *Postpartum anxiety and depression: The contribution of social support*
(Unpublished master's thesis). University of North Dakota, Grand Forks.

Haugen, E. N., Brendle, J. R., Schmutzer, P. A., & Wenzel, A. (2003, November).
*Psychopathology and its relation to sexual functioning in women during the first eight
weeks postpartum.* Poster session presented at the 36th annual meeting of the
Association for Advancement of Behavior Therapy, Boston, MA.

Haugen, E. N., Schmutzer, P. A., & Wenzel, A. (2004). Sexuality and the partner
relationship during pregnancy and the postpartum period. In J. H. Harvey,
A. Wenzel, & S. Sprecher (Eds.), *Handbook of sexuality in close relationships*
(pp. 411–435). Mahwah, NJ: Erlbaum.

Hazlett-Stevens, H., Pruitt, L. D., & Collins, A. (2009). Phenomenology of generalized anxiety disorder. In M. M. Antony & M. B. Stein (Eds.), *Oxford handbook
of anxiety and related disorders* (pp. 47–55). New York, NY: Oxford University
Press.

Heimberg, R. G., & Becker (2002). *Cognitive behavioral group therapy for social phobia:
Basic mechanisms and clinical strategies.* New York, NY: Guilford Press.

Heinrichs, M., Meinlschmidt, G., Neumann, I., Wagner, S., Kirschbaum, C., Ehlert,
U., & Hellhammer, D. H. (2001). Effects of suckling on hypothalamic-pituitary-
adrenal axis responses to psychosocial stress in postpartum lactating women. *The*

Journal of Clinical Endocrinology and Metabolism, 86, 4798–4804. doi:10.1210/jc.86.10.4798

Hendrick, V., Altshuler, L., Wertheimer, A., & Dunn, W. A. (2001). Venlafaxine and breast-feeding. *The American Journal of Psychiatry, 158,* 2089–2090. doi:10.1176/appi.ajp.158.12.2089-a

Hendrick, V., Stowe, Z. N., Altshuler, L. L., Hostetter, A., & Fukuchi, A. (2000). Paroxetine use during breast-feeding. *Journal of Clinical Psychopharmacology, 20,* 587–589. doi:10.1097/00004714-200010000-00022

Heron, J., O'Connor, T. G., Evans, J., Golding, J., Glover, V., & the ALSPAC Study Team. (2004). The course of anxiety and depression through pregnancy and the postpartum in a community sample. *Journal of Affective Disorders, 80,* 65–73. doi:10.1016/j.jad.2003.08.004

Hertzberg, T., & Wahlbeck, K. (1999). The impact of pregnancy and puerperium on panic disorder: A review. *Journal of Psychosomatic Obstetrics and Gynaecology, 20,* 59–64. doi:10.3109/01674829909075578

Hirai, M., & Clum, G. A. (2006). A meta-analytic study of self-help interventions for anxiety problems. *Behavior Therapy, 37,* 99–111. doi:10.1016/j.beth.2005.05.002

Hirshfeld-Becker, D. R., Biederman, J., Faraone, S. V., Robin, J. A., Friedman, D., Rosenthal, J. M., & Rosenbaum, J. F. (2004). Pregnancy complications associated with childhood anxiety disorders. *Depression and Anxiety, 19,* 152–162. doi:10.1002/da.20007

Hobfoll, S. E., & Leiberman, J. R. (1989). Effects of mastery and intimacy on anxiety following pregnancy: For whom is support supportive and from whom? *Anxiety Research, 1,* 327–341.

Hodgson, R. J., & Rachman, S. (1977). Obsessive-compulsive complaints. *Behaviour Research and Therapy, 15,* 389–395. doi:10.1016/0005-7967(77)90042-0

Hofberg, K., & Brockington, I. (2000). Tokophobia: An unreasoning dread of childbirth. *The British Journal of Psychiatry, 176,* 83–85. doi:10.1192/bjp.176.1.83

Holditch-Davis, D., Bartlett, T. R., Blickman, A. L., & Miles, M. S. (2003). Posttraumatic stress symptoms in mothers of premature infants. *Journal of Obstetric, Gynecologic, and Neonatal Nursing, 32,* 161–171. doi:10.1177/0884217503252035

Holtzman, M., & Glass, J. (1999). Explaining changes in mothers' job satisfaction following childbirth. *Work and Occupations, 26,* 365–404. doi:10.1177/0730888499026003005

Horowitz, M., Wilner, N., & Alvarez, W. (1979). Impact of Events Scale: A measure of subjective stress. *Psychosomatic Medicine, 41,* 209–218.

Horvath, A. O., & Symonds, D. B. (1991). Relationship between working alliance and outcome in psychotherapy: A meta-analysis. *Journal of Counseling Psychology, 38,* 139–149. doi:10.1037/0022-0167.38.2.139

Hunfeld, J. A. M., Wladimiroff, J. W., & Passchier, J. (1997). Prediction and course of grief four years after perinatal loss due to congenital abnormalities: A follow-up study. *The British Journal of Medical Psychology, 70,* 85–91.

Huppert, J. D., Simpson, H. B., Nissenson, K. J., Liebowitz, M. R., & Foa, E. B. (2009). Quality of life and functional impairment in obsessive compulsive disorder: A comparison of patients with and without comorbidity, patients in remission, and healthy controls. *Depression and Anxiety, 26,* 39–45. doi:10.1002/da.20506

Hyman, S. M., Gold, S. N., & Cott, M. A. (2003). Forms of social support that moderate PTSD in childhood sexual abuse survivors. *Journal of Family Violence, 18,* 295–300. doi:10.1023/A:1025117311660

Ichida, M. (1996). A case of posttraumatic stress disorder (PTSD), the onset of which was the complication of childbirth. *Japanese Journal of Psychosomatic Medicine, 36,* 431–434.

Ilett, K. F., Kristensen, J. H., Hackett, L. P., Paech, M., Kohan, R., & Rampono, J. (2002). Distribution of venlafaxine and its O-edsmethyl metabolite in human milk and their effects in breastfed infants. *British Journal of Clinical Pharmacology, 53,* 17–22. doi:10.1046/j.0306-5251.2001.01518.x

Ingram, R. E. (1990). Self-focused attention in clinical disorders: A review and conceptual model. *Psychological Bulletin, 107,* 156–176. doi:10.1037/0033-2909.107.2.156

Iqbal, M. M., Sobhan, T., & Ryals, T. (2002). Effects of commonly used benzodiazepines on the fetus, neonate, and the nursing infant. *Psychiatric Services, 53,* 39–49. doi:10.1176/appi.ps.53.1.39

Istvan, J. (1986). Stress, anxiety, and birth outcomes: A critical review of the evidence. *Psychological Bulletin, 100,* 331–348. doi:10.1037/0033-2909.100.3.331

Ito, S., Blajchman, A., Stephenson, M., Eliopoulos, C., & Koren, G. (1993). Prospective follow-up of adverse reactions in breastfed infants exposed to maternal medication. *American Journal of Obstetrics and Gynecology, 168,* 1393–1399.

Jacobi, F., Wittchen, H.-U., Hölting, C., Höfler, M., Pfister, H., Müller, N., & Lieb, R. (2004). Prevalence, co-morbidity, and correlates of mental disorders in the general population: Results of the German Health Interview and Examination Survey (GHS). *Psychological Medicine, 34,* 597–611. doi:10.1017/S0033291703001399

Jeffries, W. S., & Bochner, F. (1988). The effect of pregnancy on drug pharmacokinetics. *The Medical Journal of Australia, 149,* 675–677.

Jennings, K. D., Ross, S., Popper, S., & Elmore, M. (1999). Thoughts of harming infants in depressed and nondepressed mothers. *Journal of Affective Disorders, 54,* 21–28. doi:10.1016/S0165-0327(98)00185-2

Johnstone, M. (1981). Effect of maternal lorazepam on the neonate. *British Medical Journal, 282,* 1973–1974. doi:10.1136/bmj.282.6280.1973-b

Jolley, S. N., & Spach, T. (2008). Stress system dysregulation in perinatal mood disorders. In S. D. Stone & A. E. Menken (Eds.), *Perinatal and postpartum mood disorders: Perspectives and treatment guided for the health care practitioner* (pp. 133–151). New York, NY: Springer.

Jomeen, J., & Martin, C. R. (2005). The factor structure of the Cambridge Worry Scale in early pregnancy. *Journal of Prenatal & Perinatal Psychology & Health, 20,* 25–48.

Kabir, K., Sheeder, J., & Kelly, L. S. (2008). Identifying postpartum depression: Are 3 questions as good as 10? *Pediatrics, 122*, e696–e702. doi:10.1542/peds.2007-1759

Kagan, J., Snidman, N., & Arcus, D. (1998). Childhood derivatives of high and low reactivity in infancy. *Child Development, 69*, 1483–1493.

Kalil, K. M., Gruber, J. E., Conley, J. G., & LaGrandeur, R. M. (1995). Relationships among stress, anxiety, Type A, and pregnancy-related complications. *Pre- and Perinatal Psychology Journal, 9*, 221–232.

Kalil, K. M., Gruber, J. E., Conley, J., & Sytniac, M. (1993). Social and family pressures on anxiety and stress during pregnancy. *Pre- and Perinatal Psychology Journal, 8*, 113–118.

Kalra, H., Tandon, P., Trivedi, J. K., & Janca, A. (2005). Pregnancy-induced obsessive compulsive disorder: A case report. *Annals of General Psychiatry, 4*, 12. doi:10.1186/1744-859X-4-12

Katon, W. (1996). Panic disorder: Relationship to high medical utilization, unexplained physical symptoms, and medical costs. *The Journal of Clinical Psychiatry, 57*(Suppl. 10), 11–18.

Kendall-Tackett, K. (2008). Omega-3s, exercise, and St. John's wort: Three complimentary and alternative treatments for postpartum depression. In S. D. Stone & A. E. Menkin (Eds.), *Perinatal and postpartum mood disorders: Perspectives and treatment guide for the health care practitioner* (pp. 107–132). New York, NY: Springer.

Kendell, R. E., Chalmers, J., & Platz, C. (1987). Epidemiology of puerperal psychosis. *The British Journal of Psychiatry, 150*, 662–673.

Keogh, E., Ayers, S., & Francis, H. (2002). Does anxiety sensitivity predict post-traumatic stress symptoms following childbirth? A preliminary report. *Cognitive Behaviour Therapy, 31*, 145–155. doi:10.1080/16506070232113854 6

Kersting, A., Kroker, K., Steinhard, J., Hoernig-Franz, I., Wesselman, U., Luedorff, K., . . . Suslow, T. (2009). Psychological impact on women after second and third trimester termination of pregnancy due to fetal abnormalities versus women after preterm birth—a 14-month follow-up study. *Archives of Women's Mental Health, 12*, 193–201. doi:10.1007/s00737-009-0063-8

Kessler, R. C., Brandenburg, N., Lane, M., Roy-Byrne, P., Stang, P. D., Stein, D. J., & Wittchen, H.-U. (2005). Rethinking the duration requirement for generalized anxiety disorder: Evidence from the National Comorbidity Survey Replication. *Psychological Medicine, 35*, 1073–1082. doi:10.1017/S0033291705004538

Kessler, R. C., Chiu, W. T., Demler, O., & Walters, E. E. (2005). Prevalence, severity, comorbidity, and 12-month DSM-IV disorders in the National Comorbidity Survey Replication. *Archives of General Psychiatry, 62*, 617–627. doi:10.1001/archpsyc.62.6.617

Kessler, R. C., Chiu, W. T., Jin, R., Ruscio, A. M., Shear, K., & Walters, E. E. (2006). The epidemiology of panic attacks, panic disorder, and agoraphobia in the National Comorbidity Survey. *Archives of General Psychiatry, 63*, 415–424. doi:10.1001/archpsyc.63.4.415

Kessler, R. C., Ruscio, A. M., & Shear, K. (2009). Epidemiology of anxiety disorders. In M. M. Antony & M. B. Stein (Eds.), *Oxford handbook of anxiety and related disorders* (pp. 19–33). New York, NY: Oxford University Press.

Khanna, S., Rajendra, P. N., & Channabasavanna, S. M. (1988). Social adjustment in obsessive compulsive disorder. *The International Journal of Social Psychiatry, 34,* 118–122. doi:10.1177/002076408803400205

Kim, H., Bracha, Y., & Tipnis, A. (2007). Streamlining screening: EPDS by a phone automated response system. *Archives of Women's Mental Health, 10,* 163–169. doi:10.1007/s00737-007-0189-5

Kinsella, M. T., & Monk, C. E. (2009). Impact of maternal stress, depression, and anxiety on fetal neurobehavioral development. *Clinical Obstetrics and Gynecology, 52,* 425–440. doi:10.1097/GRF.0b013e3181b52df1

Kirsch, P., Esslinger, C., Chen, Q., Mier, D., Lis, S., Siddhanti, S., . . . Meyer-Lindenberg, A. (2005). Oxytocin modulates neural circuitry for social cognition and fear in humans. *The Journal of Neuroscience, 25,* 11489–11493. doi:10.1523/JNEUROSCI.3984-05.2005

Kleiman, K. (2009). *Therapy and the postpartum woman: Notes on healing postpartum depression for clinicians and the women who seek their help.* New York, NY: Routledge.

Kleiman, K. R., & Raskin, V. D. (1994). *This isn't what I expected: Overcoming postpartum depression.* New York, NY: Bantam Books.

Klein, D. F. (1994). Commentary: Pregnancy and panic disorder. *The Journal of Clinical Psychiatry, 55,* 293–294.

Klein, D. F., Skrobala, A. M., & Garfinkel, R. S. (1995). Preliminary look at the effects of pregnancy on panic disorder. *Anxiety, 1,* 227–232.

Koerner, N., & Dugas, M. J. (2008). An investigation of appraisals in individuals vulnerable to excessive worry: The role of intolerance of uncertainty. *Cognitive Therapy and Research, 32,* 619–638. doi:10.1007/s10608-007-9125-2

Kraemer, H. C., Kazdin, A. E., Offord, D. R., Kessler, R. C., Jensen, P. S., & Kupfer, D. J. (1997). Coming to terms with the terms of risk. *Archives of General Psychiatry, 54,* 337–343.

Kramer, M. S., Lydon, J., Séguin, L., Goulet, L., Kahn, S. R., McNamara, H., . . . Platt, R. W. (2009). Stress pathways to spontaneous preterm birth: The role of stressors, psychological distress, and stress hormones. *American Journal of Epidemiology, 169,* 1319–1326. doi:10.1093/aje/kwp061

Kristensen, J. H., Ilett, K. F., Hackett, L. P., Yapp, P., Paech, M., & Begg, E. J. (1999). Distribution and excretion of fluoxetine and norfluoxetine in human milk. *British Journal of Clinical Pharmacology, 48,* 521–527. doi:10.1046/j.1365-2125.1999.00040.x

Krupnick, J. L., Green, B. L., Stockton, P., Miranda, J., Krause, E., & Mete, M. (2008). Group interpersonal psychotherapy for low-income women with post-traumatic stress disorder. *Psychotherapy Research, 18,* 497–507. doi:10.1080/10503300802183678

Kulin, N. A., Pastuszak, A., Sage, S., Shick-Boschetto, B., Spivey, G., Feldkamp, M., . . . Koren, G. (1998). Pregnancy outcome following maternal use of the new selective serotonin reuptake inhibitors: A prospective controlled multicenter study. *JAMA, 279,* 609–610. doi:10.1001/jama.279.8.609

Kurki, T., Hiilesmaa, V., Raitasalo, R., Mattilla, H., & Ylikorkala, O. (2000). Depression and anxiety in early pregnancy and risk for pre-eclampsia. *Obstetrics and Gynecology, 95,* 487–490. doi:10.1016/S0029-7844(99)00602-X

Labad, J., Menchón, J. M., Alonso, P., Segalás, C., Jiménez, S., & Vellejo, J. (2005). Female reproductive cycle and obsessive-compulsive disorder. *The Journal of Clinical Psychiatry, 66,* 428–435. doi:10.4088/JCP.v66n0404

Ladouceur, R., Dugas, M. J., Freeston, M. H., Léger, E., Gagnon, F., & Thibodeau, N. (2000). Efficacy of a cognitive behavioral treatment for generalized anxiety disorder: Evaluation in a controlled clinical trial. *Journal of Consulting and Clinical Psychology, 68,* 957–964. doi:10.1037/0022-006X.68.6.957

Ladouceur, R., Talbot, F., & Dugas, M. J. (1997). Behavioral expressions of intolerance of uncertainty in worry: Experimental findings. *Behavior Modification, 21,* 355–371. doi:10.1177/01454455970213006

Laegreid, L., Hagberg, G., & Lundberg, A. (1992). The effect of benzodiazepines on the fetus and the newborn. *Neuropediatrics, 23,* 18–23. doi:10.1055/s-2008-1071305

Laegreid, L., Olegard, R., Wahlstrijm, J., & Comradi, N. (1987). Abnormalities in children exposed to benzodiazepines in utero. *The Lancet, 329,* 108–109. doi:10.1016/S0140-6736(87)91951-9

Laine, K., Hekkinen, T., Ekblad, U., & Kero, P. (2003). Effects of exposure to selective serotonin reuptake inhibitors during pregnancy on serotonergic symptoms in newborns and cord blood monoamine and prolactin concentrations. *Archives of General Psychiatry, 60,* 720–726. doi:10.1001/archpsyc.60.7.720

Lampe, L., Slade, T., Issakidis, C., & Andrews, G. (2003). Social phobia in the Australian National Survey of Mental Health and Well-Being (NSMHWB). *Psychological Medicine, 33,* 637–646. doi:10.1017/S0033291703007621

Langlois, F., Freeston, M. H., & Ladouceur, R. (2000a). Differences and similarities between obsessive intrusive thoughts in a non-clinical population: Study 1. *Behaviour Research and Therapy, 38,* 157–173. doi:10.1016/S0005-7967(99)00027-3

Langlois, F., Freeston, M. H., & Ladouceur, R. (2000b). Differences and similarities between obsessive intrusive thoughts in a non-clinical population: Study 2. *Behaviour Research and Therapy, 38,* 175–189. doi:10.1016/S0005-7967(99)00028-5

LaRocco-Cockburn, A., Melville, J., Bell, M., & Katon, W. (2003). Depression screening attitudes and practices among obstetrician-gynecologists. *Obstetrics and Gynecology, 101,* 892–898. doi:10.1016/S0029-7844(03)00171-6

Larsen, K. E., O'Hara, M. W., Brewer, K. K., & Wenzel, A. (2001). A prospective study of self-efficacy expectancies and labour pain. *Journal of Reproductive and Infant Psychology, 19,* 203–214. doi:10.1080/02646830120073215

Lavender, T., & Walkinshaw, S. A. (1998). Can midwives reduce postpartum psychological morbidity? A randomized trial. *Birth, 25*, 215–219. doi:10.1046/j.1523-536X.1998.00215.x

Lecrubier, Y., & Weiller, E. (1997). Comorbidities in social phobia. *International Clinical Psychopharmacology, 12*(Suppl. 6), S17–S21.

Lederman, R. P., Lederman, E., Work, B. A., Jr., & McCann, D. S. (1979). Relationship of psychological factors in pregnancy to progress in labor. *Nursing Research, 28*, 94–97. doi:10.1097/00006199-197903000-00012

Ledley, D. R. (2009). *Becoming a calm mom: How to manage stress and enjoy the first year of motherhood.* Washington, DC: American Psychological Association.

Leonard, L. G. (1998). Depression and anxiety disorders during multiple pregnancy and parenthood. *Journal of Obstetric, Gynecologic, and Neonatal Nursing, 27*, 329–337.

Lester, B. M., Cucca, J., Andreozzi, L., Flanagan, P., & Oh, W. (1993). Possible association between fluoxetine hydrochloride and colic in an infant. *Journal of the American Academy of Child and Adolescent Psychiatry, 32*, 1253–1255. doi:10.1097/00004583-199311000-00020

Lev-Wiesel, R., Chen, R., Daphna-Tekoah, S., & Hod, M. (2009). Past traumatic events: Are they a risk factor for high-risk pregnancy, delivery complications, and postpartum posttraumatic symptoms? *Journal of Women's Health, 18*, 119–125. doi:10.1089/jwh.2008.0774

Lev-Wiesel, R., Daphna-Tekoah, S., & Hallak, M. (2009). Childhood sexual abuse as a predictor of birth-related posttraumatic stress and postpartum posttraumatic stress. *Child Abuse & Neglect, 33*, 877–887. doi:10.1016/j.chiabu.2009.05.004

Levin, J. S. (1991). The factor structure of the Pregnancy Anxiety Scale. *Journal of Health and Social Behavior, 32*, 368–381. doi:10.2307/2137104

Levine, R. E., Oandasan, A. P., Primeau, L. A., & Berenson, A. B. (2003). Anxiety disorders during pregnancy and postpartum. *American Journal of Perinatology, 20*, 239–248. doi:10.1055/s-2003-42342

Liebowitz, M. R. (1987). Social phobia. *Modern Problems of Pharmacopsychiatry, 22*, 141–173.

Liebowitz, M. R., Heimberg, R. G., Fresco, D. M., Travers, J., & Stein, M. B. (2000). Social phobia or social anxiety disorder: What's in a name? [Letter to the editor]. *Archives of General Psychiatry, 57*, 191–192. doi:10.1001/archpsyc.57.2.191-a

Lipsitz, J. D., Gur, M., Miller, N. L., Forand, N., Vermes, D., & Fyer, A. J. (2006). An open pilot study of interpersonal psychotherapy for panic disorder (IPT-PD). *Journal of Nervous and Mental Disease, 194*, 440–445. doi:10.1097/01.nmd.0000221302.42073.a1

Lipsitz, J. D., Gur, M., Vermes, D., Petkova, E., Cheng, J., Miller, N., . . . Fyer, A. J. (2008). A randomized trial of interpersonal therapy versus supportive therapy for social anxiety disorder. *Depression and Anxiety, 25*, 542–553. doi:10.1002/da.20364

Lipsitz, J. D., Markowitz, J. C., Cherry, S., & Fyer, A. J. (1999). An open trial of interpersonal psychotherapy for the treatment of social phobia. *The American Journal of Psychiatry, 156*, 1814–1816.

Llewellyn, A., & Stowe, Z. (1998). Psychotropic medications in lactation. *The Journal of Clinical Psychiatry, 59*(Suppl. 2), 41–52.

Lobel, M., Dunkel-Schetter, C., & Scrimshaw, S. C. M. (1992). Prenatal maternal stress and prematurity: A prospective study of socioeconomically disadvantaged women. *Health Psychology, 11*, 32–40. doi:10.1037/0278-6133.11.1.32

Loveland Cook, C. A., Flick, L. H., Homan, S. M., Campbell, C., McSweeney, M. J., & Gallagher, M. E. (2004). Posttraumatic stress disorder in pregnancy: Prevalence, risk factors, and treatment. *Obstetrics and Gynecology, 103*, 710–717.

Lyons, S. (1998). A prospective study of post-traumatic stress symptoms 1 month following childbirth in a group of 42 first-time mothers. *Journal of Reproductive and Infant Psychology, 16*, 91–105. doi:10.1080/02646839808404562

Maccari, S., Darnaudery, M., Morley-Fletcher, S., Zuena, A. R., Cinque, C., & Van Reeth, O. (2003). Prenatal stress and long-term consequences: Implications of glucocorticoid hormones. *Neuroscience and Biobehavioral Reviews, 27*, 119–127. doi:10.1016/S0149-7634(03)00014-9

Maes, M., Bosmans, E., & Ombelet, W. (2004). In the puerperium, primiparae exhibit higher levels of anxiety and serum peptidase activity and greater immune responses than multiparae. *The Journal of Clinical Psychiatry, 65*, 71–76. doi:10.4088/JCP.v65n0112

Maes, M., Lin, A.-H., Ombelet, W., Stevens, K., Kenis, G., De. Jongh, R., . . . Bosmans, E. (2000). Immune activation in the early puerperium is related to postpartum anxiety and depressive symptoms. *Psychoneuroendocrinology, 25*, 121–137. doi:10.1016/S0306-4530(99)00043-8

Maes, M., Ombelet, W., De Jongh, R., Kenis, G., & Bosmans, E. (2001). The inflammatory response following delivery is amplified in women who previously suffered from major depression, suggesting that major depression is accompanied by a sensitization of the inflammatory response system. *Journal of Affective Disorders, 63*, 85–92. doi:10.1016/S0165-0327(00)00156-7

Maes, M., Verkerk, R., Bonaccorso, S., Ombelet, W., Bosmans, E., & Scharpé, S. (2002). Depressive and anxiety symptoms in the early puerperium are related to increased degradation of tryptophan into kynurenine, a phenomenon which is related to immune activation. *Life Sciences, 71*, 1837–1848. doi:10.1016/S0024-3205(02)01853-2

Magee, L., Erwin, B. A., & Heimberg, R. G. (2009). Psychological treatment of social anxiety disorder and specific phobia. In M. M. Antony & M. B. Stein (Eds.), *Oxford handbook of anxiety and related disorders* (pp. 334–349). New York, NY: Oxford University Press.

Magee, W. J., Eaton, W. W., Wittchen, H.-U., McGonagle, K. A., & Kessler, R. C. (1996). Agoraphobia, simple phobia, and social phobia in the National Comorbidity Survey. *Archives of General Psychiatry, 53*, 159–168.

Maina, G., Albert, U., Bogetto, F., Vaschetto, A., & Ravizza, L. (1999). Recent life events and obsessive-compulsive disorder (OCD): The role of pregnancy/delivery. *Psychiatry Research, 89*, 49–58. doi:10.1016/S0165-1781(99)00090-6

Malm, H., Klukka, T., & Neuvonen, P. J. (2005). Risks associated with selective serotonin reuptake inhibitors in pregnancy. *Obstetrics and Gynecology, 106,* 1289–1296.

Mantz, R., & Britton, J. R. (2007). Hospital construction and postpartum anxiety. *General Hospital Psychiatry, 29,* 562–566. doi:10.1016/j.genhosppsych.2007.08.010

March, D., & Yonkers, K. A. (2001). Panic disorder. In K. A. Yonkers & B. B. Little (Eds.), *Management of psychiatric disorders in pregnancy* (pp. 134–148). London, England: Arnold.

Markowitz, J. S., Weissman, M. M., Oullette, R., Lish, J. D., & Klerman, G. L. (1989). Quality of life in panic disorder. *Archives of General Psychiatry, 46,* 984–992.

Marks, I., Lovell, K., Noshirvani, H., Livanou, M., & Thrasher, S. (1998). Treatment of posttraumatic stress disorder by exposure and/or cognitive restructuring. *Archives of General Psychiatry, 55,* 317–325. doi:10.1001/archpsyc.55.4.317

Marrs, R. W. (1995). A meta-analysis of bibliotherapy studies. *American Journal of Community Psychology, 23,* 843–870. doi:10.1007/BF02507018

Mathew, S. J., & Hoffman, E. J. (2009). Pharmacotherapy for generalized anxiety disorder. In M. M. Antony & M. B. Stein (Eds.), *Oxford handbook of anxiety and related disorders* (pp. 350–363). New York, NY: Oxford University Press.

Matthey, S. (2008). Using the Edinburgh Postnatal Depression Scale to screen for anxiety disorders. *Depression and Anxiety, 25,* 926–931. doi:10.1002/da.20415

Matthey, S., Barnett, B., Howie, P., & Kavanagh, D. J. (2003). Diagnosing postpartum depression in mothers and fathers: Whatever happened to anxiety? *Journal of Affective Disorders, 74,* 139–147. doi:10.1016/S0165-0327(02)00012-5

Matthey, S., Barnett, B., Ungerer, J., & Waters, B. (2000). Paternal and maternal depressed mood during the transition to parenthood. *Journal of Affective Disorders, 60,* 75–85. doi:10.1016/S0165-0327(99)00159-7

Matthey, S., Silove, D., Barnett, B., Fitzgerald, M. H., & Mitchell, P. (1999). Correlates of depression and PTSD in Cambodian women with young children: A pilot study. *Stress Medicine, 15,* 103–107. doi:10.1002/(SICI)1099-1700(199904)15: 2<103::AID-SMI791>3.0.CO;2-T

Mattick, R. P., & Clarke, J. C. (1998). Development and validation of measures of social phobia scrutiny fear and social interaction anxiety. *Behaviour Research and Therapy, 36,* 455–470. doi:10.1016/S0005-7967(97)10031-6

McAuley, D. M., O'Neill, M. P., Moore, J., & Dundee, J. W. (1982). Lorazepam pre-medication for labour. *British Journal of Obstetrics and Gynaecology, 89,* 149–154.

McCabe, R. E., & Gifford, S. (2009). Psychological treatment of panic disorder and agoraphobia. In M. M. Antony & M. B. Stein (Eds.), *Oxford handbook of anxiety and related disorders* (pp. 308–320). New York, NY: Oxford University Press.

McConnell, P. J., Linn, K., & Filkins, K. (1998). Depression care update obstetrics and gynecology. *Primary Care Update for OB/GYNS, 5,* 11–15. doi:10.1016/ S1068-607X(97)00116-9

McDougle, C. J., Barr, L. C., Goodman, W. K., & Price, L. H. (1999). Possible role of neuropeptides in obsessive compulsive disorder. *Psychoneuroendocrinology, 24,* 1–4. doi:10.1016/S0306-4530(98)00046-8

McElhatton, P. R., Garbis, H. M., Elefant, E., Vial, T., Bellemin, B., Mastroiacovo, P., . . . dal Verme, S. (1996). The outcome of pregnancy in 698 women exposed to therapeutic doses of antidepressants. A collaborative study of the European network of the teratology information services (ENTIS). *Reproductive Toxicology, 10,* 285–294. doi:10.1016/0890-6238(96)00057-3

McGlinchey, J. B., & Zimmerman, M. (2007). Examining a dimensional representation of depression and anxiety disorders' comorbidity in psychiatric outpatients with item response modeling. *Journal of Abnormal Psychology, 116,* 464–474. doi:10.1037/0021-843X.116.3.464

McNally, R. J. (1989). Is anxiety sensitivity distinguishable from trait anxiety? A reply to Lilienfeld, Jacob, and Turner (1989). *Journal of Abnormal Psychology, 98,* 193–194. doi:10.1037/0021-843X.98.2.193

Melartin, T. K., Rytsälä, H. J., Leskelä, U. S., Lestelä-Mielonen, P. S., Sokero, T. P., & Isometsä, E. T. (2002). Current comorbidity of psychiatric disorders among DSM-IV major depressive disorder patients in psychiatric care in the Vantaa Depression Study. *The Journal of Clinical Psychiatry, 63,* 126–134.

Melender, H.-L. (2002). Experiences of fears associated with pregnancy and childbirth: A study of 329 pregnant women. *Birth, 29,* 101–111. doi:10.1046/j.1523-536X. 2002.00170.x

Menage, J. (1993). Post-traumatic stress disorder in women who have undergone obstetric and/or gynaecological procedures: A consecutive series of 30 cases of PTSD. *Journal of Reproductive and Infant Psychology, 11,* 221–228. doi:10.1080/02646839308403222

Mennin, D. S., Fresco, D. M., Heimberg, R. G., Schneier, F. R., Davies, S. O., & Liebowitz, M. R. (2002). Screening for social anxiety disorder in the clinical setting: Using the Liebowitz Social Anxiety Scale. *Journal of Anxiety Disorders, 16,* 661–673. doi:10.1016/S0887-6185(02)00134-2

Meshberg-Cohen, S., & Svikis, D. (2007). Panic disorder, trait anxiety, and alcohol use in pregnant and nonpregnant women. *Comprehensive Psychiatry, 48,* 504–510. doi:10.1016/j.comppsych.2007.06.004

Metz, A. Sichel, D. A., & Goff, D. C. (1988). Postpartum panic disorder. *The Journal of Clinical Psychiatry, 49,* 278–279.

Meyer, T. J., Miller, M. J., Metzger, R. L., & Borkovec, T. D. (1990). Development and validation of the Penn State Worry Questionnaire. *Behaviour Research and Therapy, 28,* 487–495. doi:10.1016/0005-7967(90)90135-6

Milgrom, J., Negri, L. M., Gemmill, A. W., McNeil, M., & Martin, P. R. (2005). A randomized controlled trial of psychological interventions for postnatal depression. *The British Journal of Clinical Psychology, 44,* 529–542. doi:10.1348/014466505X34200

Mills, J. S., Antony, M. M., Purdon, C. L., & Swinson, R. P. (2001, November). *Development of a measure of sexual fear and avoidance*. Poster session presented at the 34th annual meeting of the Association for the Advancement of Behavior Therapy, Philadelphia, PA.

Misri, S. K. (2005). *Pregnancy blues: What every woman needs to know about depression during pregnancy*. New York, NY: Bantam Dell.

Misri, S., Oberlander, T., Fairbrother, N., Carter, D., Ryan, D., Kuan, A. J., & Reebye, P. (2004). Relation between prenatal maternal mood and anxiety and neonatal health. *Canadian Journal of Psychiatry, 49,* 684–689.

Misri, S., Reebye, P., Corral, M., & Milis, L. (2004). The use of paroxetine and cognitive behavioral therapy in postpartum depression and anxiety: A randomized controlled trial. *The Journal of Clinical Psychiatry, 65,* 1236–1241. doi:10.4088/JCP.v65n0913

Misri, S., Reebye, P., Kendrick, K., Carter, D., Ryan, D., Grunau, R. E., & Oberlander, T. F. (2006). Internalizing behaviors in 4-year-old children exposed in utero to psychotropic medications. *The American Journal of Psychiatry, 163,* 1026–1032. doi:10.1176/appi.ajp.163.6.1026

Mitte, K. (2005). A meta-analysis of the efficacy of psycho- and pharmacotherapy in panic disorder with and without agoraphobia. *Journal of Affective Disorders, 88,* 27–45. doi:10.1016/j.jad.2005.05.003

Moleman, N., van der Hart, O., & van der Kolk, B. A. (1992). The partus stress reaction: A neglected etiological factor in postpartum psychiatric disorders. *Journal of Nervous and Mental Disease, 180,* 271–272. doi:10.1097/00005053-199204000-00010

Monk, C., Fifer, W. P., Myers, M. M., Sloan, R. P., Trien, L., & Hurtado, A. (2000). Maternal stress responses and anxiety during pregnancy: Effects on fetal heart rate. *Developmental Psychobiology, 36,* 67–77. doi:10.1002/(SICI)1098-2302(200001)36:1<67::AID-DEV7>3.0.CO;2-C

Morland, L., Goebert, D., Onoye, J., Frattarelli, L. A., Derauf, C., Herbst, M., . . . Friedman, M. (2007). Posttraumatic stress disorder and pregnancy health: Preliminary update and implications. *Psychosomatics, 48,* 304–308. doi:10.1176/appi.psy.48.4.304

Moscovitch, D. A., Antony, M. M., & Swinson, R. P. (2009). Exposure-based treatments for anxiety disorders: Theory and process. In M. M. Antony & M. B. Stein (Eds.), *Oxford handbook of anxiety and related disorders* (pp. 461–475). New York, NY: Oxford University Press.

Moses-Kolko, E. L., Bogen, D., Perel, J., Bregar, A., Uhl, K., Levin, B., & Wisner, K. L. (2005). Neonatal signs after late in utero exposure to serotonin reuptake inhibitors: Literature review and implications for clinical applications. *JAMA, 293,* 2372–2383. doi:10.1001/jama.293.19.2372

Mota, N., Cox, B. J., Enns, M. W., Calhoun, L., & Sareen, J. (2008). The relationship between mental disorders, quality of life, and pregnancy: Findings from a nationally representative sample. *Journal of Affective Disorders, 109,* 300–304. doi:10.1016/j.jad.2007.12.002

Murray, L., Fiori-Cowley, A., Hooper, R., Stein, A., & Cooper, P. J. (1996). The impact of postnatal depression and associated adversity on early mother-infant interaction and later infant outcome. *Child Development, 67,* 2512–2526. doi:10.2307/1131637

Navarro, P., García-Esteve, L., Ascaso, C., Aguado, J., Gelabert, E., & Martín-Santos, R. (2008). Non-psychotic psychiatric disorders after childbirth: Prevalence and comorbidity in a community sample. *Journal of Affective Disorders, 109,* 171–176. doi:10.1016/j.jad.2007.10.008

Newman, M. G., Erickson, T., Przeworski, A., & Dzus, E. (2003). Self-help and minimal-contact therapies for anxiety disorders: Is human contact necessary for therapeutic efficacy? *Journal of Clinical Psychology, 59,* 251–274. doi:10.1002/jclp.10128

Newman, M. G., Holmes, M., Zuellig, A. R., Kachin, K. E., & Behar, E. (2006). The reliability and validity of the Panic Disorder Self-Report: A new diagnostic screening measure of panic disorder. *Psychological Assessment, 18,* 49–61. doi:10.1037/1040-3590.18.1.49

Newman, M. G., Kachin, K. E., Zuellig, A. R., Constantino, M. J., & Cashman-McGrath, L. (2003). The Social Phobia Diagnostic Questionnaire: Preliminary validation of a new self-report diagnostic measure of social phobia. *Psychological Medicine, 33,* 623–635. doi:10.1017/S0033291703007669

Newman, M. G., Zuellig, A. R., Kachin, K. E., Constantino, M. J., Przeworski, A., Erickson, T., & Cashman-McGrath, L. (2002). Preliminary reliability and validity of the Generalized Anxiety Disorder Questionnaire—IV: A revised self-report diagnostic measure of generalized anxiety disorder. *Behavior Therapy, 33,* 215–233. doi:10.1016/S0005-7894(02)80026-0

Neziroglu, F., Anemone, R., & Yaryura-Tobias, J. A. (1992). Onset of obsessive compulsive disorder in pregnancy. *The American Journal of Psychiatry, 149,* 947–950.

Ninan, P. T. (2001). Generalized anxiety disorder: Why are we failing our patients? *The Journal of Clinical Psychiatry, 62*(Suppl. 19), 3–4.

Nonacs, R. M. (2005). Postpartum mood disorders. In L. S. Cohen & R. M. Nonacs (Eds.), *Mood and anxiety disorders during pregnancy and postpartum (Review of Psychiatry Series,* Vol. 24, No. 4; pp. 77–103). Washington, DC: American Psychiatric Press.

Nonacs, R., & Cohen, L. S. (1998). Postpartum mood disorders: Diagnosis and treatment guidelines. *The Journal of Clinical Psychiatry, 59*(Suppl. 2), 34–40.

Nonacs, R. M., Cohen, L. S., Viguera, A. C., & Mogielnicki, J. (2005). Diagnosis and treatment of mood and anxiety disorders in pregnancy. In L. S. Cohen & R. M. Nonacs (Eds.), *Mood and anxiety disorders during pregnancy and postpartum (Review of Psychiatry Series,* Vol. 24, No. 4; pp. 17–51). Washington, DC: American Psychiatric Press.

Norberg, M. M., Calamari, J. E., Cohen, R. J., & Riemann, B. C. (2008). Quality of life in obsessive-compulsive disorder: An evaluation of impairment and a preliminary analysis of the ameliorating effects of treatment. *Depression and Anxiety, 25,* 248–259. doi:10.1002/da.20298

Nordeng, H., Lindemann, R., Perminov, K. V., & Reikvam, A. (2001). Neonatal withdrawal syndrome after in utero exposure to selective serotonin reuptake inhibitors. *Acta Paediatrica, 90,* 288–291. doi:10.1080/080352501300067596

Northcott, C. J., & Stein, M. B. (1994). Panic disorder in pregnancy. *The Journal of Clinical Psychiatry, 55,* 539–542.

Nulman, I., & Koren, G. (1996). The safety of fluoxetine during pregnancy and lactation. *Teratology, 53,* 304–308. doi:10.1002/(SICI)1096-9926(199605)53:5<304::AID-TERA4>3.0.CO;2-0

Nulman, I., Rovert, J., Stewart, D. E., Wolpin, J., Gardner, H. A., Theis, J. G. W., & Koren, G. (1997). Neurodevelopment of children exposed in utero to antidepressant drugs. *The New England Journal of Medicine, 336,* 258–262.

Nulman, I., Rovert, J., Stewart, D. E., Wolpin, J., Pace-Asciak, P., Shuhaiber, S., & Koren, G. (2002). Child development following exposure to tricyclic antidepressant drugs. *The American Journal of Psychiatry, 336,* 258–262.

Oates, M. R. (2002). Adverse effects of maternal antenatal anxiety on children: Causal effect or developmental continuum? *The British Journal of Psychiatry, 180,* 478–479. doi:10.1192/bjp.180.6.478

Oberlander, T. F., Misri, S., Fitzgerald, C. E., Kostaras, X., Rurak, D., & Riggs, W. (2004). Pharmacologic factors associated with transient neonatal symptoms following prenatal psychotropic medication exposure. *The Journal of Clinical Psychiatry, 65,* 230–237. doi:10.4088/JCP.v65n0214

Oberlander, T. F., Warburton, W., Misri, S., Aghajanian, J., & Hertzman, C. (2006). Neonatal outcomes after prenatal exposure to selective serotonin reuptake inhibitor antidepressants and maternal depression using population-based linked health data. *Archives of General Psychiatry, 63,* 898–906. doi:10.1001/archpsyc.63.8.898

O'Connor, T. G., Ben-Shlomo, Y., Heron, J., Golding, J., Adams, D., & Glover, V. (2005). Prenatal anxiety predicts individual differences in cortisol in preadolescent children. *Biological Psychiatry, 58,* 211–217. doi:10.1016/j.biopsych.2005.03.032

O'Connor, T. G., Caprariello, P., Blackmore, E. R., Gregory, A. M., Glover, V., Fleming, P., & the ALSPAC Study Team. (2007). Prenatal mood disturbance predicts sleep problems in infancy and toddlerhood. *Early Human Development, 83,* 451–458. doi:10.1016/j.earlhumdev.2006.08.006

O'Connor, T. G., Heron, J., Glover, V., & the ALSPAC Study Team. (2002). Antenatal anxiety predicts child behavioral/emotional problems independently of postnatal depression. *Journal of the American Academy of Child and Adolescent Psychiatry, 41,* 1470–1477. doi:10.1097/00004583-200212000-00019

O'Connor, T. G., Heron, J., Golding, J., Beveridge, M., & Glover, V. (2002). Maternal antenatal anxiety and children's behavioural/emotional problems at 4 years. *The British Journal of Psychiatry, 180,* 502–508. doi:10.1192/bjp.180.6.502

O'Connor, T. G., Heron, J., Golding, J., Glover, V., & the ALSPAC Study Team. (2003). Maternal antenatal anxiety and behavioural/emotional problems in children: A test of a programming hypothesis. *Journal of Child Psychology and Psychiatry, and Allied Disciplines, 44,* 1025–1036. doi:10.1111/1469-7610.00187

O'Hara, M. W. (1995). *Postpartum depression: Causes and consequences.* New York, NY: Springer-Verlag.

O'Hara, M. W., Stuart, S., Gorman, L. L., & Wenzel, A. (2000). Efficacy of interpersonal psychotherapy for postpartum depression. *Archives of General Psychiatry, 57,* 1039–1045. doi:10.1001/archpsyc.57.11.1039

O'Hara, M. W., & Swain, A. M. (1996). Rates and risk of postpartum depression: A meta-analysis. *International Review of Psychiatry, 8,* 37–54. doi:10.3109/09540269609037816

Öhman, S. G., Grunewald, C., & Waldenström, U. (2003). Women's worries during pregnancy: Testing the Cambridge Worry Scale on 200 Swedish women. *Scandinavian Journal of Caring Sciences, 17,* 148–152. doi:10.1046/j.1471-6712.2003.00095.x

Olatunji, B. O., & Wolitzky-Taylor, K. B. (2009). Anxiety sensitivity and the anxiety disorders: A meta-analytic review and synthesis. *Psychological Bulletin, 135,* 974–999. doi:10.1037/a0017428

Olde, E., van der Hart, O., Kleber, R., & van Son, M. (2006). Posttraumatic stress following childbirth: A review. *Clinical Psychology Review, 26,* 1–16. doi:10.1016/j.cpr.2005.07.002

O'Mahen, H. A., Beach, S. R. H., & Banawan, S. (2001). Depression in marriage. In J. H. Harvey & A. Wenzel (Eds.), *Close relationships: Maintenance and enhancement* (pp. 299–319). Mahwah, NJ: Erlbaum.

Onoye, J. M., Goebert, D., Morland, L., Matsu, C., & Wright, T. (2009). PTSD and postpartum mental health in a sample of Caucasian, Asian, and Pacific Islander women. *Archives of Women's Mental Health, 12,* 393–400. doi:10.1007/s00737-009-0087-0

Orsillo, S. M. (2002a). Measures for acute stress disorder and posttraumatic stress disorder. In M. M. Antony, S. M. Orsillo, & L. Roemer (Eds.), *Practitioner's guide to empirically based measures of anxiety* (pp. 255–307). New York, NY: Kluwer Academic/Plenum. doi:10.1007/0-306-47628-2_20

Orsillo, S. M. (2002b). Measures for social phobia. In M. M. Antony, S. M. Orsillo, & L. Roemer (Eds.), *Practitioner's guide to empirically based measures of anxiety* (pp. 165–187). New York, NY: Kluwer Academic/Plenum. doi:10.1007/0-306-47628-2_14

Pastuszak, A., Schick-Boschetto, B., Zuber, C., Feldkamp, M., Pinelli, M., Sihn, S., . . . Koren, G. (1993). Pregnancy outcome following first-trimester exposure to fluoxetine (Prozac). *JAMA, 269,* 2246–2248. doi:10.1001/jama.269.17.2246

Patrick, M. J., Tilstone, W. J., & Reavey, P. (1972). Diazepam and breast-feeding. *The Lancet, 299*, 542–543. doi:10.1016/S0140-6736(72)90216-4

Perkin, M. R., Bland, J. M., Peacock, J. L., & Anderson, H. R. (1993). The effect of anxiety and depression during pregnancy on obstetric complications. *British Journal of Obstetrics and Gynaecology, 100*, 629–634.

Pini, S., Cassano, G. B., Simonini, E., Savino, M., Russo, A., & Montgomery, S. A. (1997). Prevalence of anxiety disorders comorbidity in bipolar depression, unipolar depression, and dysthymia. *Journal of Affective Disorders, 42*, 145–153. doi:10.1016/S0165-0327(96)01405-X

Piontek, C. M., Wisner, K. L., Perel, J. M., & Peindl, K. S. (2001). Serum fluvoxamine levels in breastfed infants. *The Journal of Clinical Psychiatry, 62*, 111–113.

Pleshette, N., Asch, S. S., & Chase, J. (1956). A study of anxieties during pregnancy, labor, and the early and late puerperium. *Bulletin of the New York Academy of Medicine, 32*, 436–455.

Pollack, M. H., & Simon, N. M. (2009). Pharmacotherapy for panic disorder and agoraphobia. In M. M. Antony & M. B. Stein (Eds.), *Oxford handbook of anxiety and related disorders* (pp. 295–307). New York, NY: Oxford University Press.

Priest, S. R., Henderson, J., Evans, S. F., & Hagan, R. (2003). Stress debriefing after childbirth: A randomised controlled trial. *The Medical Journal of Australia, 178*, 542–545.

Public Affairs Committee of the Teratology Society. (2007). Teratology public affairs committee position paper: Pregnancy labeling for prescription drugs: Ten years later. *Birth Defects Research Part A: Clinical and Molecular Teratology, 79*, 627–630. doi:10.1002/bdra.20389

Puryear, L. J. (2007). *Understanding your moods when you're expecting: Emotions, mental health, and happiness—before, during, and after pregnancy.* New York, NY: Houghton Mifflin.

Puscheck, E. E., & Pradhan, A. (2006, June 25). *First-trimester pregnancy loss.* Retrieved from http://emedicine.medscape.com/article/266317-print

Quine, L., Rutter, D. R., & Gowen, S. (1993). Women's satisfaction with the quality of the birth experience: A prospective study of social and psychological predictors. *Journal of Reproductive and Infant Psychology, 11*, 107–113. doi:10.1080/02646839308403202

Rachman, S. (1977). The conditioning theory of fear-acquisition: A critical examination. *Behaviour Research and Therapy, 15*, 375–387.

Radoff, L. (1977). The CES-D Scale: A self-report depression scale for research in the general population. *Journal of Applied Psychological Measurement, 1*, 385–401. doi:10.1177/014662167700100306

Ragan, K., Stowe, Z. N., & Newport, D. J. (2005). Use of antidepressants and mood stabilizers in breast-feeding women. In L. S. Cohen & R. M. Nonacs (Eds.), *Mood and anxiety disorders during pregnancy and postpartum* (*Review of Psychiatry Series*, Vol. 24, pp. 105–144). Washington, DC: American Psychiatric Press.

Rampono, J., Hackett, L. P., Kristensen, J. H., Kohan, R., Page-Sharp, M., & Ilettm, K. F. (2006). Transfer of escitalopram and its metabolite demethylescitalopram into breastmilk. *British Journal of Clinical Pharmacology, 62*, 316–322. doi:10.1111/j.1365-2125.2006.02659.x

Rampono, J., Kristensen, J. H., Hackett, L. P., Paech, M., Kohan, R., & Ilett, K. F. (2000). Citalopram and demethylcitalopram in human milk: Distribution, excretion and effects in breast fed infants. *British Journal of Clinical Pharmacology, 50*, 263–268. doi:10.1046/j.1365-2125.2000.00253.x

Rapee, R. M., & Heimberg, R. G. (1997). A cognitive behavioral model of anxiety in social phobia. *Behaviour Research and Therapy, 35*, 741–756. doi:10.1016/S0005-7967(97)00022-3

Redding, R. E., Herbert, J. D., Forman, E. M., & Gaudiano, B. A. (2008). Popular self-help books for anxiety, depression, and trauma: How scientifically grounded and useful are they? *Professional Psychology, Research and Practice, 39*, 537–545. doi:10.1037/0735-7028.39.5.537

Reich, J., Goldenberg, I., Vasile, R., Goisman, R., & Keller, M. A. (1994). A prospective follow-along study of the course of social phobia. *Psychiatry Research, 54*, 249–258. doi:10.1016/0165-1781(94)90019-1

Revicki, D. A., Brandenburg, N., Matza, L., Hornbrook, M. C., & Feeny, D. (2008). Health-related quality of life and utilities in primary-care patients with generalized anxiety disorder. *Quality of Life Research, 17*, 1285–1294. doi:10.1007/s11136-008-9406-6

Rickels, K., & Rynn, M. A. (2001). What is generalized anxiety disorder? [Discussion 13–14]. *The Journal of Clinical Psychiatry, 62*(Suppl. 11), 4–12.

Riggs, D. S., & Foa, E. B. (2009). Psychological treatment of posttraumatic stress disorder and acute stress disorder. In M. M. Antony & M. B. Stein (Eds.), *Oxford handbook of anxiety and related disorders* (pp. 417–428). New York, NY: Oxford University Press.

Rizzardo, R., Mangi, G., Cremonese, C., Rossi, R. T., & Cosentino, M. (1988). Variations in anxiety levels during pregnancy and psychosocial factors in relation to obstetric complications. *Psychotherapy and Psychosomatics, 49*, 10–16. doi:10.1159/000288060

Robertson, M., Rushton, P., Batrim, D., Moore, E., & Morris, P. (2007). Open trial of interpersonal psychotherapy for chronic posttraumatic stress disorder. *Australasian Psychiatry, 15*, 375–379. doi:10.1080/10398560701354948

Robichaud, M., & Dugas, M. J. (2009). Psychological treatment of GAD. In M. M. Antony & M. B. Stein (Eds.), *Oxford handbook of anxiety and related disorders* (pp. 364–374). New York, NY: Oxford University Press.

Robinson, L., Walker, J. R., & Anderson, D. (1992). Cognitive behavioural treatment of panic disorder during pregnancy and lactation. *Canadian Journal of Psychiatry, 37*, 623–626.

Rodriguez, M. A., Heilemann, M. S. V., Fiedler, E., Ang, A., Nevarez, F., & Mangione, C. M. (2008). Intimate partner violence, depression, and PTSD among pregnant Latina women. *Annals of Family Medicine, 6*, 44–52. doi:10.1370/afm.743

Roemer, L. (2002). Measures for generalized anxiety disorder. In M. M. Antony, S. M. Orsillo, & L. Roemer (Eds.), *Practitioner's guide to empirically based measures of anxiety* (pp. 197–210). New York, NY: Kluwer Academic/Plenum. doi:10.1007/0-306-47628-2_16

Roemer, L., & Orsillo, S. M. (2002). Expanding our conceptualizations of and treatment of generalized anxiety disorder: Integrating mindfulness/acceptance-based approaches with existing cognitive-behavioral models. *Clinical Psychology: Science and Practice, 9*, 54–68. doi:10.1093/clipsy/9.1.54

Roemer, L., Orsillo, S. M., & Salters-Pedneault, K. (2008). Efficacy of an acceptance-based behavior therapy for generalized anxiety disorder: Evaluation in a randomized controlled trial. *Journal of Consulting and Clinical Psychology, 76*, 1083–1089. doi:10.1037/a0012720

Rosen, G. M. (1987). Self-help treatment books and the commercialization of psychotherapy. *American Psychologist, 42*, 46–51. doi:10.1037/0003-066X.42.1.46

Rosenberg, L., Mitchell, A. A., Parsells, J. L., Pashayan, H., Louik, C., & Shapiro, S. (1983). Lack of relation of oral clefts to diazepam use during pregnancy. *The New England Journal of Medicine, 309*, 1282–1285.

Ross, L. E., Gilbert Evans, S. E., Sellers, E. M., & Romach, M. K. (2003). Measurement issues in postpartum depression part 1: Anxiety as a feature of postpartum depression. *Archives of Women's Mental Health, 6*, 51–57. doi:10.1007/s00737-002-0155-1

Ross, L. E., & McLean, L. M. (2006). Anxiety disorders during pregnancy and the postpartum period: A systematic review. *The Journal of Clinical Psychiatry, 67*, 1285–1298. doi:10.4088/JCP.v67n0818

Ross, L. E., Sellers, E. M., Gilbert Evans, S. E., & Romach, M. K. (2004). Mood changes during pregnancy and the postpartum period: Development of a biopsychosocial model. *Acta Psychiatrica Scandinavica, 109*, 457–466. doi:10.1111/j.1600-0047.2004.00296.x

Rowe, H. J., Fisher, J. R. W., & Loh, W. M. (2008). The Edinburgh Postnatal Depression Scale detects but does not distinguish anxiety disorders from depression in mothers of infants. *Archives of Women's Mental Health, 11*, 103–108. doi:10.1007/s00737-008-0003-z

Ruscio, A. M., Brown, T. A., Chiu, W. T., Sareen, J., Stein, M. B., & Kessler, R. C. (2008). Social fears and social phobia in the USA: Results from the National Comorbidity Survey Replication. *Psychological Medicine, 38*, 15–28. doi:10.1017/S0033291707001699

Ruscio, A. M., Chiu, W. T., Roy-Byrne, P., Stang, P. E., Stein, D. J., Wittchen, H.-U., & Kessler, R. C. (2007). Broadening the definition of generalized anxiety disorder: Effects on prevalence and associations with other disorders in the National

Comorbidity Survey Replication. *Journal of Anxiety Disorders, 21,* 662–676. doi:10.1016/j.janxdis.2006.10.004

Rush, A. J., Zimmerman, M., Wisniewski, S. R., Fava, M., Hollon, S. D., Warden, D., . . . Trivedi, M. H. (2005). Comorbid psychiatric disorders in depressed outpatients: Demographic and clinical features. *Journal of Affective Disorders, 87,* 43–55. doi:10.1016/j.jad.2005.03.005

Ryding, E. L. (1993). Investigation of 33 women who demanded a cesarean section for personal reasons. *Acta Obstetricia et Gynecologica Scandinavica, 72,* 280–285. doi:10.3109/00016349309068038

Ryding, E. L., Wijma, B., & Wijma, K. (1997). Posttraumatic stress reactions after emergency cesarean section. *Acta Obstetricia et Gynecologica Scandinavica, 76,* 856–861. doi:10.3109/00016349709024365

Ryding, E. L., Wijma, K., & Wijma, B. (1998a). Postpartum counseling after an emergency cesarean. *Clinical Psychology & Psychotherapy, 5,* 231–237. doi:10.1002/(SICI)1099-0879(199812)5:4<231::AID-CPP172>3.0.CO;2-9

Ryding, E. L., Wijma, K., & Wijma, B. (1998b). Psychological impact of emergency cesarean section in comparison with elective cesarean section, instrumental and normal vaginal delivery. *Journal of Psychosomatic Obstetrics and Gynaecology, 19,* 135–144. doi:10.3109/01674829809025691

Ryding, E. L., Wijma, B., Wijma, K., & Rydhström, H. (1998). Fear of childbirth during pregnancy may increase the risk of emergency cesarean section. *Acta Obstetricia et Gynecologica Scandinavica, 77,* 542–547. doi:10.1080/j.1600-0412.1998.770512.x

Ryding, E. L., Wirén, E., Johansson, G., Ceder, B., & Dahlström, A.-M. (2004). Group counseling for mothers after emergency cesarean section: A randomized controlled trial of intervention. *Birth, 31,* 247–253. doi:10.1111/j.0730-7659.2004.00316.x

Saisto, T., Kaaja, R., Ylikorkala, O., & Halmesmäki, E. (2001). Reduced pain tolerance during and after pregnancy in women suffering from fear of labor. *Pain, 93,* 123–127. doi:10.1016/S0304-3959(01)00302-5

Sanchis, A., Rosique, D., & Catala, J. (1991). Adverse effects of maternal lorazepam on neonates. *DICP: the Annals of Pharmacotherapy, 25,* 1137–1138.

Sanderson, W. C., DiNardo, P. A., Rapee, R. M., & Barlow, D. H. (1990). Syndrome comorbidity in patients diagnosed with a DSM-III-R anxiety disorder. *Journal of Abnormal Psychology, 99,* 308–312. doi:10.1037/0021-843X.99.3.308

Sandin, B., Chorot, P., Santed, M. A., & Valiente, R. M. (2004). Differences in negative life events between patients with anxiety disorders, depression, and hypochondriasis. *Anxiety, Stress, and Coping, 17,* 37–47. doi:10.1080/10615800310001637134

Sareen, J., Cox, B. J., Stein, M. B., Afifi, T. O., Fleet, C., & Asmundson, G. J. G. (2007). Physical and mental comorbidity, disability, and suicidal behavior associated with posttraumatic stress disorder in a large community sample. *Psychosomatic Medicine, 69,* 242–248. doi:10.1097/PSY.0b013e31803146d8

Saxen, I., & Saxen, L. (1975). Association between maternal intake of diazepam and oral clefts. *The Lancet, 306,* 498. doi:10.1016/S0140-6736(75)90567-X

Schick-Boschetto, B., & Zuber, C. (1992). Alprazolam exposure during early human pregnancy. *Teratology, 45,* 360.

Schmidt, K., Olesen, O., & Jensen, P. (2000). Citalopram and breastfeeding: Serum concentration and side effects in the infant. *British Journal of Clinical Pharmacology, 40,* 263–268.

Schmidt, N. B., Wollaway-Bickel, K., Trakowski, J., Santiago, H., Storey, J., Koselka, M., & Cook, J. (2000). Dismantling cognitive behavioral treatment for panic disorder: Questioning the utility of breathing retraining. *Journal of Consulting and Clinical Psychology, 68,* 417–424. doi:10.1037/0022-006X.68.3.417

Schmutzer, P. A., Brendle, J. R., Haugen, E. N., Jackson, L. C., & Wenzel, A. (2002, November). *A longitudinal analysis of social anxiety in postpartum women.* Poster session presented at the 35th Annual Meeting of the Association for Advancement of Behavior Therapy, Reno, NV.

Schneider, M. L., & Moore, C. F. (2000). Effect of prenatal stress on development: A nonhuman primate model. In C. Nelson (Ed.), *Minnesota Symposium on Child Psychology* (pp. 201–243). Mahwah, NJ: Erlbaum.

Schnurr, P. P., Lunney, C. A., & Sengupta, A. (2004). Risk factors for the development versus maintenance of posttraumatic stress disorder. *Journal of Traumatic Stress, 17,* 85–95. doi:10.1023/B:JOTS.0000022614.21794.f4

Schultz, L. T., & Heimberg, R. G. (2008). Attentional focus in social anxiety disorder: Potential for interactive processes. *Clinical Psychology Review, 28,* 1206–1221. doi:10.1016/j.cpr.2008.04.003

Schwartz, C. E., Snidman, N., & Kagan, J. (1999). Adolescent social anxiety as an outcome of inhibited temperament in childhood. *Journal of the American Academy of Child and Adolescent Psychiatry, 38,* 1008–1015. doi:10.1097/00004583-199908000-00017

Searle, J. (1996). Fearing the worst—Why do pregnant women feel "at risk"? *Australian and New Zealand Journal of Obstetrics and Gynaecology, 36,* 279–286. doi:10.1111/j.1479-828X.1996.tb02711.x

Sebastian, L. (1998). *Overcoming postpartum depression and anxiety.* Omaha, NE: Addicus Books.

Seng, J. S., Oakley, D. J., Sampselle, C. M., Killions, C., Graham-Bermann, S., & Liberzon, I. (2001). Posttraumatic stress disorder and pregnancy complications. *Obstetrics and Gynecology, 97,* 17–22. doi:10.1016/S0029-7844(00)01097-8

Seng, J. S., Sperlich, M., & Low, L. K. (2008). Mental health, demographic, and risk behavior profiles of pregnant survivors of childhood and adult abuse. *Journal of Midwifery & Women's Health, 53,* 511–521. doi:10.1016/j.jmwh.2008.04.013

Shafran, R., Thordarson, S., & Rachman, S. (1996). Thought-action fusion in obsessive compulsive disorder. *Journal of Anxiety Disorders, 10,* 379–391. doi:10.1016/0887-6185(96)00018-7

Shalev, A. Y., Freedman, S., Peri, T., Brandes, D., Sahar, T., Orr, S. P., & Pitman, R. K. (1998). Prospective study of posttraumatic stress disorder and depression following trauma. *The American Journal of Psychiatry, 155,* 630–637.

Sholomskas, D. E., Wickamaratne, P. J., Dogolo, L., O'Brien, D. W., Leaf, P. J., & Woods, S. W. (1993). Postpartum onset of panic disorder: A coincidental event? *The Journal of Clinical Psychiatry, 54,* 476–480.

Sichel, D. A., Cohen, L. S., Dimmock, J. A., & Rosenbaum, J. F. (1993). Postpartum obsessive compulsive disorder: A case series. *The Journal of Clinical Psychiatry, 54,* 156–159.

Sichel, D. A., Cohen, L. S., Rosenbaum, J. F., & Driscoll, J. (1993). Postpartum onset of obsessive compulsive disorder. *Psychosomatics, 34,* 277–279.

Sichel, D. A., & Driscoll, J. W. (1999). *Women's moods: What every woman must know about hormones, the brain, and emotional health.* New York, NY: HarperCollins.

Simon, G., Cunningham, M., & Davis, R. (2002). Outcomes of prenatal antidepressant exposure. *The American Journal of Psychiatry, 159,* 2055–2061. doi:10.1176/appi.ajp.159.12.2055

Sjöström, K., Valentin, L., Thelin, T., & Maršál, K. (1997). Maternal anxiety in late pregnancy and fetal hemodynamics. *European Journal of Obstetrics, Gynecology, and Reproductive Biology, 74,* 149–155. doi:10.1016/S0301-2115(97)00100-0

Small, R., Lumley, J., Donohue, L., Potter, A., & Waldenström, U. (2000). Randomised controlled trial of midwife led debriefing to reduce maternal depression after operative childbirth. *British Medical Journal, 321,* 1043–1047. doi:10.1136/bmj.321.7268.1043

Smoller, J. W., Yamaki, L. H., Fagerness, J. A., Biederman, J., Racette, S., Laird, N. M., . . . Hirshfeld-Becker, D. (2005). The corticotrophin-releasing hormone gene and behavioral inhibition in children at risk for panic disorder. *Biological Psychiatry, 57,* 1485–1492. doi:10.1016/j.biopsych.2005.02.018

Söderquist, J., Wijma, B., & Wijma, K. (2006). The longitudinal course of post-traumatic stress after childbirth. *Journal of Psychosomatic Obstetrics and Gynaecology, 27,* 113–119. doi:10.1080/01674820600712172

Söderquist, J., Wijma, K., & Wijma, B. (2004). Traumatic stress in late pregnancy. *Journal of Anxiety Disorders, 18,* 127–142. doi:10.1016/S0887-6185(02)00242-6

Soet, J. E., Brack, G. A., & DiIorio, C. (2003). Prevalence and predictors of women's experience of psychological trauma during childbirth. *Birth, 30,* 36–46. doi:10.1046/j.1523-536X.2003.00215.x

Spanier, G. B. (1976). Measuring dyadic adjustment: New scales for assessing the quality of marriage and similar dyads. *Journal of Marriage and the Family, 38,* 15–28. doi:10.2307/350547

Spielberger, C. D., Gorsuch, R. L., & Lushene, R. E. (1970). *Manual for the State-Trait Anxiety Inventory.* Palo Alto, CA: Consulting Psychologists Press.

Spigset, O. (1994). Anesthetic agents and excretion in breast milk. *Acta Anaesthesiologica Scandinavica, 38,* 94–103. doi:10.1111/j.1399-6576.1994.tb03848.x

Spinelli, M. G. (2004). Maternal infanticide associated with mental illness: Prevention and the promise of saved lives. *The American Journal of Psychiatry, 161*, 1548–1557. doi:10.1176/appi.ajp.161.9.1548

Spinelli, M. G., & Endicott, J. (2003). Controlled clinical trial of interpersonal psychotherapy versus parenting education program for depressed pregnant women. *The American Journal of Psychiatry, 160*, 555–562. doi:10.1176/appi.ajp.160.3.555

Stangier, U., Heidenreich, T., Peitz, M., Lauterbach, W., & Clark, D. M. (2003). Cognitive therapy for social phobia: Individual versus group format. *Behaviour Research and Therapy, 41*, 991–1007. doi:10.1016/S0005-7967(02)00176-6

Starcevic, V., & Berle, D. (2006). Cognitive specificity of anxiety disorders: A review of selected key constructs. *Depression and Anxiety, 23*, 51–61. doi:10.1002/da.20145

Starcevic, V., Latas, M., Kolar, D., Vucinic-Latas, D., Bogojevic, G., & Milovanovic, S. (2008). Co-occurrence of Axis I and Axis I disorders in female and male patients with panic disorder with agoraphobia. *Comprehensive Psychiatry, 49*, 537–543. doi:10.1016/j.comppsych.2008.02.009

St. Clair, S. M., & Schirmer, R. G. (1992). First trimester exposure to alprazolam. *Obstetrics and Gynecology, 80*, 843–846.

Stein, M. B., & Stein, D. J. (2008). Social anxiety disorder. *The Lancet, 371*, 1115–1125. doi:10.1016/S0140-6736(08)60488-2

Steiner, M., Dunn, E., & Born, L. (2003). Hormones and mood: From menarche to menopause and beyond. *Journal of Affective Disorders, 74*, 67–83. doi:10.1016/S0165-0327(02)00432-9

Stewart, S. E., Jenike, E., & Jenike, M. A. (2009). Biological treatment for obsessive compulsive disorder. In M. M. Antony & M. B. Stein (Eds.), *Oxford handbook of anxiety and related disorders* (pp. 375–390). New York, NY: Oxford University Press.

Stuart, S., Couser, G., Schilder, K., O'Hara, M. W., & Gorman, L. (1998). Post-partum anxiety and depression: Onset and comorbidity in a community sample. *Journal of Nervous and Mental Disease, 186*, 420–424. doi:10.1097/00005053-199807000-00006

Sugiura-Ogasawara, M., Furukawa, T. A., Nakano, Y., Hori, S., Aoki, K., & Kitamura, T. (2002). Depression as a potential causal factor in subsequent miscarriage in recurrent spontaneous aborters. *Human Reproduction, 17*, 2580–2584. doi:10.1093/humrep/17.10.2580

Sutter-Dallay, A. L., Giaconne-Marcesche, V., Glatigny-Dallay, E., & Verdoux, H. (2004). Women with anxiety disorders during pregnancy are at increased risk of intense postnatal depressive symptoms: A prospective survey of the MATQUID cohort. *European Psychiatry, 19*, 459–463. doi:10.1016/j.eurpsy.2004.09.025

Taddio, A., Ito, S., & Koren, G. (1996). Excretion of fluoxetine and its metabolite, norfluoxetine, in human breast milk. *Journal of Clinical Pharmacology, 36*, 42–47.

Taylor, J. F., Rosen, R. C., & Leiblum, S. R. (1994). Self-report assessment of female dysfunction: Psychometric evaluation of the Brief Index of Sexual Functioning for Women. *Archives of Sexual Behavior, 23,* 627–643. doi:10.1007/BF01541816

Teixeira, J. M. A., Fisk, N. M., & Glover, V. (1999). Association between maternal anxiety in pregnancy and increased uterine artery resistance index: Cohort based study. *British Medical Journal, 318,* 153–157.

Torgrud, L. J., Walker, J. R., Murray, L., Cox, B. J., Chartier, M., & Kjernisted, K. D. (2004). Deficits in perceived social support associated with generalized social phobia. *Cognitive Behaviour Therapy, 33,* 87–96. doi:10.1080/16506070410029577

Torner, L., Toschi, N., Pohlinger, A., Landgraf, R., & Neumann, I. D. (2001). Anxiolytic and anti-stress effects of brain prolactin: Improved efficacy of anti-sense targeting of the prolactin receptor by molecular modeling. *The Journal of Neuroscience, 21,* 3207–3214.

Torres, A. R., Prince, M. J., Bebbington, P. E., Bhugra, D., Brugha, T. S., Farrell, M., . . . Singleton, N. (2006). Obsessive-compulsive disorder: Prevalence, comorbidity, impact, and help-seeking in the British National Psychiatric Morbidity Survey of 2000. *The American Journal of Psychiatry, 163,* 1978–1985. doi:10.1176/appi. ajp.163.11.1978

Tükel, R., Polat, A., Özdemir, Ö., Aksüt, D., & Türksoy, N. (2002). Comorbid conditions in obsessive-compulsive disorder. *Comprehensive Psychiatry, 43,* 204–209. doi:10.1053/comp.2002.32355

Tuohy, A., & McVey, C. (2008). Subscales measuring symptoms of non-specific depression, anhedonia, and anxiety in the Edinburgh Postnatal Depression Scale. *The British Journal of Clinical Psychology, 47,* 153–169.

Turner, S. M., Beidel, D. C., & Stanley, M. A. (1992). Are obsessive thoughts and worry different cognitive phenomena? *Clinical Psychology Review, 12,* 257–270. doi:10.1016/0272-7358(92)90117-Q

Twohig, M. P., & O'Donohue, W. T. (2007). Treatment of posttraumatic stress disorder with exposure therapy during late term pregnancy. *Clinical Case Studies, 6,* 525–535. doi:10.1177/1534650107296804

Uguz, F., Akman, C., Kaya, N., & Cilli, A. S. (2007). Postpartum-onset obsessive-compulsive disorder: Incidence, clinical features, and related factors. *The Journal of Clinical Psychiatry, 68,* 132–138. doi:10.4088/JCP.v68n0118

Uguz, F., Gezginc, K., Zeytinci, I. E., Karatayli, S., Askin, R., Guler, O., . . . Gecici, O. (2007). Obsessive-compulsive disorder in pregnant women during the third trimester of pregnancy. *Comprehensive Psychiatry, 48,* 441–445. doi:10.1016/ j.comppsych.2007.05.001

Van Ameringen, M., Mancini, C., & Patterson, B. (2009). Pharmacotherapy for social anxiety disorder and specific phobia. In M. M. Antony & M. B. Stein (Eds.), *Oxford handbook of anxiety and related disorders* (pp. 321–333). New York, NY: Oxford University Press.

van Balkom, A. J. L. M., de Haan, E., van Oppen, P., Spinhoven, P., Hoogduin, K. A. L., & van Dyck, R. (1998). Cognitive and behavioral therapies alone versus in combination with fluvoxamine in their treatment of obsessive compulsive disorder. *Journal of Nervous and Mental Disease, 186,* 492–499. doi:10.1097/00005053-199808000-00007

van Balkom, A. J. L. M., van Boeijen, C. A., Boeke, A. J. P., van Oppen, P., Kempe, P. T., & van Dyck, R. (2008). Comorbid depression, but not comorbid anxiety disorders, predicts poorer outcome in anxiety disorders. *Depression and Anxiety, 25,* 408–415. doi:10.1002/da.20386

van Boeijen, C. A., van Balkom, A. J. L. M., van Oppen, P., Blankenstein, N., Cherpanath, A., & van Dyck, R. (2005). Efficacy of self-help manuals for anxiety disorders in primary care: A systematic review. *Family Practice, 22,* 192–196. doi:10.1093/fampra/cmh708

Van den Bergh, B. R. H., Van Calster, B., Smits, T., Van Huffel, S., & Lagae, L. (2008). Antenatal maternal anxiety is related to HPA-axis dysregulation and self-reported depressive symptoms in adolescence: A prospective study on the fetal origins of depressed mood. *Neuropsychopharmacology, 33,* 536–545. doi:10.1038/sj.npp.1301450

Van den Bergh, B. R. H., & Marcoen, A. (2004). High antenatal maternal anxiety is related to ADHD symptoms, externalizing problems, and anxiety in 8- and 9-year-olds. *Child Development, 75,* 1085–1097. doi:10.1111/j.1467-8624.2004.00727.x

van Pampus, M. G., Wolf, H., Schultz, W. C. W., Weijmar, N. L., & Aarnoudse, J. G. (2004). Posttraumatic stress disorder following preeclampsia and HELLP syndrome. *Journal of Psychosomatic Obstetrics and Gynaecology, 25,* 183–187. doi:10.1080/01674820400017863

van Wingen, G. A., Broekhoven, F., Verkes, R. J., Petersson, K. M., Bäckström, T., Buitelaar, J. K., & Fernandez, G. (2008). Progesterone selectively increases amygdale reactivity in women. *Molecular Psychiatry, 13,* 325–333. doi:10.1038/sj.mp.4002030

Vesga-López, O., Schneier, F. R., Wang, S., Heimberg, R. G., Liu, S.-M., Hasin, D. S., & Blanco, C. (2008). Gender differences in generalized anxiety disorder: Results from the National Epidemiologic Survey on Alcohol and Related Conditions. *The Journal of Clinical Psychiatry, 69,* 1606–1616.

Villenponteaux, V. A., Lydiard, R. B., Laraia, M. T., Stuart, G. W., & Ballenger, J. C. (1992). The effects of pregnancy on preexisting panic disorder. *The Journal of Clinical Psychiatry, 53,* 201–203.

Ware, M. R., & DeVane, C. L. (1990). Imipramine treatment of panic disorder during pregnancy. *The Journal of Clinical Psychiatry, 51,* 482–484.

Webster, P. A. C. (1973). Withdrawal symptoms in neonates associated with maternal antidepressant therapy. *The Lancet, 302,* 318–319. doi:10.1016/S0140-6736(73)90815-5

Weinstock, M. (2001). Alterations induced by gestational stress in brain morphology and behavior in the offspring. *Progress in Neurobiology, 65,* 427–451. doi:10.1016/S0301-0082(01)00018-1

Weisberg, R. B., & Paquette, J. A. (2002). Screening and treatment of anxiety disorders in pregnant and lactating women. *Women's Health Issues, 12*, 32–36.

Weisenfeld, A. R., Malatesta, C. Z., Whitman, P. B., Grannose, C., & Vile, R. (1985). Psychophysiological response of breast and bottle-feeling mothers to their infants' signals. *Psychophysiology, 22*, 79–86. doi:10.1111/j.1469-8986.1985.tb01563.x

Weissman, M. M., Markowitz, J. C., & Klerman, G. L. (2000). *Comprehensive guide to interpersonal psychotherapy*. New York, NY: Basic Books.

Wen, S. W., Yang, Q., Garner, P., Fraser, W., Olatunboson, O., Nimrod, C., & Walker. M. (2006). Selective serotonin reuptake inhibitors and risk of adverse pregnancy outcome. *American Journal of Obstetrics and Gynecology, 194*, 961–966. doi:10.1016/j.ajog.2006.02.019

Wenzel, A. (2005, March). *Anxiety disorders at eight weeks postpartum: Prevalence, predictors, and interpersonal consequences*. Paper presented at the 25th annual meeting of the Anxiety Disorders Association of America, Seattle, WA.

Wenzel, A., Gorman, L. L., O'Hara, M. W., & Stuart, S. (2001). The occurrence of panic and obsessive compulsive symptoms in women with postpartum dysphoria: A prospective study. *Archives of Women's Mental Health, 4*, 5–12. doi:10.1007/s007370170002

Wenzel, A., Haugen, E. N., & Goyette, M. (2005). Postpartum sexual adjustment in women with and without generalized anxiety disorder. *Journal of Reproductive and Infant Psychology, 23*, 365–366. doi:10.1080/02646830500273723

Wenzel, A., Haugen, E. N., Jackson, L. C., & Brendle, J. R. (2005). Anxiety disorders at eight weeks postpartum. *Journal of Anxiety Disorders, 19*, 295–311. doi:10.1016/j.janxdis.2004.04.001

Wenzel, A., Haugen, E. N., Jackson, L. C., & Robinson, K. (2003). Prevalence of generalized anxiety at eight weeks postpartum. *Archives of Women's Mental Health, 6*, 43–49. doi:10.1007/s00737-002-0154-2

Wenzel, A., & Kashdan, T. B. (2008). Emotional disturbances and the initial stages of relationship development: Processes and consequences of social anxiety and depression. In S. Sprecher, A. Wenzel, & J. H. Harvey (Eds.), *Handbook of relationship initiation* (pp. 425–450). New York, NY: Psychology Press.

Wessely, S., & Deahl, M. (2003). Psychological debriefing is a waste of time. *The British Journal of Psychiatry, 183*, 12–13.

Wesson, D. R., Camber, S., Harkey, M., & Smith, D. E. (1985). Diazepam and desmethyldiazepam in breast milk. *Journal of Psychoactive Drugs, 17*, 55–56.

Whisman, M. A. (2007). Marital distress and DSM-IV psychiatric disorders in a population-based national survey. *Journal of Abnormal Psychology, 116*, 638–643. doi:10.1037/0021-843X.116.3.638

White, T., Matthey, S., Boyd, K., & Barnett, B. (2006). Postnatal depression and post-traumatic stress after childbirth: Prevalence, course, and co-occurrence. *Journal of Reproductive and Infant Psychology, 24*, 107–120. doi:10.1080/02646830600643874

Whitelaw, A. G. L., Cummings, A. J., & McFadyen, I. R. (1981). Effect of maternal lorazepam on the neonate. *British Medical Journal, 282*, 1106–1108. doi:10.1136/bmj.282.6270.1106

Wichman, C. L., Fothergill, A., Moore, K. M., Lang, T. R., Heise, R. H., & Watson, W. J. (2008). Recent trends in selective serotonin reuptake inhibitor use in pregnancy. *Journal of Clinical Psychopharmacology, 28*, 714–716. doi:10.1097/JCP.0b013e31818b53fd

Wiederman, M. W. (2000). Women's body image self-consciousness during physical intimacy with a partner. *Journal of Sex Research, 37*, 60–68. doi:10.1080/00224490009552021

Wiegartz, P. S., & Gyoerkoe, K. L. (2009). *The pregnancy and postpartum anxiety workbook: Practical skills to help you overcome anxiety, worry, panic attacks, obsessions, and compulsions.* Oakland, CA: New Harbinger.

Wijma, K. (2003). Why focus on "fear of childbirth"? *Journal of Psychosomatic Obstetrics and Gynaecology, 24*, 141–143. doi:10.3109/01674820309039667

Wijma, K., Alehagen, S., & Wijma, B. (2002). Development of the Delivery Fear Scale. *Journal of Psychosomatic Obstetrics and Gynaecology, 23*, 97–107. doi:10.3109/01674820209042791

Wijma, K., Söderquist, J., & Wijma, B. (1997). Posttraumatic stress disorder after childbirth: A cross-sectional study. *Journal of Anxiety Disorders, 11*, 587–597. doi:10.1016/S0887-6185(97)00041-8

Wijma, K., & Wijma, B. (1992). Changes in anxiety during pregnancy and after delivery. In K. Wijma & B. von Schoulz (Eds.), *Reproductive life: Advances in psychosomatic obstetrics and gynaecology* (pp. 81–88). Lancaster, England: Parthenon Publishing Group.

Wijma, K., Wijma, B., & Zar, M. (1998). Psychometric properties of the W-DEQ; a new questionnaire for the measurement of fear of childbirth. *Journal of Psychosomatic Obstetrics and Gynaecology, 19*, 84–97. doi:10.3109/01674829809048501

Williams, K. E., & Koran, L. M. (1997). Obsessive compulsive disorder in pregnancy, the puerperium, and the premenstrum. *The Journal of Clinical Psychiatry, 58*, 330–334.

Wisner, K. L., Peindl, K. S., Gigliotti, T., & Hanusa, B. H. (1999). Obsessions and compulsions in women with postpartum depression. *The Journal of Clinical Psychiatry, 60*, 176–180.

Wisner, K. L., Peindl, K. S., & Hanusa, B. H. (1996). Effects of childbearing on the natural history of panic disorder with comorbid mood disorder. *Journal of Affective Disorders, 41*, 173–180. doi:10.1016/S0165-0327(96)00069-9

Wittchen, H.-U. (2002). Generalized anxiety disorder: Prevalence, burden, and cost to society. *Depression and Anxiety, 16*, 162–171. doi:10.1002/da.10065

Wittchen, H.-U., Carter, R. M., Pfister, H., Montgomery, S. A., & Kessler, R. C. (2000). Disabilities and quality of life in pure and comorbid generalized anxiety disorder and major depression in a national survey. *International Clinical Psychopharmacology, 15*, 319–328. doi:10.1097/00004850-200015060-00002

Wolitzky-Taylor, K. B., Horowitz, J. D., Powers, M. B., & Telch, M. J. (2008). Psychological approaches in the treatment of specific phobias: A meta-analysis. *Clinical Psychology Review, 28*, 1021–1037. doi:10.1016/j.cpr.2008.02.007

Wolk, S. I., Horwath, E., Goldstein, R. B., Wickramaratne, P., & Weissman, M. M. (1996). Comparison of RDC, *DSM-III, DSM-III-R* diagnostic criteria for generalized anxiety disorder. *Anxiety, 2*, 71–79. doi:10.1002/(SICI)1522-7154(1996)2: 2<71::AID-ANXI2>3.0.CO;2-G

Wright, J. H., Basco, M. R., & Thase, M. E. (2006). *Learning cognitive behavior therapy: An illustrated guide*. Washington, DC: American Psychiatric Association.

Wright, S., Dawling, S., & Ashford, J. J. (1991). Excretion of fluvoxamine in breast milk. *British Journal of Clinical Pharmacology, 31*, 209.

Yehuda, R. (2001). Biology of posttraumatic stress disorder. *The Journal of Clinical Psychiatry, 62*(Suppl. 17), 41–46.

Yonkers, K. A., Wisner, K. L., Stewart, D. E., Oberlander, T. F., Dell, D. L., Stotland, N., . . . Lockwood, C. (2009). The management of depression during pregnancy: A report from the American Psychiatric Association and the American College of Obstetricians and Gynecologists. *General Hospital Psychiatry, 31*, 403–413. doi:10.1016/j.genhosppsych.2009.04.003

Zaers, S., Waschke, M., & Ehlert, U. (2008). Depressive symptoms and symptoms of post-traumatic stress disorder in women after childbirth. *Journal of Psychosomatic Obstetrics and Gynaecology, 29*, 61–71. doi:10.1080/01674820701804324

Zanardo, V., Freato, F., & Zacchello, F. (2003). Maternal anxiety upon NICU discharge of high-risk infants. *Journal of Reproductive and Infant Psychology, 21*, 69–75. doi:10.1080/0264683021000060093

Zar, M., Wijma, K., & Wijma, B. (2001). Pre- and postpartum fear of childbirth in nulliparous and parous women. *Scandinavian Journal of Behaviour Therapy, 30*, 75–84. doi:10.1080/02845710152507418

Zeskind, P. S., & Stephens, L. (2004). Maternal selective serotonin reuptake inhibitor use during pregnancy and newborn neurobehavior. *Pediatrics, 113*, 368–375. doi:10.1542/peds.113.2.368

INDEX

ABOUT THE AUTHOR

Amy Wenzel received her PhD in clinical psychology from the University of Iowa and completed her psychology internship at the University of Wisconsin Medical School. She has held faculty positions at the University of North Dakota, the American College of Norway, and the University of Pennsylvania School of Medicine. She is currently on the affiliated faculty at the University of Pennsylvania School of Medicine, and she is the director of the Hope and Resiliency Clinic for high-risk patients and the founder of Wenzel Consulting, LLC. She has received grants and awards from the National Institute of Mental Health, the National Alliance for Research on Schizophrenia and Depression, the American Foundation for Suicide Prevention, the Association for Behavioral and Cognitive Therapies, and the Anxiety Disorders Association of America. She has published more than 80 journal articles and chapters and has authored or edited six books, most of which pertain to cognitive behavioral therapy, anxiety disorders, and close relationships.